DISPLAY COPY
DO NOT REMOVE

Synopsis of Pediatric Emergency Care

Synopsis of Pediatric Emergency Care

Edited by
Jagannath S. Surpure, MD, FAAP, FACEP
Clinical Professor of Pediatrics
University of Nevada, School of Medicine
Director, Pediatric Emergency Department
University Medical Center, Las Vegas, Nevada

With 43 Contributing Authors

Foreword by Martha Bushore, MD, FAAP, FACEP, FCCM,
Atlanta, Georgia

Andover Medical Publishers
Boston   London   Oxford   Singapore   Sydney   Toronto   Wellington

Andover Medical Publishers is an imprint of Butterworth–Heinemann

Copyright © 1993 by Butterworth–Heinemann, a division of Reed Publishing (USA) Inc. All rights reserved.

No part of this publication may be reproduced, stored in a retrieval system, or transmitted, in any form or by any means, electronic, mechanical, photocopying, recording, or otherwise, without the prior written permission of the publisher.

Every effort has been made to ensure that the drug dosage schedules within this text are accurate and conform to standards accepted at time of publication. However, as treatment recommendations vary in the light of continuing research and clinical experience, the reader is advised to verify drug dosage schedules herein with information found on product information sheets. This is especially true in cases of new or infrequently used drugs.

Recognizing the importance of preserving what has been written, it is the policy of Butterworth–Heinemann to have the books it publishes printed on acid-free paper, and we exert our best efforts to that end.

Library of Congress Cataloging-in-Publication Data

Synopsis of pediatric emergency care / edited by Jagannath S. Surpure
 ; with 43 contributors.
    p.   cm.
  Includes bibliographical references and index.
  ISBN 1-56372-011-6 (hardcover) :
  1. Pediatric emergencies—Handbooks, manuals, etc.   I. Surpure, Jagannath S.
  [DNLM: 1. Emergencies—in infancy & childhood—handbooks.
  2. Pediatrics—handbooks. 3. Wounds and Injuries—in infancy &
  childhood—handbooks.   WS 39 S993]
RJ370.S96 1993
618.92'0025—dc20
DNLM/DLC
for Library of Congress   92-49571
                                                                                                              CIP

British Library Cataloguing-in-Publication Data
A catalogue record for this book is available from the British Library.

Butterworth–Heinemann
80 Montvale Avenue
Stoneham, MA 02180

10 9 8 7 6 5 4 3 2 1

Printed in the United States of America

This book is dedicated to my father who inspired, encouraged, and guided my education

Contents

Contributors xiii
Foreword xix
Preface xxi
Acknowledgments xxiii

PART I

Resuscitation

1 Cardiopulmonary Resuscitation 3
  David Johnson

2 Neonatal Resuscitation 11
  K.C. Sekar

PART II

Acute Airway Management

3 Croup and Epiglottitis 23
  Narendra C. Singh
  Niranjan Kissoon

4 Asthma/Bronchiolitis 33
  William Ahrens
  Gary Strange

5 Respiratory Failure 47
  Steven M. Barrett

6 Foreign Body Aspiration 57
  Joseph D. Losek

PART III
Circulation

7 **Shock**   67
   Morris Gessouroun

8 **Dysrhythmias**   87
   Jagannath S. Surpure

9 **Congestive Heart Failure**   95
   Charles Cooper

PART IV
Poisoning

10 **Acute Pediatric Poisoning**   103
    David McCarty

PART V
Trauma/Orthopedics

11 **Acute Osteomyelitis and Septic Arthritis**   117
    William A. Herndon

12 **Major Multiple Trauma**   129
    Douglas A. Boenning
    Simon Cooper

13 **Head Trauma**   143
    David J. Gower

14 **Abdominal Trauma**   157
    E. Stevers Golladay
    Dileep R. Vyas

15 **Thoracic Trauma**   169
    E. Stevers Golladay
    Dileep R. Vyas

PART VI

Central Nervous System

16 Spine Injuries   185
    Curtis Gruel

17 Coma and Altered Mental Status   209
    James H. McCrory

18 Convulsive Status Epilepticus   221
    Jeff Biehler

19 Acute Meningitis   233
    Richard Stuntz
    Terrence Morton, Jr.
    Robert Schafermeyer

PART VII

Gastrointestinal

20 Gastrointestinal Bleeding   243
    David Fisher

21 Intussusception   249
    Phyllis T. Doerger
    Jonathan Singer

22 Hypertrophic Pyloric Stenosis   259
    David Fisher

23 Acute Appendicitis   267
    David Tuggle

24 Acute Abdominal Pain   275
    Edwin Ide Smith

PART VIII

Renal/Genitourinary

25 Dehydration and Electrolyte Problems   285
    A. Eugene Osburn

26 Acute Scrotum   293
   J. Stephen Archer
   Philip L. Jones

PART IX
Metabolic/Endocrine

27 Diabetic Ketoacidosis   303
   Pierce R. Blackett
   Adolfo D. Garnica
   David B. Domek

28 Acute Adrenal Insufficiency/Crisis   315
   Adolfo D. Garnica
   Pierce R. Blackett

PART X
Hemotology and Oncology

29 Sickle Cell Disease   327
   Dilip L. Solanki

30 Oncologic Emergencies   337
   Nirmal Bhaya

PART XI
Miscellaneous

31 The Febrile Child under Two Years of Age   351
   Roger Barkin

32 Prehospital-Emergency Medical Services   359
   George L. Foltin
   Lou E. Romig

33 Child Abuse   367
   Gwendolyn Gibson
   Robert Block

34 Sexual Abuse   373
   Gwendolyn Gibson
   Robert Block

PART XII
Environmental

35 Snake Poisoning 379
James S. Walker

36 Mammalian Bites 393
Steven C. Jackson

37 Hypothermia 403
Steven C. Jackson

38 Heat Injuries 413
James S. Walker

Index 425

Contributors

William Ahrens, MD
Assistant Professor Emergency Medicine
University of Illinois–Chicago
Chicago, Illinois

J. Stephen Archer, MD, FACS
Clinical Assistant Professor Urology–OUHSC
University of Oklahoma Health Sciences Center
Oklahoma City, Oklahoma

Roger Barkin, MD, MPH, FAAP, FACEP
Professor of Pediatrics
Chairman, Department of Pediatrics
Rose Medical Center
Denver, Colorado

Steven M. Barrett, MD, FACEP
Associate Professor of Surgery
Chief, Section of Emergency Medicine
University of Oklahoma Health Sciences Center
Oklahoma City, Oklahoma

Nirmal Bhaya, MD
Assistant Professor of Pediatrics
Wayne State University School of Medicine
Director: Pediatric Emergency Medicine Fellowship
Children's Hospital of Michigan
Detroit, Michigan

Jeff Biehler, MD
Attending Staff
Emergency Dept.
Children's Hospital of Oklahoma
University of Oklahoma Health Sciences Center
Oklahoma City, Oklahoma

Pierce R. Blackett, MD
Assistant Professor of Pediatrics
Children's Hospital of Oklahoma
University of Oklahoma Health Sciences Center
Oklahoma City, Oklahoma

Robert Block, MD
Professor of Pediatrics
Vice Chair—Department of Pediatrics
University of Oklahoma, Tulsa Campus
Tulsa, Oklahoma

Douglas A. Boenning, MD
Associate Medical Director
Emergency Medicine Trauma Center
Children's National Medical Center
Washington, District of Columbia

Charles Cooper, MD
Clinical Professor, Pediatrics
Pediatric Cardiology
Tulsa Medical College
Director, Noninvasive Pediatric Cardiology
St. Francis Hospital
Tulsa, Oklahoma

Simon Cooper
Research Assistant
Children's National Medical Center
Washington, District of Columbia

Phyllis T. Doerger, MD
Chief Resident
Wright State University School of Medicine
Department of Emergency Medicine
Dayton, Ohio

David B. Domek, MD
Assistant Professor of Pediatrics
Children's Hospital of Oklahoma
University of Oklahoma Health Sciences Center
Oklahoma City, Oklahoma

David Fisher, MD
Clinical Assistant Professor Surgery/Emergency Medicine
Staff Physician
Deaconess Hospital
Emergency Department
Oklahoma City, Oklahoma

George L. Foltin, MD, FAAP, FACEP
Assistant Professor of Clinical Pediatrics
New York University School of Medicine
Director, Pediatric Emergency Service
Bellevue Hospital Center
New York, New York

Adolfo D. Garnica, MD
Associate Professor of Pediatrics
Children's Hospital of Oklahoma
University of Oklahoma Health Sciences Center
Oklahoma City, Oklahoma

Morris Gessouroun, MD
Associate Professor, Pediatrics
Director—Pediatric Intensive Care Unit
University of Oklahoma Health Sciences Center
Oklahoma City, Oklahoma

Gwendolyn Gibson, MD
Assistant Professor of Pediatrics
University of Oklahoma College of Medicine–Tulsa
Tulsa, Oklahoma

E. Stevers Golladay, MD
Professor of Surgery
Head of the Section of Pediatric Surgery
Louisiana State University Medical Center
New Orleans, Louisiana

David J. Gower, MD
Assistant Professor of Surgery
Section of Neurosurgery
University of Oklahoma Health Sciences Center
Oklahoma City, Oklahoma

Curtis Gruel, MD
Assistant Professor Orthopedic Surgery
Children's Hospital of Oklahoma
University of Oklahoma Health Sciences Center
Oklahoma City, Oklahoma

William A. Herndon, MD
Associate Professor Orthopedic Surgery
Children's Hospital of Oklahoma
University of Oklahoma Health Sciences Center
Oklahoma City, Oklahoma

Steven C. Jackson, MD
Staff Emergency Physician
Adventist Hospital
Portland, Oregon

David Johnson, MD
Assistant Professor of Pediatrics
Divisions of Emergency Medicine & Clinical Pharmacology
The Hospital for Sick Children
Toronto, Ontario, Canada

Philip L. Jones, MD
Chief Resident
Department of Urology
University of Oklahoma College of Medicine
Oklahoma City, Oklahoma

Niranjan Kissoon, MB, BSc, FRCP(C), FAAP
Associate Professor Pediatrics
Department of Pediatrics
University of Florida–Health Sciences Center
Jacksonville, Florida

Joseph D. Losek, MD, FAAP, FACEP
Associate Professor of Pediatrics
Medical College of Wisconsin
Children's Hospital of Wisconsin
Milwaukee, Wisconsin

David McCarty, MD, FACEP
Asst. Professor of Surgery/Emergency Medicine
Emergency Medicine/Trauma Center
Oklahoma Memorial Hospital
University of Oklahoma Health Sciences Center
Oklahoma City, Oklahoma

James H. McCrory, MD, FAAP, FCCM
Attending Staff
Pediatric Critical Care Center
St. John's Regional Health Center
Springfield, Missouri

Terrence Morton, Jr., MD, FACEP
Clinical Faculty—Dept. of Emergency Medicine
Carolinas Medical Center
University of North Carolina, Chapel Hill, N.C.
Charlotte Memorial Hospital
Charlotte, North Carolina

A. Eugene Osburn, DO, FAAP, FACEP
Associate Professor of Pediatrics
Children's Hospital of Oklahoma
University of Oklahoma Health Sciences Center
Oklahoma City, Oklahoma

Lou E. Romig, MD, FAAP
Attending Physician, Emergency Services and EMS Liaison
Miami Children's Hospital
Miami, Florida

Robert Schafermeyer, MD, FACEP, FAAP
Associate Chairman, Department of Emergency Medicine
Carolinas Medical Center, Charlotte, N.C.
Clinical Associate Professor of Pediatrics
University of North Carolina, Chapel Hill, N.C.
Charlotte Memorial Hospital
Charlotte, North Carolina

K.C. Sekar, MD
Assistant Professor of Pediatrics/Neonatology
Children's Hospital of Oklahoma
Oklahoma City, Oklahoma

Narendra C. Singh, BSc, MBBS, FRCP(C), FAAP
Assistant Professor of Pediatrics
Pediatric Emergency Medicine
Children's Hospital of Western Ontario
London, Ontario, Canada

Jonathan Singer, MD
Professor of Emergency Medicine and Pediatrics
Wright State University School of Medicine
Vice-Chair and Program Director
Department of Emergency Medicine
Dayton, Ohio

Edwin Ide Smith, MD
Professor of Surgery, Chairman–Division of Pediatric Surgery, University of Texas
Southwestern Medical Center
Dallas, Texas

Dilip L. Solanki, MD
Professor of Medicine
Director of Clinical Oncology/Oklahoma Medical Center
Hematology Oncology Section
University of Oklahoma Health Sciences Center
Oklahoma City, Oklahoma

Gary Strange, MD
Associate Professor of Emergency Medicine
Residency Program Director
University of Chicago
Chicago, Illinois

Richard Stuntz, MD, FACEP
Clinical Faculty – Dept. of Emergency Medicine
Carolinas Medical Center
University of North Carolina, Chapel Hill, N.C.
Charlotte Memorial Hospital
Charlotte, North Carolina

David Tuggle, MD
Assistant Professor of Surgery
Children's Hospital of Oklahoma
University of Oklahoma Health Sciences Center
Department of Pediatric Surgery
Oklahoma City, Oklahoma

Dileep R. Vyas, MD
Assistant Professor of Pediatrics
University of Arkansas for Medical Sciences
Arkansas Children's Hospital
Little Rock, Arkansas

James S. Walker, DO, FACEP
Assistant Professor of Surgery
Residency Director, Section of Emergency Medicine & Trauma
University of Oklahoma Health Sciences Center
Oklahoma City, Oklahoma

Foreword

This book is a written response to the many physicians, including pediatricians, emergency physicians, and pediatric emergency physicians who need to review a practical approach to management of selected emergent conditions. How does this book contribute to the growing body of pediatric emergency medicine literature? There are a number of textbooks published addressing many of the conditions of illness and injury that present under the broad umbrella of pediatric emergency care but with variable depth of coverage of each condition. The comprehensive pediatric emergency texts exceed 1000 pages in length and provide in-depth coverage of numerous conditions of illness and injury with narrative descriptions of diagnosis and management guidelines. The life support courses are designed to be action-oriented with "how to" instructions for selected life-threatening conditions so that the physician with relatively little familiarity with these conditions can provide resuscitation and recognition of respiratory and circulatory failure using PALS or stabilization of selected life-threatening conditions using APLS. None of these course textbooks provide comprehensive coverage of a single diagnosis, other than the condition of cardiopulmonary arrest, and none of the course textbooks provide comprehensive coverage of the wide range of pediatric emergency conditions. Dr. Surpure has selected about 40 of the most common life-threatening conditions of illness or injury and has provided in-depth coverage of these conditions with clear diagnostic and management guidelines, often complemented by algorithms, in 423 pages. For the physician who wants to master diagnosis and management of the life-threatened child, this book can be used as a reference for immediate diagnosis and management in the emergency department, or it can be used as a study resource for expanding the provider's understanding of the important conditions selected for coverage.

Dr. Jack Surpure is distinguished in the specialty of pediatric emergency medicine because of numerous outstanding contributions. He originated and continues to serve as chief editor and manager of *Pediatric Emergency Trends*, a national monthly newsletter providing brief editorial reviews of significant contributions to the specialty literature, and he is editor of "Pep Talk" feature of *Pediatric Emergency Care*. He also coordinates numerous courses to enhance pediatric emergency provider knowledge and skills in America and abroad. The specialty of Pediatric Emergency Medicine is fortunate to have Dr. Surpure as an ongoing insightful innovator and contributor. This synopsis is his current contribution and will surely find its place in the history of the growth and development of pediatric emergency medicine.

Martha Bushore

Preface

The growth of pediatric emergency medicine has been phenomenal; there has been an explosion of new knowledge in this area in the last decade. The numerous new courses (APLS, PALS), books, journals, and newsletters are the indicators of this parameter. The advancement of new knowledge, equipment, and life-support care has resulted in children now being resuscitated and cared for more efficiently. The establishment of specialized care centers and properly trained personnel and equipment at remote and small community hospitals will further improve the emergency care of ill and injured children. Obviously the ultimate goal is improved medical care for all children.

This book attempts to provide practical clinical information on the most important emergency children's problems that are seen in the emergency department on a daily basis. Hopefully this practical knowledge will assist the frontline clinicians in approaching precise diagnosis and management. This book is not an attempt to provide a comprehensive review of all children's emergencies. Rather it presents a quick practical approach to most common and frequent childhood emergency problems faced by the clinician in daily practice. Each chapter uniformly provides a brief review of pathophysiology followed by discussion and presentation of diagnostic and therapeutic modalities. In most chapters, the clinical decisionmaking is simplified by an algorithmic approach.

We sincerely hope that this synopsis format will be of practical benefit to all health professionals who care for critically ill and injured children.

J.S. Surpure

Acknowledgments

I am indebted to the eminent clinical experts who generously contributed the chapters, and much credit is owed to them. It would not have been possible to publish this book without their help. Indeed, the book is a true synopsis of many dedicated individuals' experience, knowledge, expertise, and sensitivity toward children.

Very special thanks to Judith Gimple, Bywater Production Services, for her superb assistance in proofreading and editing the manuscript. It was a great pleasure to work with her as she kept me on my toes with frequent reminders and suggestions. Appreciation also goes to Ed Johnson for his excellent computer work, and Arlene Conrad for her assistance in editing.

Finally, I thank the readers, and hope that this book will be useful for them in daily clinical practice and will guide them in caring for ill and injured children.

Synopsis
of Pediatric
Emergency Care

PART I

Resuscitation

1

Cardiopulmonary Resuscitation

David Johnson

Cardiopulmonary arrests in children occur infrequently compared to adults (1). Of children who require resuscitation, however, the majority are young (45 to 70 percent are less than one year old and 21 to 30 percent are one to four years of age) (2). Though early reports suggested children have a better outcome than adults, recent reviews demonstrate that children who suffer *cardio*pulmonary arrests have poor outcomes with only 5 to 21 percent surviving to hospital discharge (3). In contrast, children who have just respiratory arrests have a much higher survival rate.

PATHOPHYSIOLOGY

Cardiopulmonary arrests in children are caused by a wide range of problems. The most common causes include asthma, sudden infant death syndrome, intravascular volume depletion due to traumatic hemorrhage, or illnesses such as gastroenteritis, infectious diseases such as meningitis, sepsis, pneumonia, epiglottitis, croup, and bronchiolitis. Unlike adults, cardiac arrests as a result of a primary cardiac problem (congenital heart disease, myocarditis, or dysrhythmias) occur uncommonly. Though pediatric arrests are due to a wide range of etiologies, the final common pathway is usually respiratory failure and/or circulatory collapse, resulting in end-organ anoxia. Cardiac arrest probably occurs within five minutes of complete anoxia (4). Because cardiac arrest in children is predominately caused by anoxia, most children present with bradycardia or asystole. Only about 10 percent of children with cardiac arrest present with ventricular fibrillation and commonly have ventricular rhythms with cardiac arrest (1).

CLINICAL PRESENTATION/DIFFERENTIAL DIAGNOSES

Recognition of a cardiopulmonary arrest is not difficult. Clinical characteristics are cyanosis, a grayish hue, diaphoresis, mottling, unresponsiveness, and absence of respiration or pulse. Rapid recognition and institution of advanced life support is critical. Identifying the etiology of a cardiopulmonary arrest should follow the establishment of an airway, ventilation, and circulation.

More difficult is the recognition of the prearrest state—a child who is still awake but agitated and subtly tachypneic from hypoxia, and who has normal blood pressure but is tachycardic with poor capillary refill. Given the poor outcome of children who suffer cardiopulmonary arrests, early intervention in these children can be lifesaving.

HISTORY, PHYSICAL EXAMINATION, LABORATORY AND MANAGEMENT

In an arrest situation, the classical approach of taking a history, performing a complete examination, and performing initial laboratory tests before deciding on management is obviously not applicable. Instead these elements are interwoven.

Setting Up a Team

The presentation of a young child in cardiopulmonary arrest is anxiety-provoking and often results in a chaotic resuscitation. Optimal performance is derived from having a well-trained, experienced team with members having preassigned specific roles. The ideal size of team ranges between five and eight people. Too small a team makes it difficult to move rapidly through the resuscitation algorithm; too large a team causes unnecessary confusion. The team should include a leader and a scribe as well as individuals assigned to manage the airway, perform chest compressions, establish venous access, place and maintain monitors, assess vital signs, draw up medications, and apply cardiac defibrillation. As soon as possible, an experienced team member should meet and talk with any family members available to ascertain recent and past medical history.

Establishing an Airway and Assuring Ventilation

Evaluate the airway and then the ventilation by looking quickly at the chest and abdomen for signs of movement and listening over the mouth and nose for the movement of air. If there are no signs of respiration, check the oropharynx for foreign objects, then suction the airway of excess secretions. Place the child in a "sniffing" position. If intubation cannot be accomplished immediately, patients can be ventilated temporarily with 100 percent oxygen by use of a bag and mask (most commonly a self-inflating bag with a reservoir). If placing fingers behind the angle of the jaw while bagging the child is not sufficient to maintain an open airway, either place an oropharyngeal airway or have a second person bag while the other maintains a patent, sealed oral airway. If an oral airway is placed, choose one with a tip that reaches approximately to the angle of the jaw.

Intubation should be accomplished as soon as feasible since it maximizes ventilation and minimizes the risk of aspiration (5). Children less than eight years of age should be intubated with an endotracheal (ET) tube without a cuff. The size of ET tube can best be estimated by matching the external diameter of the tube to the diameter of the child's little finger. See Table 1.1. for estimates of ET tube, laryngoscope blade, and suction catheter sizes based on age. The time required to intubate should be monitored, and prolonged efforts should be avoided by intermittent ventilation with 100 percent oxygen by mask.

Table 1.1 Sizing of ET tubes, laryngoscopes, and catheters, based on age

Age	Internal Diameter of tube, mm	Laryngoscope blade size	Suction Catheters
Newborn	3	0–1	6 F
6 months	3.5	1	8 F
18 months	4	2	8 F
3 years	4.5	2	8 F
5 years	5	2	10 F
6 years	5.5	2	10 F
8 years	6	2	10 F
12 years	6.5	2	10 F
16 years	7	3	10 F
Adult (F)	7.5–8	3	12 F
Adult (M)	8–8.5	3	14 F

Adapted with permission from Silverman BK. Advanced pediatric life support. Dallas: AAP and ACEP, 1989.

Appropriate placement of the ET tube should be promptly confirmed by auscultation and checking for condensation in the tube with exhalation. If there is any doubt about proper placement, the tube should be pulled and the patient reintubated. Ventilation rates based on age are listed in Table 1.2. Ventilation volume should be 10 to 15 ml/kg; practically this volume can be approximated by bagging sufficient to lift the chest wall visibly (5). Auscultate the chest in anterior and lateral fields bilaterally, and quickly check for asymmetry of the chest wall and deviation of the trachea. A naso- or orogastric tube should be placed after intubation to evacuate the stomach of air and of any other contents.

Cricothyroidotomy or tracheostomy are *rarely* required (PALS). Complications from these procedures are common, and ventilation can almost always be maintained with bag and mask until intubation can be accomplished.

Table 1.2 Compression/ventilation standards for pediatric resuscitation

	Infant (less than 1 year)	Child (1–7 Years)	Child (more than 7 years)
Compression (rate/min)	100–120	80–100	60–80
Depth of compression (inches)	½–1	1½	1½–2
Ventilation (rate/min)	20	16	12
Technique	Hand encircling chest or two fingers	Heel of one hand	One or two hands

Adapted with permission from Silverman BK. Advanced pediatric life support. Dallas: AAP and ACEP, 1989.

Airway and ventilation should be repeatedly reassessed throughout resuscitation. In addition, the oxygen delivery system should be double-checked to assure that 100 percent oxygen is being delivered to the patient.

Assessment of Circulation/Chest Compressions

Palpate the brachial or femoral pulse. A slow or absent pulse in an apneic, unconscious child requires the initiation of chest compressions. Place the child on a firm surface. Compressions should be performed on the lower third of the sternum, approximately 1.5 to 2 cm above the xiphoid (6). The downward stroke should last for 50 percent of the compression cycle. See Table 1.2 for a summary of technique and rates based on age. Compressions should be stopped every few minutes to check for the return of arterial pulses.

Establishing Venous Access

Venous access should be obtained rapidly to allow the provision of fluids and drugs. Peripheral venous catheters should be attempted first, preferably in the upper extremity (7). If placement is not accomplished within two minutes, however, other alternatives should be tried (5). Unless a member of the team is extensively experienced in obtaining rapid central venous access, in a child under five years of age an intraosseous needle should be placed. If neither a bone marrow nor a specifically designed intraosseous needle is available, a two-inch, 18 to 20 gauge spinal needle can be used. The preferred location is on the flat, medial surface of the proximal tibial shaft 1 to 2 cm below the tibial tuberosity. Alternately, especially in older children or adolescents, a needle can be placed in the medial surface of the tibia proximal to the medial malleolus (8). All resuscitation drugs and fluids can be delivered rapidly and safely via this route.

Central venous access is obtained most reliably and rapidly by the Seldinger guide-wire technique via the femoral vein (PALS). The use of this route does not impinge on other aspects of resuscitation. Cannulation by the open or percutaneous cutdown technique *in unexperienced hands* is difficult and slow and generally should be avoided.

Assessment of Cardiac Rhythm/Defibrillation

Place "quick look" paddles or monitor leads to assess the child's cardiac rhythm. If supraventricular tachycardia, ventricular tachycardia, or ventricular fibrillation are present, deliver countershock and medications rapidly. (For supraventricular tachycardia (SVT) or ventricular tachycardia (VT), cardiovert with synchronized 0.25 to 0.5 Wsec/kg then double if the first attempt is unsuccessful. For VF, defibrillate with nonsynchronized, 2 Wsec/kg, then double and repeat twice if the first attempt is unsuccessful.) Most cases of ventricular fibrillation occur in children with congenital heart disease. Other causes of fibrillation are hypothermia, hypoglycemia, abnormalities of potassium and calcium, and drug overdoses such as tricyclic antidepressants or digoxin (3). If a normal sinus rhythm is present, reassess the brachial and femoral

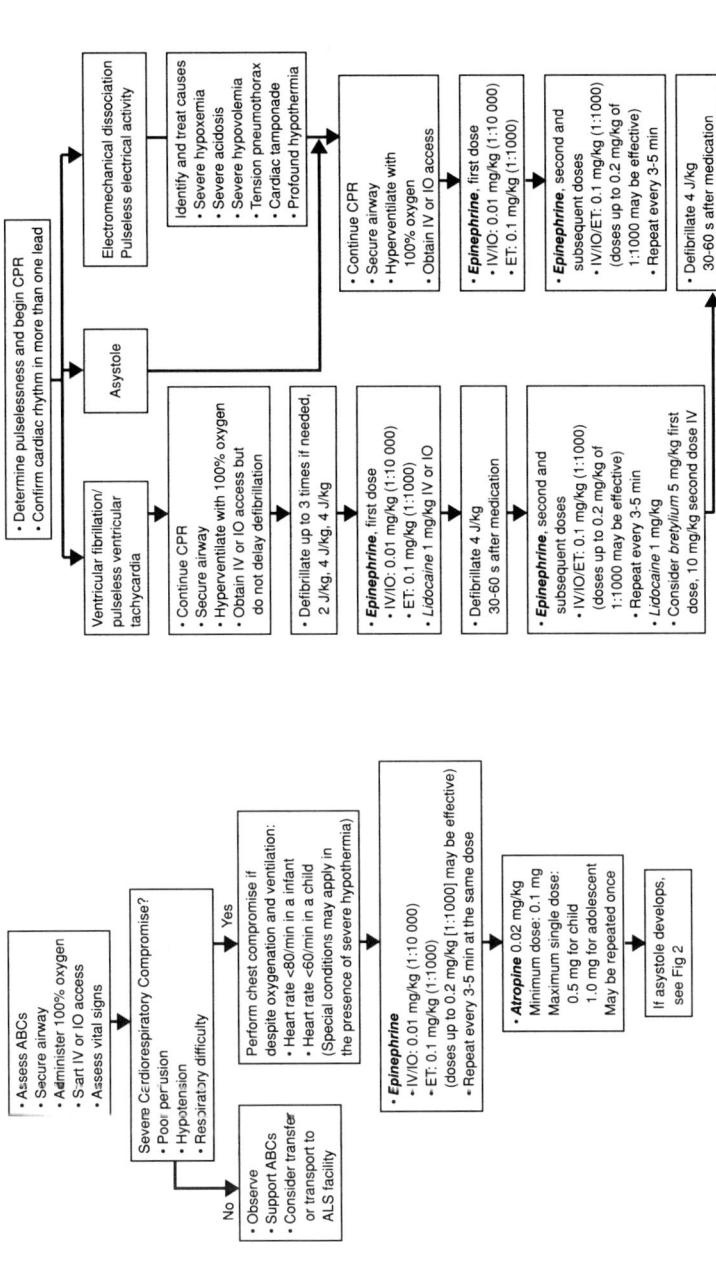

Figure 1.1 Algorithm for pediatric cardiopulmonary resuscitation: (a) bradycardia decision tree (ABCs = airway, breathing, circulation; ALS = advanced life support; IO = intraosseous; IV = intravenous) and (b) asystole and pulseless arrest decision tree (CPR = cardiopulmonary resuscitation). (Adapted with permission from Emergency Cardiac Care Committee and Subcommittee of the American Heart Association. Guidelines for cardiopulmonary resuscitation and emergency cardiac care: Part IV. Pediatric advanced life support. JAMA 1992;268:2262–2275.)

pulses. If they are not palpable, electromechanical dissociation (EMD) is present. Conditions associated with EMD are hypovolemia, tension pneumothorax, cardiac tamponade, and pulmonary embolus. By far the most common rhythm found in apneic, pulseless children will be asystole or bradycardia. Patients who survive with this rhythm will usually do so with the initiation of ventilation or with the first couple of doses of epinephrine (9,10).

Drug Therapy

Recommendations for drug therapy during pediatric resuscitation have changed significantly over the last 10 years. Several issues remain unresolved and recommendations may continue to change. See Table 1.3 for current dosing recommendations.

Oxygen. Most arrests occur as a result of inadequate delivery of oxygen to the tissues. It is therefore imperative that 100 percent oxygen be used throughout the resuscitation to minimize tissue hypoxia.

Epinephrine. After oxygen, epinephrine is widely considered to be the most effective drug in resuscitation. It is indicated for asystole, bradycardia, EMD, and ventricular fibrillation. The mechanism of action appears to be largely due to its effects, which result in increased coronary perfusion

Table 1.3 Principle drugs used in pediatric resuscitation

Drug	Dose	Concentration	Comments
Atropine	0.02 mg/kg/dose	Range .1 mg to 1.2 mg/ml	Recommended minimum dose .1 mg
Bretyllum	5–10 mg/kg/dose	50 mg/ml	For Rx of V Fib, give undiluted rapid IV push
Calcium chloride	20 mg/kg/dose	100 mg/ml (10%)	Use with central venous access
Calcium gluconate	100 mg/kg/dose	100 mg/ml (10%)	Use with peripheral venous access
Dopamine	2–20 µg/kg/min	40, 80 and 160 mg/ml	Titrate to desired effect
Epinephrine (infusion)	.01 mg/kg/dose .1–1.5 µg/kg/min	.1 mg/ml (1:10,000)	Consider using 20-fold larger dose Titrate to desired effect
Glucose	250 mg/kg/dose	250 mg/ml (25%)	Probably important in neonates. If glucose is low, give on one bolus dose, then start infusion of 5% glucose.
Lidocaine (infusion)	1 mg/kg/dose 20–50 µg/kg/min	10 & 20 mg/ml (1 & 2%)	Give bolus undiluted over 2–4 min
Sodium bicarbonate	1 mEq/kg/dose	.5–1 mEq/mi (4.2 & 8.4%)	Use only if ventilation is established

Adapted with permission from Silverman BK. Advanced pediatric life support. Dallas: AAP and ACEP, 1989.

pressure and cerebral blood flow. Considerable data in animals suggest that doses of 0.1 to 0.2 mg/kg/dose are more effective than is the standard recommended dose—0.01 mg/kg/dose. High-dose epinephrine appears promising, its efficacy and safety has now been established in humans, especially in children (11).

Glucose. The neonatal myocardium uses glucose as its major energy substrate, and infants, especially those who are chronically ill, have limited glycogen stores. Consequently early assessment of a child's serum glucose by rapid chemstick is essential. Blind or repeated administration of glucose is not warranted, however, as it may result in a hyperosmolar state (3).

Atropine. This is generally recommended for both asystole or bradycardia. Since bradycardia most commonly stems from hypoxia, however, attention should be directed toward adequacy of airway and ventilation before atropine is given (3).

Sodium bicarbonate. Controversy surrounds the use of bicarbonate in an arrest situation. Evidence is accumulating that the administration of bicarbonate can cause a *lowering* of intracellular pH. To date, a consensus has formed that bicarbonate should not be given until adequate ventilation has been established, and arterial blood gases drawn subsequently demonstrate a residual metabolic acidosis (3).

Calcium. No longer recommended in an arrest situation unless hypocalcemia is demonstrated or unless there is a specific therapeutic indication such as hyperkalemia, hypermagnesemia, or calcium channel blocker overdose (PALS).

Lidocaine. Ventricular fibrillation or unstable tachycardia that does not respond to defibrillation are indications for the use of lidocaine. If one bolus dose is not effective, a repeat bolus dose may be given in 10 to 15 minutes. Start a continuous infusion immediately. A third bolus may be needed 10 to 15 minutes later while the infusion is reaching steady-state concentrations.

Bretyllium. This should be considered if lidocaine fails to convert ventricular fibrillation. A bolus of 5 mg/kg should be given, followed by defibrillation. If not effective, a second dose of 10 mg/kg can be administered, followed again by defibrillation.

Guidelines for Stopping Resuscitation Efforts

There are no established standards for terminating resuscitative efforts in an emergency setting. Based on epidemiologic studies of cardiopulmonary resuscitation, however, some general statements and broad guidelines can be derived. Unwitnessed cardiopulmonary arrests or patients who have a delay of greater than 12 minutes before cardiopulmonary resuscitation (CPR) is initiated have a poor prognosis (12). Children presenting with asystole do much worse than do children presenting with other types of rhythm (1). Children who develop sinus rhythm and perfusion after more than two doses of epinephrine also have low long-term survival (10). The exception is children who are hypothermic, most commonly from cold-water drowning. Establishing brain death by strict criteria takes time, however, and is impossible to do in an emergency setting.

Based on this set of facts, it is reasonable to intubate, ventilate, and perform compressions on all children who present in cardiopulmonary arrest until their hypoxia and respiratory acidosis is reversed, their core temperature is raised to 35°C, and they have been given at least two doses of epinephrine and *as indicated* counter shocked or given drugs such as glucose. Resuscitative efforts should be continued on children who intermittently restore perfusion or demonstrate supraventricular tachycardia or a ventricular rhythm. Regardless of the duration of suspected anoxia, any child who restores perfusion should continue to be treated. Though the prognosis for some of these children will be poor, termination can only be medicolegally carried out in an intensive care setting and should not be terminated in the field. Resuscitation can be stopped, however, on children who remain unresponsive without pulse and rhythm after the resuscitative efforts outlined above have been completed (13).

CONCLUSIONS

Survival rates from cardiopulmonary resuscitation in children are low. Hence vigilant monitoring of children with potentially fatal diseases is essential. Early intervention prior to arrest will result in the highest possible rates of recovery. Since all cardiopulmonary arrests are not completely preventable, however, the highest survival rates will result from prompt, well-organized resuscitative efforts.

Last, the physiology and pharmacology of cardiopulmonary resuscitation are evolving sciences. Changes in approach and outcome can be expected to continue to occur over the next decade.

REFERENCES

1. Eisenberg M, Bergner L, Hallstrom A. Epidemiology of cardiac arrest and resuscitation in children. Ann Emerg Med 1983;12:672.
2. Ludwig S, Fleisher G. Pediatric cardiopulmonary resuscitation: a review and a proposal. Pediatr Emerg Care 1985;1:40.
3. Zaritsky A. Drug therapy of cardiopulmonary resuscitation in children. Drugs 1989; 37:356.
4. Caputo G, Delgado-Paredes C, Swedlow D, et al. Anoxic cardiopulmonary arrest in a pediatric animal model: Clinical and laboratory correlates of duration. Pediatr Emerg Care 1978;1:57.
5. Silverman BK. Advanced pediatric life support. Dallas: American Academy of Pediatrics & American College of Emergency Physicians, 1989;1–14.
6. Orlowski JP. Optimum position for external cardiac compression in infants and young children. Ann Emerg Med 1986;15:667.
7. Hedges JR, Barsan WB, Doan LA, et al. Central versus peripheral intravenous routes in cardiopulmonary resuscitation. Am J Emerg Med 1984;2:385.
8. Spivery WH. Intraosseous infusions. J Peds 1987;111:639.
9. Gillis J, Dickson D, Rieder M, et al. Results of inpatient pediatric resuscitation. Crit Care Med 1979;14:469.
10. Zaritsky A, Nadkarni V, Getson P, et al. CPR in children. Ann Emerg Med 1987;16:1107.
11. Emergency Cardiac Care Committee and Subcommittee of the American Heart Association. Guidelines for cardiopulmonary resuscitation and emergency cardiac care: Part IV. Pediatric advanced life support. JAMA 1992;268:2262–2275.
12. Smith JP, Bodai MI. Guidelines for discontinuing prehospital CPR in the emergency department—a review. Ann Emerg Med 1985;14:1093.
13. Dieckmann RA. Cardiopulmonary arrest and resuscitation. In Grossman M, Dieckmann RA, eds. Pediatric emergency medicine. Philadelphia: Lippincott, 1991.

2

Neonatal Resuscitation

K.C. Sekar

Resuscitation of the newborn infant is a medical emergency. It is required for any neonate who, in the first few minutes of life, cannot establish adequate effective ventilation to meet the needs for oxygenation and carbon dioxide excretion or whose cardiovascular status is inadequate to perfuse the central nervous system (CNS), heart, and other vital organs. Ineffective oxygenation and inadequate perfusion in the newborn may start at a variable period before delivery secondary to conditions that interrupt the placenta's ability to remove carbon dioxide and hydrogen ions or to supply oxygen (fetal asphyxia). This may progress through the intrapartum and the immediate postpartum period. Conditions that reduce the neonate's ability to initiate and/or maintain breathing at birth, however, will also regularly result in asphyxia.

Transition from fetal to neonatal life requires many adjustments that the newborn must accomplish in order to function normally at birth. Some infants have difficulty making this transition and require resuscitation in the first few minutes after birth. An effective resuscitation requires, besides capable personnel and a smooth working team, an understanding of the physiology of progressive asphyxia, temperature regulation, and appropriate ventilatory and monitoring equipment, drugs, and fluids. In the emergency department, good communication should be maintained between obstetrics, pediatrics, anaesthesiology, and the nursing service. At least two persons are required to perform proper neonatal resuscitation. High-risk conditions that may result in an asphyxiated newborn infant are given in Table 2.1. If possible these conditions should be anticipated and preparation made well in advance.

PATHOPHYSIOLOGY OF ASPHYXIA

An understanding of the pathophysiology of asphyxia is a prerequisite to anyone performing neonatal resuscitation. Much of the information about the physiological changes associated with asphyxia comes from experiments on animals. Although differences exist among the diverse species studied, the species that is most closely analogous to the human fetus when it is subjected to total asphyxia is the Rhesus monkey fetus. A Rhesus monkey fetus was delivered via caeserian section with catheters placed in the fetal vessels prior to delivery; it prevented from gasping with a saline-filled rubber bag placed over its head.[3] The animal was observed over a period of several minutes and the physiological changes that occurred were recorded during

Table 2.1 Conditions of high risk for the newborn

Prenatal	Natal	Postnatal
Maternal age more than 35 years	Abnormal presentation	Birth asphyxia
Diabetes	Premature delivery	Respiratory distress
Hypertension	Multiple births	Hypothermia
Hemorrhage	Maternal hypertension	Meconium staining
Infection	Prolonged labor	Premature infant
Prolonged rupture of membranes	Prolapse of the cord	Intrauterine growth retardation (IUGR)
Drug therapy	Maternal anesthesia	
Drug dependency	Caesarean section	
Heroin	Abnormal fetal heart rate	
Methadone	Meconium-stained amniotic fluid	
Cocaine	Polyhydramnios	
Anemia		
Isoimmunization		

this "total asphyxia." Rapid gasps occurred shortly after the onset of asphyxia accompanied by muscular efforts producing thrashing movements of the arms and legs. This ceased after little more than a minute and heralded the onset of *primary apnea*. During primary apnea, spontaneous respirations could still be induced by appropriate sensory stimuli. This apnea lasted for about a minute. The heart rate dropped but was still above 100 per minute. A series of spontaneous deep gasps then followed for the next four or five minutes, gradually becoming weaker and terminating at the last gasp followed by *secondary apnea*. This occurred after approximately eight minutes of total anoxia. During secondary apnea, respirations could not be induced by sensory stimuli, and death would occur if secondary apnea was not reversed within several minutes. The longer the delay in resuscitation after the last gasp, the longer the time to the first gasp after resuscitation.

When an asphyxiated newborn is encountered in the emergency department, it is extremely difficult to determine whether primary or secondary apnea is present. In all situations, secondary apnea must be assumed and resuscitative efforts should be initiated immediately.

Dramatic changes in the acid base parameters of the Rhesus monkey occurred during asphyxia. During 10 minutes of asphyxia pH dropped from 7.3 to 6.8, PCO_2 rose from 45 to 150 mmHg and PO_2 fell from 25 to almost 0 mmHg. Associated with this was an increase in the blood lactate level (anaerobic glycolysis), free fatty acid and glycerol (release of epinephrine and norepinephrine), and mobilization of hepatic glycogen. This mobilization of glycogen makes it an unusual event to find hypoglycemia in an asphyxiated newborn infant. Therefore infusion of hypertonic glucose solutions are not recommended during resuscitation.

During the course of asphyxia blood pressure fell gradually after an initial transient rise. The skin became blotchy and blue in response to circulatory failure. Blood was preferentially redistributed, however, to vital organs like the heart, the brain, and the adrenal glands at the expense of less vital organs like the kidneys, the spleen, and the lungs (*diving reflex*). This situation resulted in asphyxial damage to virtually every organ in the body like necrotizing enterocolitis in the gastrointestinal tract, postasphyxial icterus, shock lung, persistent pulmonary hypertension, renal failure, and sclerema of the skin secondary to asphyxial injury to the dermal capillaries.

The most common antecedent of persistent neurologic dysfunction in a newborn infant is perinatal asphyxia. This is true because, although the brain is less than 2 percent of the body weight, it accounts for almost 20 percent of the total oxygen consumption. Thus the brain is dependent on a continuous, uninterrupted supply of oxygen and glucose in order for it to function normally. Asphyxia also leads to a loss of the brain's ability to control its own blood supply (*auto regulation*). Such a loss in the brain's ability to control circulation exposes the brain to fluctuations in systemic blood pressure. This could result in intracranial hemorrhage. A wide array of typical pathological lesions have been described in the brain of asphyxiated newborn infants. The asphyxiated neuronal cell membrane becomes vulnerable to cation and water flux since acidosis alters its intrinsic ion pumping mechanisms. Potassium leaks out and sodium enters the neuron. This is the biochemical basis for the brain swelling found in postasphyxia.

Newborn infants have some protective mechanisms to tolerate asphyxia such as a lower metabolic rate of any particular tissue than the adults do, availability of substrates for anaerobic degradation, and an intact circulation to redistribute lactate and hydrogen ion to tissues still being perfused. Severe sustained asphyxia, however, will overcome these protective mechanisms, and severe brain damage and death will occur if asphyxia is not reversed.

The description of asphyxia and its consequences described above generally refers to severe total asphyxia. In practice, various grades of asphyxia much milder than this will be encountered. Also modern obstetrical management with fetal monitoring and determination of fetal acid base status with scalp blood sampling can detect impending asphyxia *in utero*, and preventive measures can be undertaken before delivery.

CLINICAL PRESENTATION

In the emergency department, neonatal resuscitation should be an infrequent event. In the few situations that require resuscitation, however, both skill and quick response is required to prevent the damaging effects of prolonged asphyxia. Clinical presentation could vary from mild asphyxia, where an infant presents with slight disturbances in the stability of cardiorespiratory system, to complete cardiac and respiratory arrest associated with shock, severe hypothermia, and metabolic acidosis.

Table 2.2 Resuscitation equipment

Radiant warmer	Laryngoscope blades, nos. 0 and 1
EKG/respiration monitor	Umbilical catheters 3.5 and 5 Fr
Suction with manometer	Three-way stopcock
Wall oxygen with flow meter	Sterile umbilical catherization tray
Suction catheters, sizes 5, 6, and 8 Fr	ET tube adaptor for meconium suctioning
Resuscitation bag with manometer	Gloves
Face masks—small, medium, and large	Stethoscope
Oral airways	Warm towels
ET tube, sizes 2.5, 3, and 3.5 mm	Cap to cover the scalp
ET tube stylette	Umbilical cord clamp
Laryngoscope	

Therefore the worst situation should be anticipated, and preparation should be made in the emergency department. All the necessary equipment for performing neonatal resuscitation should be available at all times (Table 2.2). A radiant warmer should be ready with proper lighting. All resuscitative procedures should be performed with gloved hands, as the physician invariably has to respond to infants with very little knowledge of their prenatal history. All ancillary services should be informed of the arrival of the asphyxiated newborn infant.

EVALUATION OF THE NEWBORN INFANT

Immediately after arrival, infants should be placed under a radiant warmer and Apgar scores should be determined. The components of the Apgar scores are given in Table 2.3. These parameters can be assessed very easily at the bedside within a few seconds. Traditionally Apgar Scores are given in the delivery room at one and five minutes after birth. The one-minute Apgar score determines the need to intervene. The five-minute Apgar score assesses the efficacy of resuscitation and perhaps later mortality and morbidity. If the five-minute Apgar score is less than seven, additional scores should be obtained every five minutes up to twenty minutes unless two successive scores are eight or greater. Apgar scores should be given by a person not directly involved in the resuscitation (for example, a nurse). Apgar scores, particularly when they indicate delay in return of tone, indentify neonates who have sustained significant CNS insults. Low Apgar scores at ten, fifteen, and twenty minutes are useful in predicting neonatal, and later, mortality and morbidity. Based on Apgar scores, asphyxia can be classified as

0–2 (severe asphyxia)—these infants will require aggressive resuscitation
3–6—these infants will respond to stimulation, suctioning, and oxygen
More than 7—these infants will rarely require resuscitation

Table 2.3 Apgar Scores

Sign	Score		
	0	1	2
Heart rate	Absent	Less than 100	More than 100
Respiratory effort	Absent	Weak, irregular	Good, crying
Muscle tone	Flaccid	Some flexion	Well flexed
Reflex irritability	No response	Grimace	Cry
Color	Pale	Blue	Pink

LABORATORY EVALUATION

Generally laboratory evaluation will not be of any benefit in the immediate management of the newborn infant. Besides obtaining the vital signs, the temperature, and the acid base status, no other laboratory evaluation will be necessary. As time becomes the limiting factor, quick clinical assessment and immediate action should be carried out. Biochemical markers of asphyxia other than acid base status have been described in the literature. These markers are generally not useful in the immediate management of the infant.

MANAGEMENT
Goals of Resuscitation

The major objectives of resuscitation of the newborn infant are (1) to maintain neutral thermal environment, (2) to provide adequate ventilatory support, (3) to maintain adequate circulation that will provide adequate oxygen-carrying capacity and blood supply to the brain, (4) to minimize fluid and electrolyte shifts within the brain, and (5) to provide sufficient calories for optimal brain metabolism. The process of resuscitation is a continuum and the person involved in resuscitation should stop at every step of the process and reassess whether the objective has been achieved. If the objective has been achieved, resuscitative efforts should be stopped, the infant should be observed briefly, and efforts should be resumed as indicated. Overzealous attempts at resuscitation without close attention to the infant's condition will lead to complications. An algorithm for management is given in Figure 2.1. As can be seen, heart rate and respiratory efforts should be the guide to the resuscitative process.

Thermal Environment

All infants should be maintained under neutral thermal environment where metabolic demands are minimal. Infants who are asphyxiated have a particularly unstable thermoregulatory system, and recovery from acidosis will be delayed if hypothermia is present. Immediately after its arrival in the emergency department or delivery, the infant should be placed under a radiant warmer and completely dried.

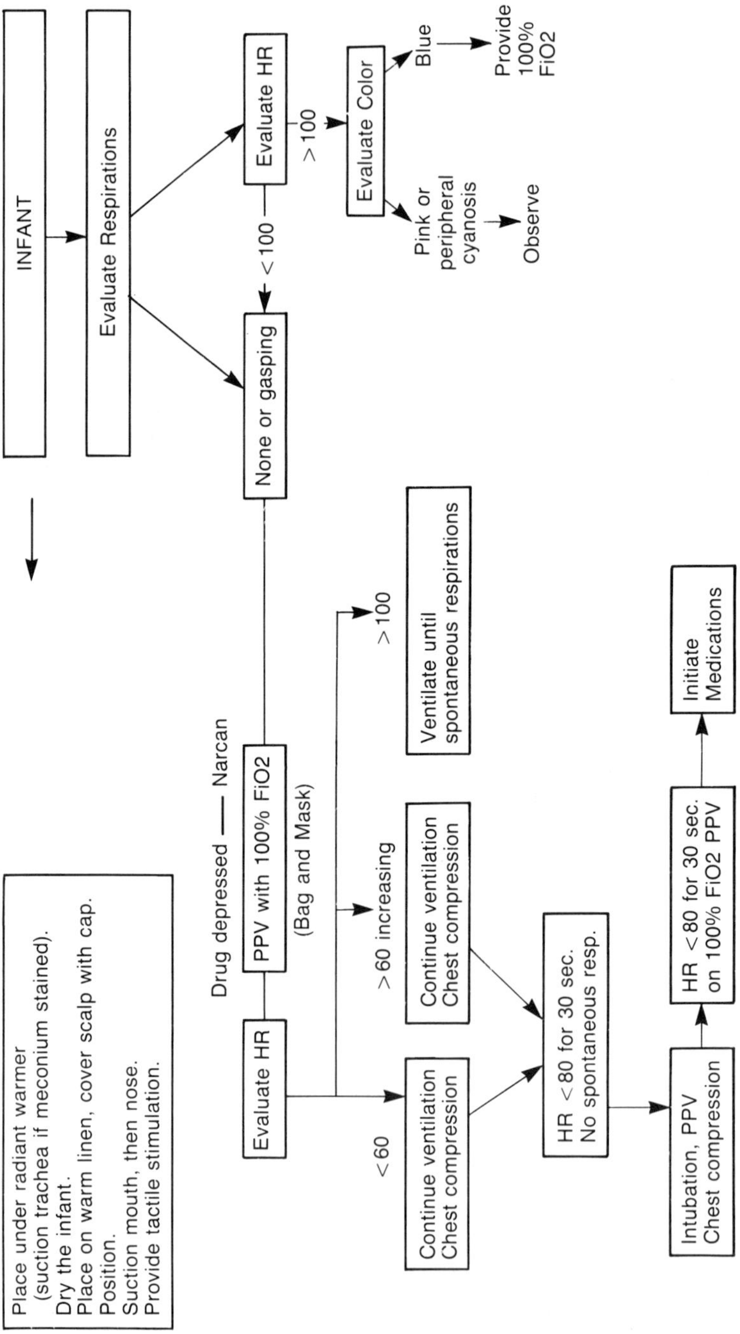

Figure 2.1 Management of an asphyxiated newborn infant

Skin temperature should be maintained between 36.2 and 36.8 C. Under the radiant warmer, heat losses are markedly reduced and the infant is readily accessible for resuscitative efforts.

Establishment of Adequate Ventilation and Circulation

After it has been dried, the infant should be placed in a slight Trendelenburg position with the neck slightly extended. Care should be taken to not hyper or underextend the neck as this may affect the entry of air. First the mouth is suctioned then the nose with either a bulb syringe, a DeLee suction catheter, or a mechanical suction catheter. Irrespective of the suction device used, the mouth should always be suctioned first in order to avoid aspirating the material from the mouth into the trachea. Special precautions to be followed when meconium is present in the amniotic fluid are described at the end of this chapter. This procedure itself will provide some stimulation. If the infant is breathing, evaluate the heart rate, and if it is above 100/min, evaluate color. If the infant is pink, continue to observe. If the heart rate is below 100/min, initiate bag and mask ventilation. If the infant has central cyanosis, administer 100 percent oxygen, lowering the concentration as the infant gradually improves, or continue to administer it if cyanosis persists. If the infant is apneic, provide stimulation with a gentle slapping of the foot or by rubbing the back, and re-evaluate breathing. If the infant is breathing, proceed as before with the evaluation of heart rate and color. If the infant is apneic, initiate bag and mask ventilation.

Bag and Mask Ventilation

A clear understanding of the operation of the type of bag used is mandatory for the person performing resuscitation. The two types of bags used for resuscitation are an anesthesia bag (flow-inflating bag) and a self-inflating bag. A pressure release valve set to release at 30 to 35 cm H_2O is a common feature in most self-inflating bags. More pressure can be achieved when necessary by occlusion, bypassing the pressure release valve in some bags. Extreme caution should be used when this is used as excessive pressure may be transmitted to the lungs. A pressure manometer attached to bag may help to control the pressure in this situation.

When bag and mask ventilation becomes necessary, select the appropriate bag and mask, and check to make sure the connections and the pressure release mechanisms are working properly. Connect the bag to an oxygen source capable of delivering 90 percent to 100 percent. Then position the bag and mask on the infant and ventilate, observing chest wall movement. If there is a rise, ventilate for 15 to 30 seconds. If there is no rise, check for leaks and/or blocked airways, and if nothing is found, increase ventilation pressure and ventilate as before. The ventilation rate should be 40 to 60/min at a pressure of 15 to 20 cm for normal lungs. After this, stop and evaluate the heart rate. If the heart rate is below 60/min, continue to ventilate and initiate chest compressions. If the heart rate is above 60/min, and increasing, continue to ventilate until it reaches 100/min, then stop, evaluate the infant, and provide tactile stimulation.

Chest Compressions

The indication for chest compressions is a heart rate of 60/min and one that does not increase after 30 seconds of bag and mask ventilation. During chest compressions, ventilation should continue as before except during heart rate checks. This maneuver is usually performed using two fingers in the lower one third of the sternum just above the xiphoid. The compressions are performed at a rate of 120/min. Chest compressions interposed with ventilation in a 3:1 ratio may be more effective than simultaneous ventilation and compressions. The three compressions are followed by a pause to allow delivery of an effective breath. This will result in provision of 90 compressions and 30 breaths in each minute (5). After 30 seconds of the procedure, stop and count the heart rate. If it is increasing and is above 80/min, stop compression, and continue to ventilate until respiration is established. If it is still below 80/min, continue chest compressions and ventilation, and prepare for endotracheal intubation.

Endotracheal (ET) Intubation

The infant should be intubated if bag and mask ventilation is ineffective in establishing heart rate and respiration. The infant should also be intubated if prolonged positive pressure ventilation is anticipated (prematures), tracheal suctioning is required (meconium stained amniotic fluid), or diaphragmatic hernia is suspected. Intubation should be accomplished within a short period of time (20 seconds) with free flow of 100 percent oxygen provided close to the infants nostrils. The infant should be bagged, making certain that the rise in chest movement is equal, that breath sounds are equal on both sides, and that there is no gastric distention. The infant should be ventilated for 30 seconds, and if the heart rate is still below 80/min, medications should be considered.

Medications during Resuscitation

Medications during resuscitation are indicated if the heart rate remains below 80/min after adequate ventilation for 30 seconds with 100 percent oxygen and chest compressions or if the heart rate is zero. Medications during resuscitation are rarely required. Resuscitation medications, route of administration, and indications for their use are given in Table 2.4. Quick access for intravenous medications can be achieved by insertion of an umbilical venous catheter. Special circumstances include

> *Meconium stained amniotic fluid.* If thick particulate stained amniotic fluid is encountered, ideally the infant's hypopharynx should be suctioned with a Delee suction catheter immediately after the infant's head is delivered in the mother's perineum. After the delivery of the infant, residual meconium from the hypopharynx should be suctioned, the trachea intubated, and meconium suctioned until the returns are free of meconium. Suction can be applied directly to the ET tube by the use of an adapter and a wall suction device. In a very active infant, clinical judgment has to be made about whether the difficulty of intubating outweighs the advantages of full meconium removal. It should be noted that it may not be possible to

Table 2.4 Resuscitation Medications

Drug	Indications	Dose	Route
Epinephrine 1:10,000	Bradycardia	0.1 to 0.3 ml/kg	IV or IT give rapidly
Sodium bicarbonate (0.5 mEq/ml, 4.2% solution)	Metabolic acidosis	2 mEq/kg	IV slowly (1 mEq/kg/min)
Narcan neonatal (1.0 mg/ml)	Respiratory depression secondary to narcotics	0.1 mg/kg	IV, IM, SQ, IT
Volume expanders 5% albumin Normal saline Ringer's lactate	Hypotension	10 ml/kg	IV over 5–10 min.
Dopamine	Shock	5 to 20 µg/kg/min	IV continuous pump infusion, monitor HR & BP closely

IM = intramuscular
IT = intratracheal
IV = intravenous
SQ = subcutaneous

remove all meconium. In a severely asphyxiated infant, the number of reintubations should be minimized, and positive pressure ventilation should be initiated without further delay. After the trachea has been suctioned, the stomach should be suctioned to prevent aspiration of meconium containing gastric contents.

Asphyxial myocardiopathy. With severe and prolonged perinatal asphyxia, myocardial ischemia can occur with resulting congestive heart failure, systemic hypotension, and hypoperfusion. These babies present with hepatomegaly, the electrocardiogram (EKG) showing ischemic pattern and hypoglycemia. The specific treatment in this situation is to administer digitalis and a positive inotropic agent such as isoproterenol.

Hydrops fetalis. Two skilled resuscitators are needed in this situation. One person manages the airway as before. The second person catheterizes the umbilical vein, performs abdominal paracentesis, and takes the steps to maintain adequate circulation. These infants have severe anasarca with very low serum protein levels. Rh negative blood, cross-matched against the mother's blood, is used to isovolumetrically exchange the blood volume to improve the hematocrit and oxygen carrying capacity.

SUGGESTED READING

1. American Heart Association. Advanced Cardiac Life-Support for Neonates. JAMA 1980; 244:495–500.
2. Bloom RS, Cropley C. Textbook of neonatal resuscitation, Dallas: American Heart Association, American Academy of Pediatrics, 1991.
3. Klaus MH, Fanaroff AA. Care of the high-risk neonate, 3d ed. Philadelphia: Saunders, 1986.
4. Scanlon JW. Neonatal resuscitation: An overview neonatology letter. Wyeth Laboratories 1983;1:1–3.
5. Emergency Cardiac Care Committee and Subcommittee of the American Heart Association. Guidelines for cardiopulmonary resuscitation and emergency cardiac care: Part VII. Neonatal resuscitation. JAMA 1992;268:2276–2281.

PART II

Acute Airway Management

3

Croup and Epiglottitis

Narendra C. Singh
Niranjan Kissoon

Acute airway obstruction in children is one of the most common life-threatening emergencies in pediatric practice. It usually generates a great deal of anxiety since there is little time for deliberation, and it may lead to significant morbidity and indeed mortality. Protocols outlining the management of airway obstruction are useful in facilitating the care of these patients and should be readily available.

Obstructions of the upper airway can be divided into those that involve the supraglottic structures and the subglottic structures themselves. In addition to the anatomic classification, airway obstruction may also be categorized etiologically as either infectious or noninfectious. Infections causing narrowing of the upper airway have been collectively referred to as croup syndrome. More commonly, however, the term croup has been used to describe viral croup. The attack rate of viral croup is between three and fifteen per thousand children per year between six months and five years of age with the highest incidence being in children between six and eighteen months of age. Of these, approximately one percent require hospitalization, and a significantly lower number require airway intervention. Epiglottitis is of bacterial etiology and accounts for one in every thousand pediatric admissions to a hospital with the peak incidence occurring in children between two and six years of age.

PATHOPHYSIOLOGY

The anatomy of the upper airway renders the child at a considerable disadvantage when compared to the adult and predisposes children to upper airway obstruction. For example, the larger occiput in the infant is more likely to compromise the airway by flexion of the cervical spine while the relatively large tongue with less muscle tone increases the likelihood of posterior displacement and obstruction of the airway. Epiglottic enlargement is also more hazardous in children since the epiglottis is relatively longer and stiffer and projects more posteriorly as compared to adults. In addition, the submucosa in the subglottic area is more loosely attached, facilitating accumulation of fluid and development of edema, while the soft, cartilaginous airway in infants may collapse during inspiration.

Since resistance to airflow is related to the fourth power of the radius (Poisslle's Law), small changes in the airway diameter can have profound effects on airway resistance in the pediatric patient. Flow of air into the airway during inspiration results from the generation of a negative intrathoracic pressure (that is, a drop in intrathoracic and intratracheal [IT] pressure below extrathoracic pressure) (Figure 3.1). Since the difference in intrathoracic and extrathoracic pressures necessary to maintain flow is proportional to the fourth power of the airway radius, a 50 percent decrease in radius may increase the pressure by a factor of 32. Attempts to generate this high negative intrathoracic pressure result in the typical physical findings of retraction of the chest wall and pulsus paradoxus. The high negative pressure also results in collapse of the soft extrathoracic airway and worsening of the obstruction.

Parainfluenza virus Type 1 accounts for most cases of viral croup followed by Type 2, Type 3, Influenza A and B, and respiratory syncytial viruses. Parainfluenza primarily infects the celiated respiratory epithelium thus the ventricular and subglottic regions are the chief sites involved in viral croup. In addition to edema, laryngeal muscle spasm as a result of Type 1 hypersensitivity response to parainfluenza virus with the release of spasmogenic mediators may also contribute to airway obstruction.

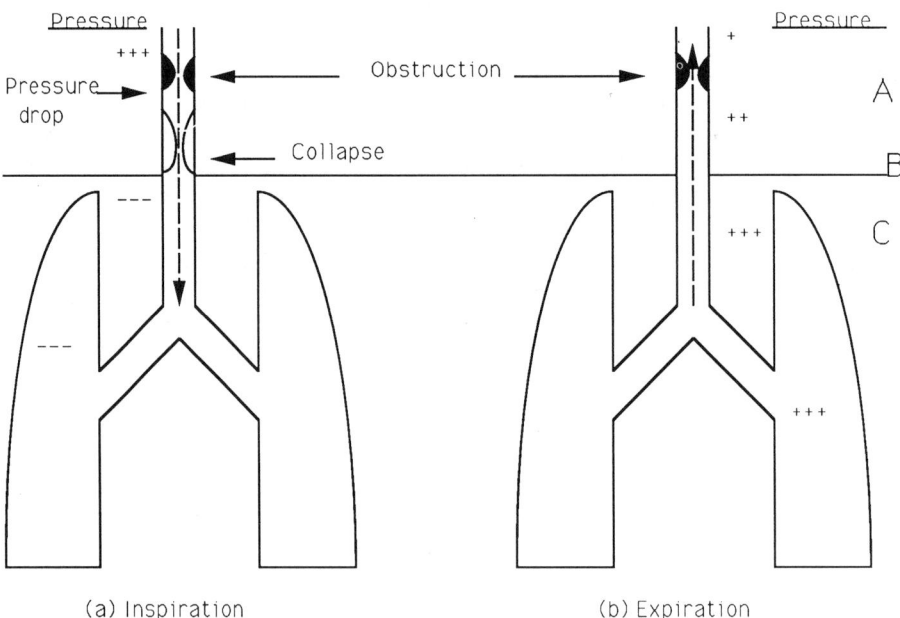

Figure 3.1 A = extrathoracic airway; B = intrathoracic structures including the lung; C = thoracic inlet. During inspiration, there is greater negative intrathoracic pressure conducted to the lungs and major intrathoracic airways. There is airflow from the upper airway, which is at atmospheric pressure, causing a net pressure differential (pressure drop) to further collapse the extrathoracic airway and hence causing further airway narrowing. During expiration, the positive pressure in the airway exceeds atmospheric pressure, and hence the airway is held open.

H. influenza Type B is responsible for almost all cases of epiglottitis in otherwise healthy children. *H. influenza* is carried in the nasopharynx of five percent of asymptomatic children. Invasive disease occurs, however, in one percent of these carriers. The organism is believed to spread hematogenously to the epiglottis, resulting in local inflammation and the typical cherry red edematous epiglottis. Less commonly *S. pneumonia* may be the causative organism; a variety of other agents, however, may be responsible in the immunocompromised patients.

CLINICAL PRESENTATION

The child with viral croup often has an antecedent viral upper respiratory tract infection and may be mildly febrile. After a few days, the child develops a barky or seal-like cough that is accompanied by an inspiratory stridor that is worse at night and is more pronounced during agitation. The course tends to be insidious peaking at three to four days and resolving over a one week period. Most patients will follow this typical course without significant respiratory difficulty. Severe disease is usually indicated by marked tachypnea, the use of accessory muscles and supraclavicular, intercostal and subcostal indrawing. In severe disease, stridor may be marked, however, a decrease in stridor may be an ominous sign of critical airway obstruction on impending respiratory failure.

Epiglottitis, unlike croup, is sudden in onset and rapidly progressive in symptomatology. The preceding illness, unlike viral croup, may only be a few hours in duration. The initial symptoms are sore throat, fever, and cough followed by dysphagia, drooling, and respiratory distress. On examination the child is drooling, anxious, looks acutely ill, and is typically sitting forward with the neck hyperextended, occasionally in a tripod position. Attempts at direct visualization of the pharynx and epiglottis in this situation may induce complete obstruction and is therefore not recommended. Febrile dysphagia in children should always be considered to be epiglottitis until proven otherwise.

DIAGNOSIS AND DIFFERENTIAL DIAGNOSIS

In most cases, the clinical presentation of viral croup and epiglottitis are quite classical with distinctive differences making them often relatively easy to differentiate (Table 3.1). Few investigations are required to support the clinical impression. Hematologic and radiologic evaluation are often unnecessary and may exacerbate the anxiety and delay appropriate treatment. Sending an acutely ill patient to the X-ray department delays treatment and increases the likelihood of airway obstruction with supine positioning especially in patients with epiglottitis. Less than ten percent of patients with croup or epiglottitis remain a diagnostic dilemma. If this group is stable, they may be accompanied to the X-ray department by a physician who is competent in providing airway support. The two classical X-ray findings of epiglottitis are enlargement of the epiglottis and distention of the hypopharynx (Figure 3.2).

Radiologic evaluation of the patient with classical signs and symptoms of croup is unnecessary. If, however, the symptoms are causes of obstruction, the lateral view

Table 3.1 Differentiating features between croup and epiglottitis

	Croup	Epiglottitis
Incidence	More common	Less common
Etiology	Viral	H. influenza Type B
Site of Obstruction	Subglottic	Supraglottic
Age	6 months to 3 years	2 to 6 years
Recurrence	5%	Rare
Clinical features		
Symptoms		
Onset	Gradual (days)	Sudden (hours)
Fever	Low grade	High
Cough	Barky	Minimal
Dysphagia	None	Severe
Drooling	None	Present
Voice	Hoarse	Clear or muffled
Sore throat	Common	Common
Signs		
Posture	Recumbent	Sitting (tripod)
Toxic	Absent	Present
Temperature	Normal/low grade	High
RR	Rapid	Initially normal
Retractions	Present	Absent early
Cyanosis	Absent early	Absent early
Investigations		
CBC (total WBC)	12,000	24,000
(differential count)	60% PMN	85% PMN
X-ray*		
LAT	Subglottic narrowing (1 cm below the glottis)	Enlarged epiglottis Distended hypopharynx
PA	Distention of hypopharynx Tapering of trachea (Steeple Sign)	

*X-rays should not be attempted when the diagnosis of epiglottitis is strongly suspected on clinical grounds.

CBC = complete blood count
WBC = white blood cell
LAT = lateral
PA = postanterior
PMN = polymorphonuclear neutrophil leukocytes

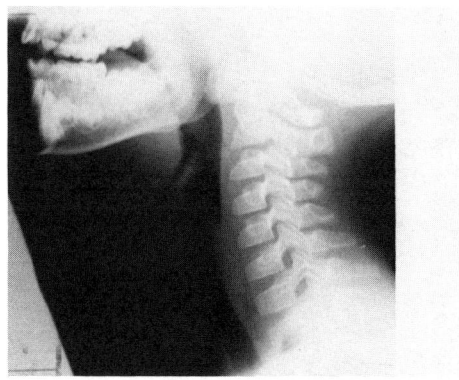 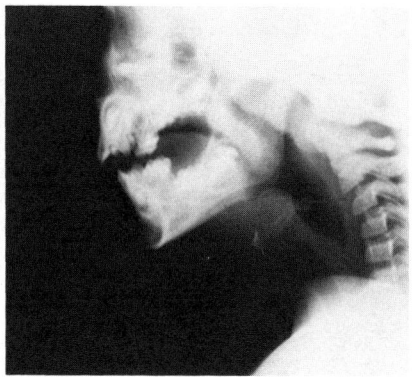

Figure 3.2 The normal radiograph of the upper airway is demonstrated on the left with the well-defined epiglottis. On the right radiograph, the epiglottis is swollen and thumb-like in appearance.

of the neck often demonstrates subglottic narrowing, usually extending one cm below the demonstrated narrowing of the subglottic region, the Steeple Sign (Figure 3.3).

There are a number of other, less common causes of airway obstruction in children. The most common noninfectious etiology of airway obstruction in children is foreign body aspiration followed by the common obstructions: tracheomalacia and angioneurotic edema. Other infectious causes include enlarged tonsils or adenoids, retropharyngeal abscess, peritonsillitis abscess, and bacterial tracheitis. Children who have been intubated in the neonatal period may develop mild subglottic stenosis and are predisposed to airway obstruction even with mild viral infections.

Management of Croup

In the assessment of the child with croup, determination of the severity and the anticipated progression needs to be made in order to determine further management. The croup score (Table 3.2) has been recommended as a tool to aid in the decision-making process but should not be used to replace good clinical judgement. In making decisions regarding triage of patients with croup, emphasis should be placed on the age of the child and on the ability of the parents to assess and respond appropriately if the child's condition deteriorates. The younger the child, the lower should be the threshold for hospitalization. Management of the various levels of severity in croup is illustrated in Figure 3.4 and discussed in more detail in the following subsections.

Mild Croup

Children with mild disease are usually not stridorous at rest; they often have a barky cough, however, and may become stridorous with agitation. These children have a croup score of less than two. If the parents are reliable and will react appropriately to increasing distress, the child may be discharged home with the recommendation to use a cool mist vaporizer.

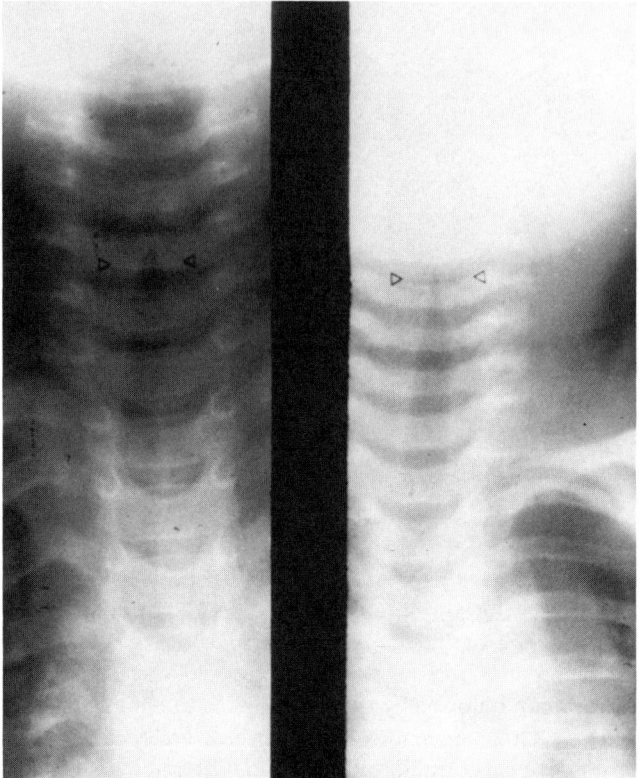

Figure 3.3 The radiograph on the left demonstrates the normal anatomy of the upper airway with normal tapering in the subglottic region. On the right is the radiograph of a child with croup. This demonstrates the manifested narrowing in the subglottic region, the Steeple Sign.

Mild to Moderate

These children have very mild stridor at rest; this may become more pronounced, however, with agitation (croup score 2 to 4). These children may be observed in the emergency department in a humidified tent. If in the physician's judgement the parents are reliable and will return to the hospital if deterioration occurs, the child can be discharged. In that event, the parents would be advised to continue cold mist therapy. These children may also benefit from a stroll outside in cold weather.

Moderately Severe

Children with easily audible stridor at rest without the use of a stethoscope (croup score greater than 5) should be admitted to the hospital. These children should be placed in a humidified tent with oxygen. Further deterioration of the child's

Table 3.2 Clinical croup score

Parameter	0	1	2
Inspiratory breath sounds	Normal	Harsh, with rhonchi	Delayed
Stridor	None	Inspiratory	Inspiratory and expiratory
Cough	None	Hoarse cry	Bark
Retractions Flaring	None	Flaring and suprasternal retractions	Flaring, suprasternal intercostal retractions
Cyanosis	None	In air	In 40% oxygen

Reprinted with permission from Downes JJ, Raphaely RC. Anaesthesiology. Pediatric Intensive Care 1975;43:238–250.

condition may require the use of racemic epinephrine. Nebulized racemic epinephrine (0.25 to 0.5 cc in 2 cc normal saline) can be given as often as is required clinically; after repeated doses, however, the child should be considered for intensive care monitoring and an ear, nose, and throat (ENT) and anaesthesia evaluation. Steroids have been demonstrated to be beneficial in alleviating the signs and symptoms and may be used with this group of patients.

Severe Croup

These patients are in significant distress and clinically there is decreased air entry, use of accessory muscles, subcostal and intercostal indrawing, and possibly cyanosis (Figure 3.5). These patients are considered in the same context as are acute epiglottitis and constitute medical emergencies. Any maneuvers that would agitate the child should be avoided. Oxygen is provided in a nonthreatening manner with the child in the parents arms. Racemic epinephrine should be attempted to provide relief of the obstruction. If there is a favorable response, the child should be transferred to the critical care unit for further management (NPO [*nil per OS*—nothing by mouth], humidity, and oxygen) and close monitoring. Children who do not respond to racemic epinephrine and are becoming exhausted and obtunded should be considered for emergency intubation. It is preferable to intubate the child electively in a controlled fashion rather than to perform a crisis intubation at the time of cardiopulmonary collapse. Intubation is best conducted in the operating room, following inhalation anaesthesia with ENT and with anaesthesia present.

If the child with epiglottitis or severe croup becomes obtunded or is unable to ventilate adequately, bag and mask ventilation should be initiated. In spite of the degree of obstruction, many of these patients can be effectively bag and mask ventilated. If this is effective, then awaiting more experienced personnel is advisable since inexperienced manipulation of the airway may cause further trauma and increase the degree of obstruction. If bag and mask ventilation is ineffective, intubation should be attempted by the physician who is most skilled in the procedure. If this fails, a needle cricothyrotomy should be performed.

30 | SYNOPSIS OF PEDIATRIC EMERGENCY CARE

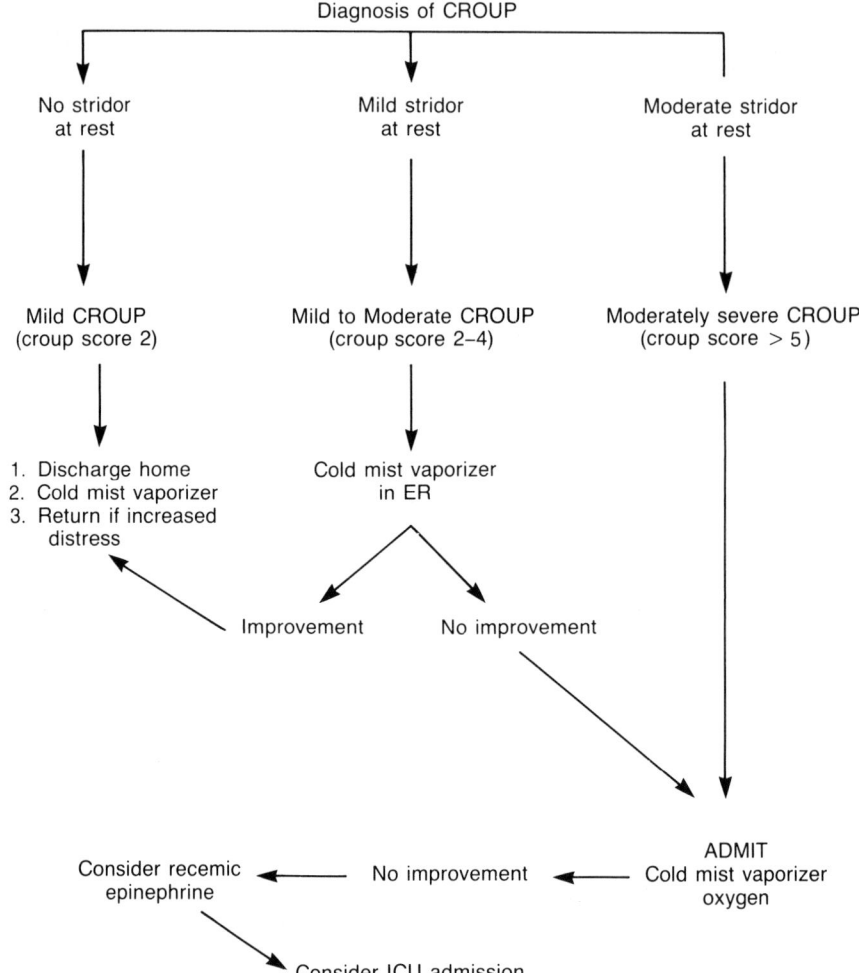

Figure 3.4 Algorithm for the treatment of mild to moderately severe croup.

Management of Epiglottitis

The management of the child who presents with epiglottitis (see Figure 3.5) is anxiety-provoking, and therefore all emergency departments involved with the care of children should have a management protocol with which their medical staff is familiar. Once the diagnosis is strongly suspected depending on the institution, a combination of otolaryngology, anaesthesia, and critical care should be notified. Oxygen is provided to the child in a nonthreatening manner. Aggressive examination of the patient, especially oral examination, as well as hematological and radiological investigations should be avoided. The child should be transported to the operating room accom-

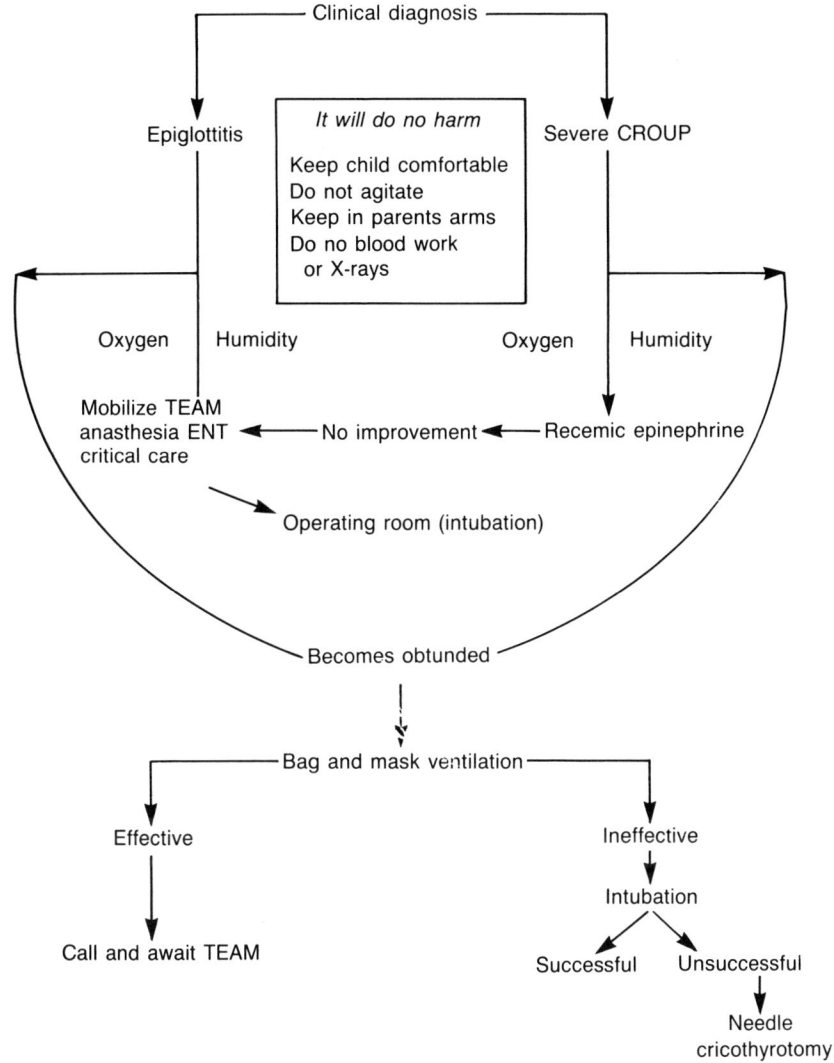

Figure 3.5 Algorithm for the management of epiglottitis and severe croup.

panied by the parent as well as by the appropriate personnel and equipment necessary to secure an emergency airway if necessary.

In the operating room, following an inhalation anaesthetic, nasotracheal intubation will be performed and antibiotics administered (Ampicillin and Chloramphenicol or Cefuroxime). Blood and supraglottic specimens are sent for culture. After securing the endotracheal (ET) tube and proper restraints and sedation, the child will be transported to the pediatric critical care unit for further therapy. Close monitoring for complications (pulmonary edema, pneumonia, metabolic abnormalities, and infection) is required. The child is usually extubated in 24 to 48 hours. Prophylactic Rifampin (20 mg/kg/dose [max 600 mg]) orally once daily for four days) is recommended for all contacts in households with at least one contact younger than 48 months. The patient with epiglottitis should also be given a course of Rifampin.

In recent years, mortality and morbidity as a result of severe croup and epiglottitis has significantly decreased. Much of this is attributed to a better understanding of the pathophysiology of the disease and to an appreciation of the rapidity with which patients can deteriorate. The major impact is as a result of medical personnel being familiar with appropriate protocols for the management of these children and because of subsequent skilled airway management.

SUGGESTED READING

1. Backofen JE, Rogers NC. Upper airway disease. In Rogers MC, ed. Textbook of pediatric intensive care. Baltimore: Williams & Wilkins, 1987;171-197.
2. Committee on Infectious Disease, Report of the committee on infectious disease, 22d ed. Elk Grove Village, Ill.: American Academy of Pediatrics, 1991;222-223.
3. Grad R, Taussig LN. Acute infections producing upper airway obstruction. In Chernick V, ed. Kendig's disorders of the respiratory tract in children, 4th ed. Philadelphia: Saunders, 1989;336-348.
4. Kairys SW, Obnstead EM, O'Connor GT. Steroid treatment of laryngotracheitis. A meta-analysis of the evidence from randomized trials. Pediatrics 1989;83:683-693.
5. Mauro RD, Poole SR, Lockhard CH. Differentiation of epiglottis from laryngotracheitis in the child with stridor. AJDC 1988;142:679-682.
6. Rapkin RH. Epiglottitis and Severe Croup. In Dickerman JD, ed. The critically ill child, diagnosis and medical management, 3d ed. Philadelphia: Saunders, 1985;1-17.
7. Travis KW, Todres ID, Shannon DC. Pulmonary edema associated with croup and epiglottitis. Pediatrics 1977;59:695-698.

4

Asthma/Bronchiolitis

William Ahrens
Gary Strange

ASTHMA

Asthma afflicts up to 10 percent of all children. Epidemiologic evidence indicates that this disease is becoming more frequent and more severe with a marked increase in emergency visits, hospital admissions, and deaths. Evidence also suggests that underdiagnosis and undertreatment contribute to asthma's morbidity and mortality. Children come to the emergency department for exacerbations of asthma that range from chronic, aggravating cough to respiratory failure. The clinician must recognize and manage this wide spectrum of disease with the goal of relieving symptoms and averting disaster (1–4).

Pathophysiology

The clinical pathology of asthma results from a reversible obstruction of the large and small airways that impedes the egress of gas on exhalation. The trapping of intrapulmonary air causes areas both of hyperexpansion and of postobstructive atelectasis, resulting in ventilation-perfusion mismatch. Airway obstruction appears to arise from two separate but interrelated processes:

1. Muscular induced constriction of the tracheobronchial tree
2. Obstruction of the lumen of the airways with mucosal edema, secretions, and other products of inflammation.

Tracheobronchial muscle tone is controlled by the competing activity of acetylcholine and endogenous sympathomimetic agents. Drugs that stimulate sympathomimetic beta-acceptors or inhibit acetylcholine can reverse tracheobronchial constriction and obstruction of airflow. This phenomenon forms the basis of the treatment of asthma with beta-agonist and anticholinergic agents.

Airway inflammation is a complex process controlled by a multitude of mediators, many of which are potent bronchoconstrictors. If it is allowed to proceed unchecked, inflammation ultimately leads to intraluminal airway obstruction from mucosal edema and thick, tenacious secretions. Because they have relatively narrow peripheral airways and underdeveloped alveolar capacity, infants and young children are especially vulnerable to the effect of airway obstruction. Autopsies of children dying from asthma show greatly overdistended lungs with severe mucus plugging of larger and smaller airways (Figure 4.1) (1-4,5,7,8).

Clinical Presentation

The most common clinical manifestation of asthma is expiratory wheezing. Most children will have a history of reactive airway disease and will be receiving outpatient treatment. The diagnosis can be difficult in the "first-time wheezer" or in a child with atypical symptoms. In infants, bronchiolitis is the most common cause of wheezing. Congenital anomalies also tend to present in younger patients, and it is in this group that the greatest danger of a tracheal or esophageal foreign body exists. While on an emergent basis there is no diagnostic test for asthma, a family history of reactive airway disease, a history of recurrent symptoms, and a good response to therapy all support the diagnosis. While it has been said that "all that wheezes is not asthma," most that wheezes is indeed reactive airway disease. Indeed, asthma tends to suffer more from underdiagnosis than it does from overdiagnosis. Asthma can cause vague complaints such as decreased exercise tolerance or atypical chest pain, but the most common clinical manifestation other than wheezing is cough. Patients or parents often describe the cough as harsh, chronic, and worse at night. Small children often suffer posttussive regurgitation from gagging on thick, tenacious secretions. These patients are often misdiagnosed as having pneumonia, especially when small areas of atelectasis that are seen on a chest X-ray are interpreted as infectious infiltrates. Children with "cough equivalent asthma" are often treated with multiple courses of

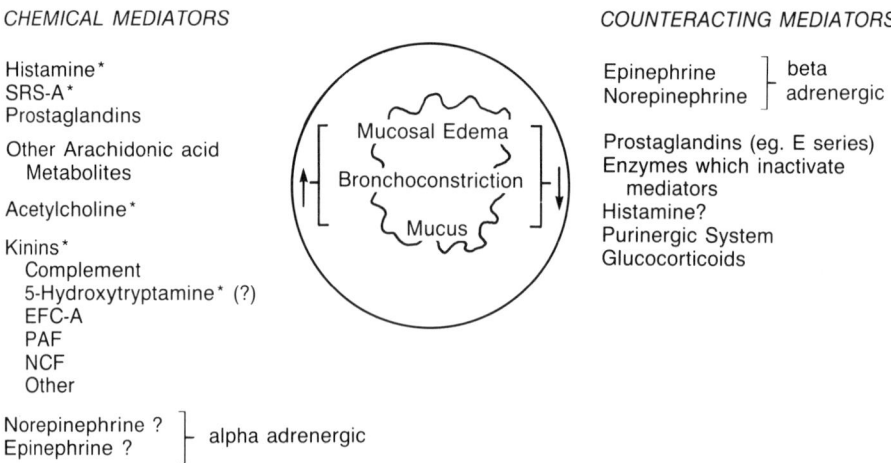

Figure 4.1 The pharmacologic basis of asthma. (Asterisk(*) = hypersensity (10-7000-fold) shown in asthmatics.

Table 4.1 Differential diagnosis of wheezing

Infancy
  Bronchiolitis, viral upper respiratory tract infection, pertussis, cystic fibrosis, bronchopulmonary dysplasia, congenital malformation (vascular ring, choanal atresia, tracheoesophageal fistula, web), gastroesophageal reflux, laryngotracheomalacia, immunodeficiency syndromes, congenital heart disease

Childhood
  Aspiration (foreign body or incompetent lower esophageal sphincter), epiglottitis, croup, gastroesophageal reflux, cystic fibrosis, hypersensitivity pneumonitis, tuberculosis, tumor, allergic bronchopulmonary aspergillosis, ciliary defects, parasitic pneumonitis, immunodeficiency syndromes, habit or imitation cough

Adolescence
  Aspiration (particularly with neurologic disorder), cystic fibrosis, gastroesophageal reflux, α_1-antitrypsin deficiency, ciliary defects, immunodeficiency or autoimmune collagen disorders, tuberculosis, tumor, allergic bronchopulmonary pneumonitis, cardiac disease, hyperventilation syndrome, sighing dyspnea, vocal cord dysfunction

---

antibiotics. Any child diagnosed as having more than one episode of pneumonia or labeled as suffering from "chronic bronchitis" must be strongly suspected of having an underlying problem. Most commonly these patients suffer from asthma (Table 4.1).

Evaluation

The evaluation of a child with an acute exacerbation of asthma begins with an assessment of the severity of the respiratory distress. Several factors are important in determining the degree of airway obstruction:

Mental status. The patient's mental status should be noted—a happy or calm patient usually denotes, at most, mild distress, while an anxious asthmatic indicates severe airway obstruction and probably hypoxia. Increasing lethargy or obtundation signals imminent respiratory arrest.

Accessory muscle use. After assessment of mental status, the patient should be observed for the presence or absence of chest wall retractions and for nasal flaring. The use of accessory muscles of respiration implies moderate to severe airway obstruction. The more pronounced the retractions the more severe the respiratory distress.

Respiratory rate. Tachypnea is an important part of the response to airway obstruction and is virtually always present in acute asthma. Especially in infants and young children, careful attention must be given to the respiratory rate since their limited alveolar capacity demands that they increase minute ventilation mainly through breathing faster.

Auscultation. Auscultation of the chest can be helpful in determining the effectiveness of air exchange. In most patients, airway obstruction results in prolonged expiration. The loudness of wheezing should be noted but must be evaluated in the context of air exchange. The absence of wheezing implies inadequate air exchange and indicates severe airway obstruction—the "silent chest" demands urgent attention. Symmetry of breath sounds should also be noted. Unilateral diminished breath sounds can indicate severe postobstructive atelectasis or can be a manifestation of a pneumothorax.

Peak flow and spirometry. In older children, peak flow and spirometry provide useful information regarding the degrees of airway obstruction. This is especially true if the patient's baseline is known. These physiologic measurements often indicate a higher degree of airway obstruction than is predicted by the physical examination and thus may help to avoid underestimating a patient's illness. Peak flow predominantly measures obstruction in larger airways, while spirometry is useful in assessing the more peripheral airways.

Oxygen saturation. Another useful adjunct in determining the degree of illness is oxygen saturation, which can now be measured transcutaneously. While some degree of hypoxia occurs in virtually all acute asthma, a decrease in oxygen saturation (probably below 93 to 95 percent) implies significant ventilation-perfusion mismatch (35–37).

Chest X-ray. The chest X-ray is usually not helpful in an acute asthma episode. It commonly shows small areas of atelectasis that are easily confused with pneumonia. In some cases, however, an X-ray may be useful in excluding a foreign body, pneumothorax, or severe atelectasis (9).

History

Concomitant with the physical exam, a history should be obtained regarding the potential trigger of the acute attack, the duration of symptoms, and the use of medications. Short episodes provoked by known irritants are often easily reversed, while a patient with prolonged symptoms often has more resistant airway obstruction. This is especially true in patients who have either been compliant with, or have increased the frequency of, therapy with inhalational beta-agonists. A crescendo pattern of inhaler use implies a relatively severe and potentially resistant attack with a significant inflammatory component. The dose and timing of administration of theophylline should be ascertained. Some patients inappropriately increase their dosage during an acute attack and are therefore at risk of toxicity. A history regarding past or present use of steroids must be obtained. An asthmatic who deteriorates while on steroid therapy has a particularly refractory attack and is at risk for respiratory failure.

Risk Factors

It is vital to identify those patients most likely to progress to a life-threatening episode. These patients represent a population that can be considered as "high risk"

Table 4.2 Risk factors for life-threatening asthma

1. Early onset of severe asthma, particularly less than one year of age
2. Frequent need for hospitalization to control asthma
3. Dependence on corticosteroids, either oral or inhaled
4. Noncompliance or abuse of medication
5. Labile asthma with pronounced "morning dipping" diurnal airway obstruction
6. Brittle asthma with unexpected rapid deterioration of pulmonary function
7. Teenager with long-standing asthma of early onset
8. Depressive symptoms with chronic asthma

---

collectively and mandate a cautious approach to management and disposition. Patients who are steroid dependent or require frequent steroid therapy fall into this category as do patients requiring frequent emergency department visits or hospitalization. Especially ominous is a history of admission to an intensive care unit (ICU), or a history of mechanical ventilation. While any episode of acute asthma can progress to respiratory failure, patients with a history of frequent or severe attacks are at relatively greater risk for deterioration than are patients with infrequent, mild attacks.

The patients at greatest risk for fatal asthma appear to be urban adolescents of African-American descent who have a long history of severe disease. These patients may suffer from lack of access to health care as well as from the noncompliance common to adolescence. Both they and their physicians, however, often tend to underestimate the potential severity of their acute asthma attacks and therefore undermanage the illness with potentially catastrophic results (Table 4.2) (4–8).

Management
Drugs

Bronchodilators   The most important drugs used to reverse the acute bronchospastic component of airway obstruction are beta-receptor agonists. For many years, the most commonly used drug for acute asthma was epinephrine, which is a potent bronchodilator that is usually administered subcutaneously. Because it stimulates both pulmonary and cardiac betareceptors, epinephrine often causes tachycardia, and its use has been supplanted by inhaled beta-agonists with a high degree of specificity for pulmonary tissue. During nebulization, little systemic absorption occurs; thus systemic side-effects are minimized. Recent studies have focused on increasing the frequency and the dosage at which nebulized beta-agonists can be safely administered; these studies have demonstrated that cardiac toxicity is not a limiting factor. In the United States, the most commonly used bronchodilators are albuterol and metaproteronol. Some institutions also use nebulized terbutaline. These drugs are available in metered dose inhalers for home use, and for young children, they can be given as a oral suspension (Table 4.3) (1,2,10–14).

SYNOPSIS OF PEDIATRIC EMERGENCY CARE

Table 4.3 Adrenergic drugs for treatment of acute attack

Drug	Administration*	Dosage Child	Dosage Adult	Frequency	Notes
Terbutaline	Subcutaneous	0.01 mg/kg	0.25 ml	20 min (×2)	
Epinephrine aqueous 1:1000 sol (1 mg/ml)	Subcutaneous	0.01 mg/kg	0.3 ml	20 min (×3)	
Suspension epinephrine 1:200 (Sus-Phrine) 5 mg/ml	Subcutaneous	0.005 ml/kg	0.2 ml	Single dose	To follow treatment, if appropriate (see text).
Isoetharine 1:100 (10 mg/ml)	Nebulized aerosol	0.25 to 0.60 ml in 2.0 ml saline	0.25 to 1.0 ml in 2.0 ml saline	30 min (×3)	
Metaproterenol 1:20 (50 mg/ml)	Nebulized aerosol	0.1 to 0.2 ml in 2.5 ml saline	0.2 to 0.3 ml in 2.5 ml saline	30 min (×3)	‡
Albuterol 1:200 (5 mg/ml)	Nebulized aerosol	0.02 ml/kg up to 0.5 ml (100 µg/kg)	0.5 to 1.0 ml in 2.0 ml saline	30 min (×3)	‡
Terbutaline 1:1000 (1 mg/ml)	Nebulized aerosol	1 ml in 1 ml saline†	2.0 ml in 1.0 ml saline	30 min (×3)	‡

*In moderately severe or severe attack, it is best to administer drug via, or concomitant with, oxygen.
†Authors' recommendation.
‡Safety and effectiveness of the inhaled solution in patients younger than 12 years have not been established.
(Reprinted with permission from Bierman CW and Pearlman DS [eds]: Allergic Diseases from Infancy to Adulthood. 2nd ed. Philadelphia, WB Saunders Co. 1988.)

Anticholinergic drugs also function as bronchodilators, with their primary effect probably being on larger airways. Some studies have found these agents useful in acute asthma and recommend they be used concomitantly with beta-agonists. Atropine and ipatropium bromide are available for use as nebulized agents and in metered dose inhalers (2,15).

Theophylline, a methylxanthine derivative that functions at least in part as a bronchodilator, has been used for many years in the treatment of acute asthma. Recent evaluation of this drug has cast doubt on its efficacy in acute asthma, suggesting that the potential for toxicity outweighs the therapeutic benefits. However, many would consider it worth trying in a severe attack. Side effects of theophylline include vomiting and tremulousness. Higher levels can cause tachydysrythmias and, in severe cases, seizures. The metabolism of theophylline is notoriously erratic. It is wise to obtain a serum level on a patient taking theophylline prior to giving a "loading dose." Levels must be monitored closely on patients who are placed on theophylline infusions (16–17).

Corticosteroids Corticosteroids are the mainstay of therapy for the inflammatory component of airway obstruction. Their early use in an acute attack can prevent the need for hospital admission, and their use as outpatient therapy can reduce symptoms and prevent the need for a return visit to the emergency department. More importantly, by suppressing the inflammation that produces the mucus plugging, atelectasis, and ventilation-perfusion mismatch characteristic of a severe attack, steroids can prevent an episode of asthma from progressing to respiratory failure. Steroids can be administered intravenously, intramuscularly, or orally. While no definite guidelines have been derived regarding the dose, duration, or method of delivery of steroids during an acute asthma attack, most patients are treated with short, intensive bursts. Children appear to tolerate up to four one-week courses of steroid therapy during the course of a year with minimal risk of adrenal suppression. A common practice is to administer methylprednisolone 1–2mg/kg IV (intravenous) every six hours to an ill asthmatic. A patient discharged from the emergency department can be treated with prednisone 1mg/kg/day for five to seven days.

Corticosteroids should be administered immediately to any asthmatic in moderate or severe distress and should be strongly considered in any acutely ill patient with a history of severe attacks, frequent hospitalizations, or multiple courses of steroid use in the past. Patients with a history of prolonged, debilitating symptoms, especially those who have been resistant to aggressive inhalational therapy, are also candidates for steroids. A decrease in oxygen saturation implies significant ventilation-perfusion mismatch and is an indication for administering steroids. Certainly not every child suffering from acute asthma needs treatment with steroids. However, failure to treat those patients aggressively, with a significant inflammatory component to their illness can result in unnecessary morbidity (23–28).

Management of the Severe Attack

Most children with mild, episodic asthma with acute symptoms will respond well to one or two nebulized treatments. Patients with more severe respiratory distress must receive very aggressive management. If nebulizer therapy is not immediately available, subcutaneous epinephrine should be administered. Steroids should be given at once. Patients in moderate to severe distress should receive nebulizer therapy at least every 20 to 30 minutes until improvement is noted. Oxygen should be administered continuously.

The asthmatic in severe respiratory distress who does not respond to treatment with frequent nebulized beta-agonists presents a management challenge. In such patients, IV beta-agonists have been used successfully to reverse bronchospasm and avert the need for mechanical ventilation. Continuous IV isoproterenol has been found to be effective in severe refractory asthma, but it has been associated with myocardial ischemia and is not readily recommended for use in older children. Albuterol and terbutaline are used intravenously at some centers. These drugs are less active on the myocardium than isoproterenol is and to date have not been reported to cause myocardial ischemia in children. Beta-agonists can also be administered as continuous nebulized treatment on a milligram per hour basis, avoiding the potential complications of IV therapy. Further studies are needed before definite recommendations can be made regarding IV or continuous nebulized beta-agonist therapy. Both modalities are in use at many pediatric centers, however, where they play an important role in the treatment of critically ill asthmatics, and it is likely that they will soon play a major role in the emergency department (17–23).

Occasionally an asthmatic will not respond to the most aggressive therapy and will require mechanical ventilation. Intubation should be considered in the patient who develops a deteriorating mental status or progressive muscle fatigue. No absolute blood gas value mandates mechanical ventilation, but it must be considered in the setting of a rising pCO_2 or of refractory hypoxia. Most pediatric asthmatics tolerate moderate hypercarbia, but hypoxia can become lethal rapidly and must not be allowed to persist.

Most patients will need sedation prior to and following intubation. Benzodiazapines have hypnotic and anxiolytic properties and are often used to initiate sedation, but may not allow sufficient relaxation. Ketamine, a dissociative anesthetic agent, has been advocated as an induction agent in the intubation of children in status asthmaticus. In addition to sedation, ketamine causes bronchodilation and thus has some potential therapeutic benefit. Since it does not cause muscle paralysis, ketamine allows the patient to maintain some respiratory effort in the event that endotracheal tube placement is difficult. Ketamine can cause increased secretions, which can be reduced by prior treatment with an anticholinergic such as atropine or glycopyrrolate. Occasionally hallucinations can occur, and ketamine has infrequently been associated with laryngospasm. The recommended dose of ketamine is 0.5 to 2mg/kg IV. Occasionally a patient may require paralysis in order for intubation to be achieved. The use of paralytic agents carries the obvious risk of producing a patient with no spontaneous respirations in whom an airway cannot be obtained and whose disease precludes effective bag-mask ventilation. If paralysis is deemed necessary the depolarizing agent, succinylcholine, has the advantage of a very short duration of action, but it can release histamine and therefore potentiate bronchospasm. Nondepolarizing agents, such as pancuronium and vecuronium have the advantage of not releasing histamine, but have a much longer duration of action than does succinylcholine (29–31).

Disposition

No clinical scoring system predicts perfectly those patients who absolutely require admission. Even patients who have a resolution of wheezing and feel better after treatment can have significant residual airway obstruction and can relapse after responding well to initial therapy. A clinical improvement in air-exchange should be noted, and in infants, an improvement in respiratory rate and in the ability to take the bottle well should be documented. Peak expiratory flow rate, which reflects obstruction in larger airways, can provide useful information but has been unreliable in predicting relapse. Recently a decrease in oxygen saturation has been correlated with a need for hospital admission. Values between 91 to 93 percent have been associated with relapse, even in patients who appeared to improve with treatment. Oxygen saturation may reflect abnormalities in the smaller airways that result in ventilation-perfusion mismatch and that are not as quickly reversed as obstruction in larger airways. In at least one study, oxygen saturation was more sensitive than peak flow in predicting relapse.

Historical factors play an important role in determining disposition. Any patient with severe disease or a history of noncompliance should be discharged only with extreme caution. Patients or their parents must demonstrate an understanding of the illness and medical regimen, including how to use metered dose inhalers, and must have transportation to the hospital in the event of a relapse (32–37).

Summary

Fortunately the vast majority of asthmatics will not progress to respiratory failure, but by treating each episode of acute bronchospasm as a potentially life-threatening event, the emergency physician can avoid the pitfall of undermanagement that plagues this disorder. Recognition of the high-risk patient, aggressive management of patients with significant respiratory distress, and the judicious use of steroids are the current cornerstones of management.

BRONCHIOLITIS

Bronchiolitis is an extremely common cause of emergency department visits and hospital admissions. It is the most common cause of wheezing in infants less than one year of age. Pathologically the term bronchiolitis refers to inflammation in the peripheral airways. Clinically the term applies to a syndrome most often seen in young infants that is characterized by rhinorrhea, cough, retractions, and wheezing. Bronchiolitis is most often caused by respiratory syncytial virus (RSV), the most common infectious cause of lower airway disease in infants and young children. RSV infection results in 95,000 hospitalizations every year with 4500 deaths. Less commonly, bronchiolitis is caused by influenza, parainfluenza, or adenoviruses (38–42).

Epidemiology and Pathology

Bronchiolitis most commonly affects infants between two and six months of age. The disease appears during the yearly epidemics of RSV infections that occur between

October and June. By the time they reach the age of two, the vast majority of children show evidence of having been infected by RSV. Manifestations of infection range from mild lower airway disease to fulminant pneumonia with diffuse parenchymal involvement. Only a minority of children infected with RSV develop bronchiolitis. Why some children develop the characteristic bronchiolar inflammation and others do not is not well understood. Current research focuses on various immunologic mechanisms (38–39).

In infants who develop bronchiolitis, RSV infection results in necrosis of respiratory epithelium and destruction of ciliated epithelial cells in the lower airways. The airway lumen becomes obstructed with cellular debris and edema in an uneven fashion, producing areas of air trapping and atelectasis. The diffuse inflammatory response may also produce bronchospasm, especially in infants with a tendency toward reactive airway disease. While the role of bronchospasm in bronchiolitis is not yet clear, up to 30 percent of children who wheeze in association with RSV infection go on to develop reactive airway disease. Thus bronchiolitis can be thought of as a virally induced pneumonia with asthmalike features. The diffuse airway obstruction produces ventilation-perfusion mismatch and can cause significant hypoxemia. Less commonly, air trapping can result in hypercarbia and respiratory failure. Most of the morbidity and mortality in bronchiolitis occurs in infants who are less than six months of age, where underdeveloped alveolar capacity and relatively narrow airways enhance the effect of any intraluminal obstruction. This illness tends to be especially severe in infants with underlying cardiopulmonary disease. Infants with congestive heart failure, cystic fibrosis, or immunosuppression are especially likely to develop respiratory compromise. However, patients at greatest risk for respiratory failure during the course of bronchiolitis are those infants with a history of prematurity who suffer from bronchopulmonary dysplasia (BPD), a condition that often results in chronic hypoxemia, hypercarbia, and brittle reactive airway disease. In these patients bronchiolitis can lead to respiratory failure quickly (38–42).

Clinical Presentation and Diagnosis

Early findings in bronchiolitis include an upper respiratory prodrome with copious nasal discharge, restlessness, cough, and fever. The onset of lower airway involvement is characterized by tachypnea, tachycardia, and chest retractions. Auscultation of the lungs reveals wheezing with occasional fine rales. Lower airway obstruction results in prolonged expiration. Occasionally depression of the diaphragm can result in abdominal distension and the illusion of hepatosplenomegaly. Some infants develop conjunctivitis and pharyngitis (38–40).

Bronchiolitis must be distinguished from other causes of lower airway disease. These include bacterial pneumonia, chlamydia pneumonitis, anatomic anomalies such as vascular rings, and airway or esophogael foreign bodies. Congestive heart failure often presents with respiratory distress and wheezing in young infants and can easily be confused with bronchiolitis. Asthma can be difficult to distinguish from bronchiolitis, especially in the first-time wheezer; however, careful questioning often reveals prior pulmonary complaints. Although no bedside test accurately distinguishes between the two diseases, it is common clinical practice to administer a trial of beta-agonist therapy and to label patients with an unequivocal response as having *asthma* while those that do not seem to respond are considered to have *bronchiolitis*.

A definitive diagnosis of bronchiolitis can be made by culturing RSV from nasopharyngeal secretions or more rapidly by demonstrating the presence of RSV by immunofluorescent techniques. The chest X-ray is nondiagnostic. It can demonstrate diffuse hyperexpansion of the lungs, or it may show areas of patchy infiltrate that result from atelectasis (38–41).

Assessment

In the average healthy infant significant respiratory distress is indicated by pronounced tachypnea (respiratory rate of 60 to 80), poor retractions, air entry, anxiety or restlessness, and refusal to feed. Inability to bottle feed is a manifestation of exertional dyspnea and an important clue to clinically significant respiratory insufficiency in an infant. Cyanosis is uncommon, but hypoxia is often present. Transcutaneous measurement is useful in revealing oxygen saturation. In severe cases, bronchiolitis can result in hypercarbia and respiratory failure. In patients who have significant respiratory distress or underlying cardiopulmonary disease, a blood gas should be obtained to assess respiratory status definitively.

Disposition

Bronchiolitis is a self-limited illness that, in the majority of healthy infants, can be managed safely at home. Patients who are unable to tolerate feeding require hospital admission and IV fluids to maintain hydration. Patients with hypoxia require hospital admission for supplemental oxygen therapy. Any patient with significant hypercarbia is at risk for respiratory failure and should be considered a candidate for admission to a pediatric ICU.

Hospitalization should be strongly considered in patients with underlying cardiopulmonary disease, especially infants with bronchopulmonary dysplasia. Bronchiolitis is especially dangerous in infants with these risk factors. Infants less than two to three months of age with bronchiolitis should be discharged from the emergency department with extreme caution and only in the hands of an adequate caretaker. A next-day follow-up visit or phone call is a good idea in these patients.

Treatment

The definitive mainstays of treatment for bronchiolitis are the maintainance of adequate hydration and oxygenation. Because of the asthma-like qualities of bronchiolitis and because it is thought that bronchoconstriction may play some role in the illness, common clinical practice also includes the use of beta-agonist therapy. Patients often receive nebulized treatment in the emergency department, and those discharged are often treated with oral therapy. Despite their wide use in the treatment of bronchiolitis, the efficacy of beta-agonists is controversial. This is especially true in young infants in whom improvement in pulmonary function is difficult to measure. Theophylline therapy is not felt to be effective, nor have steroids been found to be useful.

In seriously ill patients, the antiviral agent ribavirin has been found to shorten the course of bronchiolitis and to reduce the time that mechanical ventilation is required in those patients who suffer respiratory failure. Currently ribavirin therapy is reserved for patients with underlying cardiopulmonary disease or for those who develop severe disease.

Apnea and Bronchiolitis

A common complication of RSV infection is apnea, which is especially likely to occur in very young infants or in those with a history of prematurity. The etiology of RSV-associated apnea is not known but it is felt to require assisted ventilation more often than is respiratory failure resulting from severe bronchiolitis. Any infant with a history of apnea requires hospital admission and close monitoring even if their bronchiolitis appears mild. Other viral infections can also cause apnea, but bacterial sepsis must be ruled out (51).

REFERENCES

1. Bierman CW, Pearlman D. Asthma. In Kendig V, Chernick EL, eds. Disorders of the respiratory tract in children, 5th ed. Philadelphia: Saunders, 1990; Chapter 41.
2. Rubin B, Marcushamer S, Priel I, et al. Emergency management of the child with asthma. Pediatric Pulmonology. 1990;8:45–57.
3. Friday G, Fireman P. Morbidity and mortality of asthma. Pediatric Clinics of North America 1988;35:1149–1162.
4. Goldenhersh MJ, Rachelefsky GS. Childhood asthma: Overview. Pediatrics in Review 1989;10:227–234.
5. Kravis L, Kolski G. Unexpected death in childhood asthma. Am J Dis Child 1985; 139:558–563.
6. Westerman DE, Bentar SR, Potgieter MB, et al. Identification of the high-risk asthmatic patient. Am J Med 1979;66:565–572.
7. Buranakul B, Washington J, Hilman B, et al. Causes of death during acute asthma in children. Am J Dis Child 1974;128:343–350.
8. Kravis L. An analysis of fifteen childhood asthma fatalities. J Allergy Clin Immunol 1987; 80:467–472.
9. Rushton A. The role of the chest radiograph in the management of childhood asthma. Clinical Pediatrics 1982;21:325–328.
10. Taussig LM, Smith SM, Blumfield R. Chronic bronchitis in childhood—what is it? Pediatrics 1981;67(1):1–5.
11. Becker A, Nelson N, Simons FER. Inhaled salbutamol vs injected epinephrine in the treatment of acute asthma in children. J Pediatr 1983;102:465–469.
12. Ruddy R, Kolski G, Scarpa N, et al. Aerosolized Metaproterenol compared to subcutaneous epinephrine in the emergency treatment of acute childhood asthma. Pediatric Pulmonology 1986;2:230–236.
13. Robertson C, Smith F, Beck R, et al. Response to frequent low doses of nebulized salbutamol in acute asthma. J Pediatr 1985;106:672–674.

14. Schuh S, Parkin P, Rajan A, et al. High- versus low-dose, frequently administered, nebulized albuterol in children with severe, acute asthma. Pediatrics 1989;83:513–518.
15. Reisman J, Galdes-Sebalt M, Kazim F, et al. Frequent administration by ingalation of salbutamol and ipratropium bromide in the initial management of severe acute asthma in children. J All Clin Immunol 1988;81:16–20.
16. Littenberg B. Aminophylline treatment in severe, acute asthma. JAMA 1988;259:1678–1684.
17. Siegal D, Sheppard D, Gelb A, et al. Aminophylline increases the toxicity but not the efficacy of an inhaled beta-adrenergic agonist in the treatment of acute exacerbations of asthma. Am Rev Respir Dis 1985;132:283–286.
18. Bohn D, Kalloghlian A, Jenkins J, et al. Intravenous salbutamol in the treatment of status asthmaticus in children. Critical Care Med 1984;12:892–896.
19. Parry W, Martorano F, Cotton E. Management of life-threatening asthma with intravenous isoproterenol infusions. Am J Dis Child 1976;13039–13042.
20. Downes J, Wood D, Harwood I, et al. Intravenous isoproterenol infusion in children with severe hypercapnia due to status asthmaticus. Critical Care Med 1973;1:63–68.
21. Matson J, Loughlin G, Strunk R. Myocardial ischemia complicating the use of isoproterenol in asthmatic children. J Pediatr 1978;92:776–778.
22. Moler F, Hurwitz, Custer J. Improvement in clinical asthma score and $PaCO_2$ in children with severe asthma treated with continuously nebulized terbutaline. J Allergy Clin Immunol 1988;81:1101–1108.
23. Tipton WR, Nelson HS. Frequent parenteral terbutaline in the treatment of status asthmaticus in children. Annals of Allergy. 1987;58:252–256.
24. Harris J, Weinberger M, Nassif, et al. Early intervention with short courses of prednisone to prevent the progression of asthma in ambulatory patients incompletely responsive to bronchodilators. J Pediatr 1987;110:627–633.
25. Younger R, Gerber P, Herrod H, et al. Intravenous methylprednisolone efficacy in status asthmaticus of childhood. Pediatrics 1987;80:225–230.
26. Tal A, Levy N, Bearman J. Methylprednisolone therapy for acute asthma in infants and toddlers: A controlled clinical trial. Pediatrics 1990;86:350–356.
27. Harfi H, Hanissian A, Crawford L. Treatment of status asthmaticus in children with high doses and conventional doses of methylprednisolone. Pediatrics 1978;61:829–831.
28. Dolan L, Kesarwala H, Holroyde J, et al. Short-term, high-dose, systemic steroids in children with asthma: The effect on the hypothalamic-pituitary-adrenal axis. J Allergy Clin Immunol 1987;80:81–87.
29. Rogers, MC: Lower airway disease: Bronchiolitis and asthma. In Rogers, MC, ed. Textbook of Pediatric Intensive Care. Baltimore: Williams & Wilkins, 1987; Chapter 7.
30. L'Hommedieu CS, Arens JJ. The use of ketamine for emergency intubation of patients with status asthmaticus. Ann Emerg Med 1987;16:568–71.
31. Rock MJ, Reyes de la Rocha SR, L'Hommedieu CS, et al. Use of ketamine in asthmatic children to treat respiratory failure refractory to conventional therapy. Crit Care Med 1986;14:514–516.
32. Ownby D, Abarzua J, Anderxon J. Attempting to predict hospital admission in acute asthma. Am J Dis Child 1984;138:1062–1066.
33. Skoner D, Fischer T, Gormley C, et al. Pediatric predictive index for hospitalization in acute asthma. Ann of Em Med 1987;16:25–31.
34. Silver R, Ginsburg C. Early prediction of the need for hospitalization in children with acute asthma. Clinical Pediatrics 1984;23:81–84.
35. Geelhoed G, Landau L, LeSouef P. Predictive value of oxygen saturation in emergency evaluation of asthmatic children. Br Med J 1988;297:395–396.
36. Geelhoed G, Landau L, Lesouef P. Oxymitry and peak expiratory flow in assessment of acute childhood asthma. J Pediatr 1990;117:907–909.
37. Roca J, Ramis LI, Rodriguez-Roisin R, et al. Serial relationships between ventilation-perfusion inequality and spirometry in acute severe asthma requiring hospitalization. Am Rev Respir Dis 1988;137:1055–1061.

38. Welliver R, Cherry J. Bronchiolitis and infectious asthma. In Feign R, Cherry J, eds. Textbook of pediatric infectious diseases, 2d ed. Philadelphia: Saunders, 1987; Chapter 10.
39. Hall CB. Respiratory syncytial virus. In Feigin R, Cherry J, eds. Textbook of pediatric infectious diseases, 2d ed. Philadelphia: Saunders, 1987; Chapter 29.
40. Wohl ME. Bronchiolitis. In Kendig EL, Chernick V, eds. Disorders of the respiratory tract in children, 5th ed. Philadelphia: Saunders, 1990; Chapter 18.
41. Hall CB, McBride JT. Respiratory syncytial virus—from chimps with colds to conundrums and cures. NEJM;1991:57–58.
42. Wohl ME. Bronchiolitis. Pediatric Annals 1986;15:307–313.
43. Brooks LJ, Cropp GJ. Theophylline therapy in bronchiolitis. Am J Dis Child 1981; 135:934–936.
44. Lenny W, Milner AD. At what age do bronchodilator drugs work? Arch Dis Child 1978; 53:532–535.
45. Silverman M. Bronchodilators for wheezy infants. Arch Dis Child 1984;59:84–87.
46. Sly PD, Lanteri CJ, Raven JM. Do wheezy infants recovering from bronchiolitis respond to inhaled salbutamol? Pediatric Pulmonology 1991;10:36–39.
47. Hughes DM Lesouef PN, Landau LI. Effect of salbutamol on respiratory mechanics in bronchiolitis. Pediatric Research 1987;22:83–87.
48. Tal A, Bavilski C, Yohai D, et al. Dexamethasone and salbutamol in the treatment of acute wheezing in infants. Pediatrics 1983;71:13–16.
49. Leer JA, Green J, Heimlich EM, et al. Corticosteroid treatment in bronchiolitis: A controlled collaborative study in 297 infants and children. Am J Dis Child 1969;117:495.
50. Smith DW, Frankel Lr, Mathers LH, et al. A controlled trial of aerosolized ribavirin in infants receiving mechanical ventilation for severe respiratory syncytial virus infection. NEJM 1991;325:24–29.
51. Church NR, Anas NG, Hall CB, et al. Respiratory syncytial virus related apnea in infants. Am J Dis Child 1984;138:247–250.

5

Respiratory Failure

Steven M. Barrett

Disorders of the respiratory system are the most common childhood emergencies (1). Deaths from respiratory disorders account for one third of all mortality in children under fifteen years of age and for almost one half of all deaths under one year of age (2). Most pediatric cardiac arrests are secondary to a respiratory etiology.

PATHOPHYSIOLOGY

Respiratory failure is defined as an impairment of adequate oxygen absorption for the body's metabolic requirements or of adequate carbon dioxide excretion. Hypercapnia, hypoxemia, or both result from one or more of three mechanisms: (1) inadequate alveolar ventilation, (2) mismatching of alveolar ventilation and pulmonary perfusion, or (3) abnormal diffusion of gases across the alveolar-capillary interface. Respiratory distress is the clinical state characterized by an abnormal respiratory rate or by increased work of breathing. Respiratory distress may progress to respiratory failure. Some patients in respiratory failure, however, (for example, from certain neuromuscular disorders or respiratory muscle exhaustion) may have little or no evidence of respiratory distress such as tachypnea or other clues of increased respiratory effort.

Alveolar ventilation depends on input from the central nervous system (CNS) and the function of the thoracic pump (peripheral nerves, intercostal and accessory muscles, diaphragm, and rib cage) and the lungs (3). The lung can be divided into conducting airways (the trachea and bronchi) and the alveoli. The conducting airways constitute anatomic dead space since the air in these airways does not participate in gas exchange. Anatomic dead space differs from physiologic dead space, which is defined as those areas of abnormal lung in which ventilation-perfusion (V/Q) mismatch prevents normal gas exchange. *Tidal volume* is the amount of air inspired in a single breath and includes both the anatomic dead space volume and the alveolar volume. Tidal volume is a function of respiratory effort, airways resistance, alveolar compliance, and chest wall elasticity. The product of tidal volume and respiratory rate is the minute ventilation. The product of dead space volume and respiratory rate is the dead space ventilation. Subtracting dead space ventilation from minute ventilation yields alveolar ventilation. A reduction in alveolar ventilation results in hypercapnic respiratory failure ($PaCO_2 > 55$ mmHg) (3).

Table 5.1 Causes of respiratory failure

Hypercapnic (PaCO$_2$ > 55 mmHg)
1. Decreased alveolar ventilation
   a. CNS depression from head injury, coma, status epilepticus, drug overdose
   b. Peripheral nervous system dysfunction from spinal cord trauma, Guillain-Barre syndrome, botulism, myasthenia gravis
   c. Upper airway obstruction from foreign bodies, epiglottitis, croup, aspiration, thermal injury, tracheomalacia
   d. Increased airway resistance from asthma, bronchiolitis, cystic fibrosis, organophosphate poisoning
   e. Decreased lung compliance from pulmonary edema, interstitial fibrosis
   f. Increased chest wall compliance from flail chest
   g. Pleural space dysfunction from pneumothorax, hemothorax, pleural effusion
   h. Respiratory muscle fatigue from excessive work of breathing, shock states
   i. Respiratory muscle failure from muscular dystrophies
2. Increased dead space ventilation
   a. Decreased pulmonary blood flow from multiple pulmonary emboli, pulmonary hypertension syndromes, decreased cardiac output states
   b. Air trapping and alveolar overdistention from asthma, bronchopulmonary dysplasia (BPD)
3. Increased production of CO$_2$
   a. Increased metabolic rate with major burns
   b. Altered respiratory quotient from excessive glucose administration

Hypoxemic (PaO$_2$ < 50 mmHg)
1. Decreased F$_i$O$_2$
   Alveolar hypoxia, for example, from altitude illness
2. Intrapulmonary shunting with increased pulmonary vascular resistance
   a. Diffuse alveolar flooding with pulmonary vascular obliteration from adult respiratory distress syndrome (for example, due to shock states, sepsis, disseminated intravascular coagulation, fat embolism)
3. Intrapulmonary shunting without increased pulmonary vascular resistance
   a. Local alveolar flooding from pneumonia, lung contusion
4. Low V/Q match with increased pulmonary vascular resistance
   a. Bronchospasm with increased pulmonary artery tone from meconium aspiration syndrome
5. Low V/Q match without increased pulmonary vascular resistance
   a. Alveolar flooding from cardiogenic or noncardiogenic pulmonary edema (for example, due to smoke inhalation, toxic gas inhalation, near-drowning, salicylate or opiate toxicity, gastric juice aspiration)
6. Intracardiac shunting with increased pulmonary vascular resistance
   a. Right-to-left shunting with increased pulmonary artery tone from endocardial cushion defect
7. Intracardiac shunting without increased pulmonary vascular resistance
   a. Right-to-left shunting without pulmonary vascular disease from pulmonic stenosis with a ventricular septal defect
8. Hypoventilation
   a. Decreased alveolar ventilation from upper airway obstruction, congenital lobar emphysema, diaphragmatic hernia, gastric distention, abdominal distention
9. Diffusion impairment
   a. Interstitial space dysfunction from pulmonary fibrosis
10. Decreased mixed venous oxygen tension
    a. Increased oxygen extraction by tissues in cardiogenic shock

Source: Anas NG. Respiratory failure. In Leven DL, Morriss FC, eds. Essentials of pediatric emergency care. St. Louis: Quality Medical Publishing, 1990;64–71.

The normal tidal volume in most children is 5 to 7 ml/kg. In the young patient, the thoracic cage is pliable and may fail to support the lung adequately during respiratory distress. The clinical manifestation of this compromised lung expansion is paradoxical chest wall movement (sternal and intercostal retractions) during inspiration. Furthermore, air movement in the pediatric patient is more dependent on diaphragmatic motion than it is in the adult. When diaphragmatic movement is impeded by pressure from above (for example, air trapping in obstructive airways disease) or from below (for example, abdominal distention), effective respiration is threatened because the pliable chest wall may not be able to compensate (4).

The upper airways in infants and children are small and more easily obstructed by foreign bodies, local swelling, or the tongue than is the case in adults. In addition, an upper respiratory infection or rhinitis may cause significant respiratory compromise in the infant less than 4 months old who is an obligate nose breather. The lower airways in children are also smaller and have incompletely developed supporting cartilage. Therefore alveolar ventilation may also be easily compromised at this level if the lower airways become obstructed by mucus, blood, pus, edema, or bronchoconstriction (4).

The adequacy of V/Q matching is determined by the composition of alveolar gas (oxygen and carbon dioxide) and the degree to which alveolar ventilation and pulmonary perfusion are balanced (3). A difference exists between the alveolar and arterial oxygen levels (A-aDO$_2$); this value is 10 to 20 mmHg and is due to venous admixture from anatomic shunts through the bronchial and the besian circulation. Abnormalities in gas exchange that occur as a result of changes in the composition of alveolar gas include a reduced inspired oxygen fraction (F_iO_2) (for example, high altitude), an increased arterial carbon dioxide tension (PaCO$_2$) (for example, hypoventilation), and alterations in the respiratory exchange ratio (for example, increased CO$_2$ production from excessive glucose metabolism). These causes of respiratory failure are characterized by hypoxemia (PaO$_2$ < 50 mmHg) with a normal A-aDO$_2$ and generally with hypercapnia (PaCO$_2$ > 55 mmHg) (3).

In addition to the composition of alveolar gas, the adequacy of gas exchange is determined by the balance of alveolar ventilation and pulmonary perfusion. The ideal V/Q match is altered by a reduction in alveolar ventilation (for example, pulmonary edema or atelectasis) or by a reduction in pulmonary blood flow (for example, pulmonary embolism). The extreme example of reduced ventilation (V/Q = 0) is defined as intrapulmonary shunting; the extreme of reduced perfusion is dead space ventilation (V/Q = ∞). The shunt refers to that fraction of blood that passes through the lungs and is not oxygenated. A low V/Q is greater than zero but less than the ideal. In most clinical disorders of V/Q balance, the V/Q ratios are between the extreme values along a spectrum. Most of these patients will have a mixture of both V/Q mismatch and absolute shunt. The actual V/Q ratio is influenced by protective reflexes, such as hypoxic vasoconstriction in areas of reduced ventilation (3).

Respiratory failure as a result of V/Q mismatch is manifested by hypoxemia with an increased A-aDO$_2$ (that is, > 20 mmHg). Increasing the F_iO_2 will usually improve hypoxemia caused mainly by V/Q mismatch but will not significantly raise the PaO$_2$ when hypoxemia is caused mainly by an absolute shunt. Any condition that reduces the mixed venous oxygen tension (for example, reduced cardiac output) or that increases oxygen consumption (for example, increased metabolic rate) will worsen hypoxemia in the presence of V/Q imbalance. Hypoxemia is a stimulus to increase minute ventilation; thus the patient with hypoxemic respiratory failure from low or zero V/Q balance will usually present with hypocapnia ($PaCO_2$ < 35 mmHg) as long as the respiratory muscles can sustain the hyperventilation.

Increased dead space ventilation occurs when pulmonary perfusion is reduced relative to alveolar ventilation. This situation may be present as the result of pulmonary vasoconstriction (for example, pulmonary hypertension in the newborn), obliteration of small vessels in the pulmonary arterial bed (for example, adult respiratory distress syndrome), or multiple pulmonary emboli (for example, secondary to endocarditis) (3).

The third influence on gas exchange is the ability of oxygen and carbon dioxide to diffuse across the alveolar-capillary membrane. In general, a blood-gas tension abnormality results from abnormal diffusion of gases only when at least two of the following three factors are present: (1) decreased PaO_2 which reduces the driving pressure of O_2; (2) increased thickness of the alveolar-capillary membrane, which increases the resistance to gas diffusion (for example, interstitial edema or fibrosis); (3) either a reduction in the cross-sectional area of the pulmonary capillary bed (for example, adult respiratory distress syndrome) or a reduction in the time for red blood cell oxygen loading in the capillary bed (for example, high cardiac output states) (3).

Pediatric patients are also at greater risk than are adults for respiratory compromise because of their generally higher metabolic rate and, therefore, their increased oxygen consumption and carbon dioxide elimination. Respiratory distress adds to this metabolic demand on the ventilatory system by increasing the work of breathing, thus exacerbating the disparity between demand and supply (4). Causes of respiratory failure are categorized in Table 5.1.

CLINICAL PRESENTATION

During the initial history and physical examination, certain symptoms and signs may suggest the presence of hypercapnia (Table 5.2) or hypoxemia (Table 5.3). Patients with primary hypercapnic respiratory failure will generally be hypoxemic, and those with primary hypoxemic respiratory failure will usually have normal or decreased values of $PaCO_2$. Immediate evidence for the presence of respiratory failure includes severe respiratory distress in an agitated or anxious patient or inadequate air exchange in an obtunded patient.

The child who is not critically ill should be allowed to remain in the parent's lap or arms in a comfortable position. The respiratory rate, rhythm, and effort should be observed. Normal respiratory rates are age-related. In general, rates above 40 per minute are abnormal for an infant, and rates above 30 per minute are abnormal for a child (4). Other signs of increased work of breathing include the use of accessory neck muscles (sternocleidomastoid and scalene muscles), retractions (intercostal, subcostal, lower sternum, or supraclavicular), nasal flaring, and paradoxical chest or abdominal wall motion. Chest retractions and nasal flaring are more specific for

Table 5.2 Evidence for hypercapnia

Headache	Wheezing
Drowsiness, coma	Decreased air entry by auscultation
Sweating	Asymmetric air entry by auscultation
Tachycardia	Excessive work of breathing
Hypertension	Paradoxical chest wall motion
Peripheral vasodilation	Paradoxical abdominal wall motion
Stridor	Apneic episodes

respiratory tract disorders than is tachypnea. Retractions of different parts of the thorax are often striking in infants and young children with respiratory distress because of the highly compliant chest wall (1).

Dysphagia and drooling suggest upper airway obstruction. Stridor is an inspiratory crowing sound that is present in upper respiratory tract obstruction. Stridor has a high-pitched quality with croup and laryngeal foreign body aspiration and a low-pitched muffled quality with epiglottitis. A harsh, brassy cough, particularly when it is associated with inspiratory stridor, likewise suggests the presence of laryngeal or subglottic obstruction (for example, foreign body or croup). Grunting is caused by early closure of the glottis during exhalation. Grunting increases expiratory airway pressure, thus preventing airway collapse in a manner similar to the mechanism of positive end expiratory pressure (PEEP). Grunting may occur in patients with lower respiratory tract diseases (for example, pneumonia, asthma, or bronchiolitis), especially if diminished lung compliance is present (for example, pulmonary edema). Children suffering pain from any illness or injury, however, may also have grunting (4).

The adequacy of tidal volume can be assessed by inspection of abdominal excursions in the infant and chest filling in the child and by auscultation of breath

Table 5.3 Evidence for hypoxemia

Dyspnea	Tachycardia
Confusion	Hypertension
Agitation	Peripheral vasoconstriction
Restlessness	Rales by auscultation
Tachypnea	Murmur by auscultation
Retractions	Dysrhythmias
Nasal flaring	Bradycardia
Grunting	Hypotension
Sweating	Cyanosis

sounds bilaterally. Wheezing bilaterally suggests asthma or bronchiolitis (or occasionally congestive heart failure); foreign body aspiration may induce unilateral wheezing. Restlessness and irritability in an infant may be due to hypoxemia, hypercapnia, shock, or pain. Bradycardia is ominous in patients with respiratory failure and can occur in infants in response to hypoxemia (4). The presence of cyanosis in central tissues such as the tongue and the face should be noted. Peripheral cyanosis without central cyanosis can result from peripheral vasoconstriction in shock states or hypothermia or as a normal physiologic response in infants. The absence of cyanosis does not imply that oxygenation is adequate (1).

Disorders that lead to respiratory distress or failure may be progressive, sometimes acutely progressive. Patients may present with impending respiratory failure, or they may be at risk for respiratory compromise. These patients must be examined repeatedly for evidence of developing respiratory distress so that respiratory failure can be anticipated and possibly prevented with timely medical management decisions.

LABORATORY EVALUATION

Respiratory distress with tachypnea may be present in patients with disorders that are not primarily related to the respiratory system—such as sepsis, congenital heart disease, or metabolic acidosis (due to salicylate toxicity, diabetic ketoacidosis, or gastroenteritis with dehydration). Therefore confirmation of the clinical diagnosis of respiratory failure or impending failure generally requires arterial blood-gas and pH measurements. Respiratory failure is present if the $PaCO_2$ is greater than 55 mmHg (assuming no preexisting lung disease with chronic CO_2 elevation) in the presence of acidosis or if the PaO_2 is less than 50 mmHg (assuming no cyanotic congenital heart disease) in a patient breathing room air.

The alveolar-arterial oxygen difference ($A\text{-}aDO_2$) can be estimated in a patient with normal cardiac output who is breathing room air (ideally at sea level). In this situation, the alveolar O_2 tension added to the alveolar CO_2 tension equals approximately 145 mmHg. Assuming intact diffusion of blood gases at the alveolar-capillary interface, the alveolar CO_2 tension is essentially the same as the measured arterial CO_2 tension. Therefore the alveolar O_2 tension is approximately equal to 145 minus the measured $PaCO_2$. The measured PaO_2 is now subtracted from the calculated alveolar O_2 tension to yield $A\text{-}aDO_2$. An $A\text{-}aDO_2$ value of less than 20 mmHg is normal, 20 to 30 mmHg represents mild pulmonary dysfunction, 30 to 50 mmHg moderate dysfunction, and greater than 50 implies severe respiratory decompensation (5). Hypoxemia with a normal $A\text{-}aDO_2$ results from hypoventilation. Hypoxemia with an increased $A\text{-}aDO_2$ suggests either an intrapulmonary shunt, a low V/Q match, or a diffusion impairment (3).

If the patient is breathing oxygen, the PaO_2/F_iO_2 ratio can be calculated. The normal value for this ratio is about 500 to 600, and a ratio of 200 (for example, PaO_2 of 80 mmHg with F_iO_2 of 40 percent or 80/0.4) corresponds to an intrapulmonary shunt of about 20 percent, which generally indicates a need for ventilatory support (5). Further information may be gained by administering 100 percent O_2 to the hypoxemic patient. If the PaO_2 value increases to over 100 mmHg, either a low V/Q match or a diffusion impairment is present; if the PaO_2 value remains below 100 mmHg, an intrapulmonary shunt is the cause of hypoxemia (3). Even temporary administration of 100 percent O_2, however, is not completely innocuous; it can induce absorption atelectasis resulting in the measurement of a falsely elevated shunt fraction (6).

Pulse oximetry is useful for continuous measurement of O_2 saturation of hemoglobin. The relationship between PaO_2 and oxygen saturation of hemoglobin is expressed by the sigmoid-shaped oxygen-hemoglobin dissociation curves. When the $PaCO_2$, pH, and body temperature are normal, an oxyhemoglobin saturation of 90 percent correlates with a PaO_2 of about 60 mmHg. Hypercarbia, acidosis, or hyperthermia will shift the dissociation curve to the right so that an oxyhemoglobin saturation of 90 percent then correlates with a PaO_2 greater than 60 mmHg.

A chest roentgenogram is indicated and may reveal abnormalities that require intervention such as a pneumothorax or a malpositioned endotracheal tube. Furthermore the chest film can help with diagnosis of certain causes of respiratory failure. Other evaluations that may be indicated include a soft tissue lateral neck roentgenogram, electrocardiogram (EKG), complete blood count, electrolytes, glucose, and toxicology screen. A lateral decubitus chest roentgenogram is useful for evaluation of the dependent side for free pleural fluid or evidence of air trapping and the nondependent side for pneumothorax, air-fluid levels or basilar infiltrates hidden behind the diaphragm, or behind pleural effusion. Air trapping on the dependent side suggests that an ipsilateral endobronchial foreign body is not allowing the dependent lung to deflate as expected.

MANAGEMENT

Respiratory failure must be anticipated and prevented, if possible, with appropriate therapy. The goals of management of the patient with impending or fully developed respiratory failure include reestablishing adequate gas exchange in the lung and oxygen delivery to tissues. The etiology of failure should be identified, and the patient should be monitored so that the course of the disease process and the adequacy of therapy can be followed.

The patient's upper airway patency, respiratory rate and effort, vital signs, level of consciousness, color, and status of peripheral perfusion (skin temperature and capillary refill time) should be initially assessed and repeatedly monitored. Available monitoring devices include continuous pulse oximetry, indwelling arterial catheters, end-tidal CO_2 samples (capnography), transcutaneous oxygen and carbon dioxide tension electrodes, and conjunctival oxygen and carbon dioxide tension electrodes (5). Serial measurements of arterial blood gases and pH may be indicated. The patient should be reassessed repeatedly and after any therapeutic maneuver.

Sufficient oxygen should be administered to produce a hemoglobin-saturating PaO_2, that is, about 70 mmHg. In the patient with shock, an even higher PaO_2 should be attained if possible so that distal tissue watershed areas can be protected from hypoxia. A PaO_2 of less than 40 mmHg is a profound stimulus to the development of pulmonary hypertension and right heart failure. A continually high F_iO_2 can eventually cause oxygen toxicity in the lung, but the duration of this exposure necessary to produce toxicity is uncertain, and patients vary in susceptibility. Furthermore the use of positive pressure ventilation itself may play a role in the production of lung damage. Concerns about oxygen toxicity should not prevent adequate oxygenation of the patient, and a high F_iO_2 is occasionally necessary for temporary periods. The overall management protocol, however, should allow reduction of the F_iO_2 to 60 percent or lower as soon as this is practical (6).

If a hemoglobin-saturating PaO_2 cannot be achieved in a patient who is spontaneously breathing oxygen by mask, more advanced airway support may be required. Most children in respiratory distress or failure can be managed initially with bag-valve-mask ventilation and oxygenation. If early respiratory support efforts prove inadequate, endotracheal (ET) intubation and mechanically assisted ventilation may be indicated to reduce a possible low V/Q match or intrapulmonary shunt (4,6). The amount of assisted ventilation required is that which produces adequate chest wall expansion, usually a tidal volume of 10 to 15 ml/kg. In general, pressure-cycle ventilators are used for children less than 10 kg in weight (2).

Other therapeutic options depend on the type of respiratory failure identified and the specific etiology of failure (Tables 5.4 and 5.5). For example, bronchodilator therapy is indicated when hypercapnic respiratory failure from increased airways resistance is diagnosed. Response to bronchodilators is poor in most patients under 18 months of age, even in those patients later diagnosed with asthma, so that a bronchodilator therapeutic trial may be an unreliable test to differentiate asthma from bronchiolitis (1). Especially in patients with hypoxemic respiratory failure, careful fluid balance is important so that crystalloid overload can be avoided (6).

Table 5.4 Examples of management options for hypercapnic respiratory failure

Disorder	Goal	Treatment
CNS or peripheral nervous system hypoventilation	Increase alveolar ventilation	Assisted ventilation
Upper airway obstruction	Relieve or bypass obstruction	Endotracheal intubation, laryngoscopy, bronchoscopy
Increased airways resistance	Bronchodilation	Beta-adrenergic agonists, theophylline, steroids
Decreased lung compliance	Correct lung volume	Assisted lung ventilation, PEEP, diuretics
Respiratory muscle fatigue	Muscle rest	Assisted ventilation
	Improve muscle function	Beta-adrenergic agonists, theophylline
Increased dead space ventilation	Improve pulmonary blood flow	Vasodilators, reduced PEEP, inotropes, heparin

Reprinted with permission from Anas NG. Respiratory failure. In Leven DL, Morriss FC, eds. Essentials of pediatric emergency care. St. Louis: Quality Medical Publishing, 1990;64–71.

Table 5.5 Examples of management options for hypoxemic respiratory failure

Disorder	Goal	Treatment
Intrapulmonary shunt	Convert shunt to low or normal V/Q	Bronchodilators, diuretics, PEEP
Low V/Q	Correct hypoxemia	Increase F_iO_2
	Correct lung volume	Bronchodilators, diuretics, PEEP, surfactant replacement
Intracardiac shunt		
Ductus arteriosus-dependent lesions	Maintain patency of ductus	PGE_1 infusion
Tetralogy of Fallot	Relax pulmonary infundibulum	Morphine sulfate, propranolol
Hypoventilation	Increase alveolar ventilation	Assisted ventilation, racemic epinephrine
Diffusion impairment	Increased alveolar O_2	Increase F_iO_2
	Reduce resistance to diffusion	Diuretics, steroids

Reprinted with permission from Anas NG. Respiratory failure. In Leven DL, Morriss FC, eds. Essentials of pediatric emergency care. St. Louis: Quality Medical Publishing, 1990;64–71.

CONCLUSIONS

An understanding of the pathophysiology and appropriate initial assessment and management of infants and children with acute respiratory distress and failure will enable optimal care for these patients. Some causes of distress and failure are rapidly reversible with prompt recognition and proper therapy. Other disorders will follow a prolonged course to eventual improvement and recovery or to progressive deterioration and mortality despite optimal management decisions. Decompensation in these patients can occur rapidly, thus continual reevaluation and continuous monitoring are critical.

REFERENCES

1. Stokes DC. Respiratory disorders. In Ehrlich FE, Heldrich FJ, Tepas JJ III, eds. Pediatric emergency medicine. Rockville, Md.: Aspen Publishers, 1987;47–49.
2. Baker MD, Ruddy RM. Pulmonary emergencies. In Fleisher GR, Ludwig S, eds. Textbook of pediatric emergency medicine. Baltimore: Williams and Wilkins, 1988;665–668.
3. Anas NG. Respiratory failure. In Levin DL, Morriss FC, eds. Essentials of pediatric emergency care. St. Louis: Quality Medical Publishing, 1990;64–71.
4. APLS Task Force. Respiratory distress. In APLS Task Force, ed. Advanced pediatric life support textbook. Dallas: AAP/ACEP, 1989;18–23.
5. Wilson RF. Blood gases: Pathophysiology and interpretation. In Tintinalli JE, Krome RL, Ruiz E eds. Emergency medicine, a comprehensive study guide. New York: McGraw-Hill, 1992;56–60.
6. King EG. Respiratory failure in the critically ill. In Sibbald WJ, ed. Synopsis of critical care. 3rd ed. Baltimore: Williams and Wilkins;55–65.

6

Foreign Body Aspiration

Joseph D. Losek

Foreign body aspiration most commonly occurs in children six months to six years of age with the majority less than 3 years of age. Aspiration occurs approximately twice as often in boys as it does in girls (1–12). Food objects such as hot dogs, candies, nuts, and grapes are more commonly aspirated than nonfood objects (Table 6.1) (3). Young children do not have molars and cannot adequately chew these foods. In addition, they do not have a perfectly coordinated swallowing mechanism, leaving ingested foods at the laryngeal inlet when the child inspires. Combining this with the facts that children put objects in their mouths out of curiosity, habit, or carelessness and that children often eat while playing and talking explains the etiology of foreign body aspiration. Approximately 300 to 400 deaths occur each year in the United States secondary to aspiration. This is half the mortality rate prior to the Consumer Products Safety Act of 1979. This act mandated that toys and toy pieces designated for children up to 3 years of age must be at least 1¼ inches in diameter and 2¼ inches in depth (14). Despite this, recent cases illustrate the variety of nonfood objects aspirated. These include balloons, earrings, straight pin during an attempt to blow the pin through a straw, aluminum foil tab from a juice container, Barbie™ doll curler and plastic sales tag holder (15–20). Balloons are now the leading cause of pediatric choking deaths from children's products (20).

PATHOPHYSIOLOGY

The pathophysiology of foreign body aspiration is related to the degree of airway obstruction. Factors determining the degree of obstruction include age of patient, size of foreign body, organic versus nonorganic, duration, and location of foreign body. Most reviews have found the right mainstem bronchus to be the most common location, probably because its angle with the trachea is less than the left mainstem. The remaining foreign bodies are lodged in the trachea or larynx, the later being the least common location (see Table 6.1) (1–12).

Degrees of bronchial obstruction include partial obstruction on both inspiration and expiration and partial obstruction on inspiration but total obstruction on expiration and on inspiration and expiration. Total obstruction on expiration and not inspiration occurs secondary to intrathoracic negative pressure. This degree of obstruction results in air trapping and obstructive emphysema. Total obstruction causes

Table 6.1 Foreign body aspiration

	Number	Age Less Than 3 Years	M:F	Nature* Organic	Nature* Inorganic	Location† Bronchus	Location† Right	Location† Left	Location† Laryngotracheal
Laks, Barzilay (1)	149	90	94:55	141	8		73	52	24
Kim, Brummitt, Humphry, et al. (2)	202	131	135:67	156	46		99	63	19
Moazam, Talbert, Rodgers (3)	40	33	26:14	27	13				
Daniilidis, Symeonidis, Triaridis, et al. (4)	79		48:31				22	39	18
Harboyan, Nassif (5)	213			197	16		121	55	36
Aytac, Yurdakul, Ikizler, et al. (6)	462	329	351:111	358	94		327	86	45
Merchant, Kirtane, Shah, et al. (7)	132	91	81:51	108	24		68	61	13
Puhakka, Svedstrom, Kero, et al. (8)	83	46	56:27	49	34		41	25	3
Losek (9)	42		26:16	32	10		24	15	
Blazer, Naveh, Friedman (10)	200	170	133:67	187	8		83	69	35
Abdulmajid, Ebeid, Motaweh, et al. (11)	250		110:140	212	38		175	32	43
Pyman (12)	230		150:80	155	75		117	74	33
TOTAL	2082	890/1268 (70%)	1210:659 (1.8:1)	1622 (82%)	366 (18%)	1721 (86%)	1150 (67%)	571 (33%)	269 (14%)

*The nature of some foreign bodies was unknown.
†Some patients had multiple foreign bodies in more than one location.
Note: Blanks indicate no report.

atelectasis. Organic versus nonorganic foreign bodies more commonly cause a local inflammatory reaction. Thus with time, a partial obstruction can progress to a total obstruction. If total obstruction is not corrected, trapped secretions dilate the bronchioles and result in bronchiectasis and fibrosis.

CLINICAL MANIFESTATIONS

The factors that determined the pathophysiology (the degree of airway obstruction) also determine the clinical manifestations. Initially the child may have cough, gagging, choking, stridor, wheezing, hoarseness, dysphonia, drooling, or cyanosis. The caretaker may not witness these initial symptoms, and if the child is too young to verbally report the aspiration, there will be no history of foreign body aspiration. This is not uncommon, as great as 62 percent of children in one review had no history of foreign body aspiration (11). Combining the studies referred to in Table 6.1, 81 percent of the children gave a history of foreign body aspiration (1–12).

Initial symptoms may resolve, and if so, a symptomless interval occurs (12,21–23). This interval may last hours, days, or months. In a review by Laks and Barzilay of 149 patients, 41 (27 percent) were asymptomatic at presentation (1). When a foreign body becomes lodged in a fixed position, the surface sensory receptors of the respiratory tract adapt to the constant pressure. The defense cough reflex stops with this adaptation of the surface receptors. Combining studies, cough was the most common symptom but still occurred in only 76 percent of the patients (1–12). Unless the foreign body moves or secretions stimulate new surface receptors, cough will not occur. The production of secretions is dependent on the inflammatory nature of the foreign body and on the length of time it has been lodged. This adaptive quality of the airway surface receptors accounts for the symptomless interval and is one of the factors that can lead to a subsequent delay in diagnosis.

Manifested symptoms are determined by the location of the foreign body in the respiratory tract and the degree of obstruction. Total obstruction at the level of the trachea or larynx will rapidly produce respiratory failure and an inability to ventilate with resuscitative breathing. Partial obstruction at the larynx may cause inspiratory stridor, drooling, gagging, and voice change. Whereas partial obstruction at the trachea may manifest as inspiratory stridor, choking, and cough. If obstruction is nearly complete at the trachea, expiratory wheeze may also occur. Partial obstruction of the bronchus results in wheezing and cough. The degree of obstruction will determine the degree of respiratory distress. For these reasons, symptoms can be quite variable. Combining studies, symptoms of foreign body aspiration include cough (76 percent), wheezing (50 percent), respiratory difficulty (36 percent), history of cyanosis (30 percent), and choking (30 percent) (1–12). Eleven percent of the patients were asymptomatic. Location, duration, and nature of the foreign body also determine the signs of foreign body aspiration. Fever and rales support pneumonia and are more commonly found when patients present more than 24 hours postaspiration. Patients with laryngotracheal foreign bodies have significantly less wheezing, unilateral decreased air entry, and fever compared to patients with bronchial foreign bodies. Laryngotracheal foreign body patients, however, are more likely to have stridor and hoarseness. The classical physical finding of bronchial foreign body aspiration is

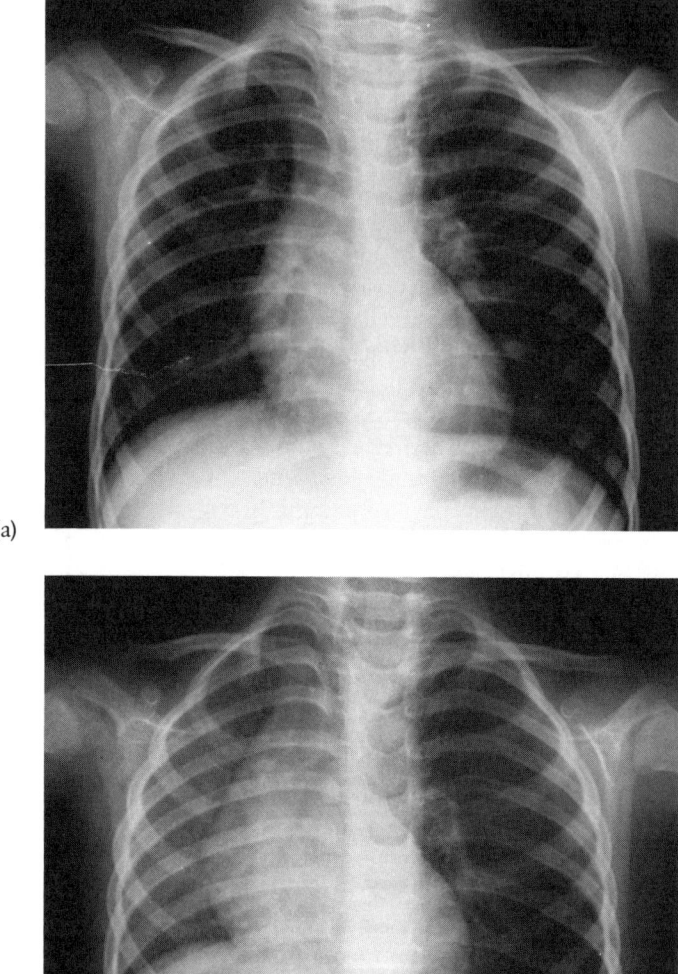

Figure 6.1 Left mainstem bronchus foreign body causes the ball-valve effects illustrated in the inspiratory (a) and expiratory (b) chest X-rays. The expiratory film shows the depression of the diaphragm and hyperinflation of the involved left side, and the shift of the mediastinum and heart to the uninvolved right side.

unilateral decrease of air entry on the affected side. Combining studies, 61 percent of patients had unequal air entry (1-12). Other signs include wheezing (34 percent), tachypnea (30 percent), and rales (18 percent). Seven percent of the patients had normal examinations (1-12).

The initial roentgenograms for suspected foreign body aspiration are inspiratory/expiratory chest X-rays (Figures 6.1a and b). The affected side will be hyperinflated on the expiratory X-ray. The degree of hyperinflation is dependent on the degree of obstruction. Obstructive emphysema was the most common abnormal finding of previous reviews, occurring in 35 percent of the patients with foreign body aspiration (1-12). Since the majority of foreign bodies are organic, and thus radiolucent, only 8 percent of the foreign bodies were seen on chest X-rays. Other findings include infiltrate (15 percent) and atelectasis (11 percent). These findings, particularly infiltrate were more commonly found when the diagnosis of foreign body aspiration was delayed. In addition, discovering an infiltrate may further delay the correct diagnosis. Overall 31 percent of the chest X-rays were normal (1-12). For laryngotracheal foreign body, chest X-rays were normal in 60 percent of the patients reported by Blazer (10).

These limitations of plain chest roentgenograms in the diagnosis of foreign body aspiration are disturbing. An additional diagnostic procedure is fluoroscopy. The behavior of the mediastinal shadow is examined during the respiratory cycle. Widening of the mediastinal shadow during inspiration is a diagnostic sign of laryngeal, tracheal, or both main bronchi obstruction. This widening, however, can also occur during forced inspiration as happens with crying. Shift of the mediastinal shadow with inspiration indicates an unilateral bronchial obstruction. Combining previous reports, fluoroscopy was performed in 429 children and 317 of them (74 percent) were supportive of a foreign body aspiration (1,5,10). Fluoroscopy, lung scan, or CT (computerized tomography), however, do not improve diagnostic accuracy compared to history, physical examination, and chest X-rays.

MANAGEMENT

The diagnosis of foreign body aspiration is often delayed. Combining studies, 169 (18 percent) patients had a diagnostic delay of greater than 30 days (1-12). Delay is often caused by the physician attributing the patient's signs and symptoms to other, more common pediatric respiratory tract disorders. Pneumonia or asthma is often the initial misdiagnosis for foreign body aspiration. Antibiotic or bronchodilator treatment can result in improvement, therefore, a high suspicion for foreign body aspiration should be present in cases of recurrent pneumonia and prolonged bronchospasm. In addition, an esophageal foreign body may result in cough, respiratory distress, and stridor similar to the symptoms caused by a laryngotracheal foreign body (24).

Bronchoscopy is the treatment of choice. Combining studies, 2032 (98 percent) children with foreign body aspiration, had the foreign body removed via bronchoscopy, 10 (0.5 percent) spontaneously coughed the foreign body out, and 34 (1.6 percent) required thoracotomy (1-12). Complications from bronchoscopy include laryngeal edema needing tracheostomy (1.4 percent to 17 percent), pneumomediastinum-pneumothorax (1 percent to 2.3 percent) and cardiac arrest (1 percent to 2.3 percent) (5,6). Prednisolone (1 to 2 mg/kg) is given prior to bronchoscopy to prevent laryngeal edema and subsequent need for possible tracheostomy. Cardiac arrest may be caused by the combination of hypoxia and reflex vagal stimulation, therefore, prebronchoscopy atropine treatment is routine.

Bronchoscopy should be performed without delay for children with foreign body aspiration. A 24-hour trial of bronchodilator therapy, postural drainage, and chest physiotherapy in hopes of the patient spontaneously coughing up the foreign body are not recommended. Movement of the foreign body may convert a partial obstruction or one bronchus obstruction to a total tracheal obstruction. Deaths secondary to foreign body airway obstruction have occurred in children with asymptomatic intervals (25,26). Blazer found that a second or a third bronchoscopy was needed in 15 percent of the children with foreign body aspiration, either because the foreign body was not found in a previous procedure (9 percent) or because an incomplete removal was made (6 percent) (10). A second, third, or fourth bronchoscopy was needed in 16 percent of the patients reported by Merchant (7). A negative bronchoscopy may also occur with an unsuspected esophageal foreign body (24).

In the emergent situation of respiratory failure secondary to foreign body aspiration, near-total or total obstruction at the level of the larynx or trachea is the most likely cause. Basic life-support therapy, including abdominal thrusts for the child one year of age and older or back blows and chest compressions for the child less than one year of age, can be initially attempted. In an emergency department, however, direct visualization with a laryngoscope and removal with McGill's forceps is recommended. If a foreign body is not visualized, a tracheal foreign body can be assumed. Endotracheal intubation is suggested with the intention of pushing the foreign body into one of the bronchi, thus permitting ventilation and oxygenation of at least one lung. Emergency tracheostomy or cricothyrotomy are final alternatives if endotracheal intubation is unsuccessful.

CONCLUSION

Foreign body aspiration occurs most commonly in children less than six years of age with the majority less than three years. Organic food materials are the most commonly aspirated foreign bodies. Prevention of the majority of cases is possible if young children are not permitted to eat peanuts, grapes, hot dogs, and other foods that require complete chewing. The presenting signs and symptoms of foreign body aspiration are variable, ranging from none to respiratory failure. Delay in diagnosis is not uncommon because the aspiration may be unwitnessed, airway adaption to the foreign body can result in an asymptomatic interval, 30 percent of chest roentgenograms are normal, and a more common pediatric respiratory disorder (asthma or pneumonia) is often diagnosed. Bronchoscopy without delay is the treatment of choice.

REFERENCES

1. Laks Y, Barzilay Z. Foreign body aspiration in childhood. Pediatr Emerg Care 1988;4:102–106.
2. Kim IG, Brummitt WM, Humphry A, et al. Foreign body in the airway: A review of 202 cases. Laryngoscope 1973;83:347–354.
3. Moazam F, Talbert JL, Rodgers BM. Foreign bodies in the pediatric tracheo-bronchial tree. Clin Pediatr 1983;22:148–150.
4. Daniilidis J, Symeonidis B, Triaridis K, et al. Foreign body in the airways. Arch Otolaryngol 1977;103:570–573.
5. Harboyan G, Nassif R. Tracheobronchial foreign bodies—A review of 14 years' experience. J Laryngol Otol 1970;84:403–412.
6. Aytac A, Yurdakul Y, Ikizler C, et al. Inhalation of foreign bodies in children. Report of 500 cases. J Thorac Cardiovasc Surg 1977;74:145–151.
7. Merchant SN, Kirtane MV, Shah KL, et al. Foreign bodies in the bronchi. (A 10 year review of 132 cases) J Postgrad Med 1984;30:219–223.
8. Puhakka H, Svedstrom E, Kero P, et al. Tracheobronchial foreign bodies. A persistent problem in pediatric patients. AJDC 1989;143:543–545.
9. Losek JD. Diagnostic difficulties of foreign body aspiration in children. Am J Emerg Med 1990;8:348–350.
10. Blazer S, Naveh Y, Friedman A. Foreign body in the airway. A review of 200 cases. Am J Dis Child 1980;134:68–71.
11. Abdulmajid OA, Ebeid AM, Motaweh MM, et al. Aspirated foreign bodies in the tracheobronchial tree: Report of 250 cases. Thorax 1976;31:635–640.
12. Pyman C. Inhaled foreign bodies in childhood. Med J Aust 1971;1:62–68.
13. Harris CS, Baker SP, Smith GA, et al. Childhood asphyxiation by food. JAMA 1984;251:2231–2235.
14. Kenna MA, Bluestone CD. Foreign bodies in the air and food passages. Pediatr in Rvw 1988;10:25–30.
15. Becker PG, Turow J. Earring aspiration and other jewelry hazards. Pediatrics 1986;78:494–496.
16. Press S, Liberman JG. Aspiration through a 'sip-up' straw. AJDC 1986;140:1090–1091.
17. Ross MN, Janik JS. 'Foil Tab' aspiration and retropharyngeal abscess in a toddler. JAMA 1988;260:3130.
18. Arnold RW, Hoffman AD, Brutinel WM, et al. 'Barbie' doll curler aspiration into the upper trachea. AJDC 1987;141:1325–1326.
19. Myer CM. Foreign body aspiration. AJDC 1988;142:485–486.
20. Ryan CA, Yacoub W, Paton T, et al. Childhood deaths from toy balloons. AJDC 1990;144:1221–1224.
21. Banks W, Potsic WP. Elusive unsuspected foreign bodies in the tracheo-bronchial tree. Clin Pediatr 1977;16:31–35.
22. Blumhagen JD, Wesenberg RL, Brooks JG, et al. Endotracheal foreign bodies. Difficulties in diagnosis. Clin Pediatr 1980;19:480–484.
23. Benjamin B, Vandeleur T. Inhaled foreign bodies in children. Med J Aust 1974;1:355–358.
24. Swischuk LE. Acute respiratory distress and stridor. Pediatr Emerg Care 1991;7:61–63.
25. Humphries CT, Wagener JS, Morgan WJ. Fatal prolonged foreign body aspiration following an asymptomatic interval. Am J Emerg Med 1988;6:611–613.
26. Walls RM: Fatal, prolonged foreign body aspiration (letter to the editor). Am J Emerg Med 1989;7:669–670.

PART III
Circulation

7

Shock

Morris Gessouroun

Shock is a systemic disorder producing a state of circulatory dysfunction that results in a failure to provide adequate supplies of oxygen and nutrients to meet the demands of the tissue beds. It is commonly perceived that shock is a state of low cardiac output heralded by the development of hypotension. It is becoming increasingly clear that such a view of shock is too simplistic. Shock occurs as a consequence of a complex intermixture of cellular, biochemical, and neuroendocrine responses interacting with local and circulating vasoactive mediators, products of cellular breakdown and exogenous agents such as endotoxin, to produce the resulting physiological state. The clinical manifestations of shock in any particular individual are the result of a complex combination of these factors, the precipitating etiologic agent, the preexisting state of health, and the effects and timing of therapeutic actions.

PATHOPHYSIOLOGY
Oxygen Derived Variables

To understand shock, it is helpful to define several factors associated with oxygen transport and utilization (Table 7.1). Oxygen availability is a direct function of cardiac index (CI) and arterial oxygen content (CaO_2), the sum of hemoglobin-bound oxygen and dissolved oxygen in arterial blood. The volume of hemoglobin-bound oxygen is the product of the hemoglobin concentration, oxygen saturation, and the binding coefficient of oxygen to hemoglobin (1.34). Dissolved oxygen is the product of arterial oxygen tension (PaO_2) and the solubility coefficient of oxygen in plasma (0.003).

Oxygen uptake (VO_2) is a direct function of CI and the difference in oxygen content between arterial and mixed-venous blood. Oxygen extraction (ER) is the ratio of VO_2 to oxygen availability. Normally VO_2 by the tissues is determined by metabolic demand and is not determined or limited by the oxygen availability. Should oxygen availability fall, in the face of constant metabolic demand, ER increases as needed to maintain constant VO_2. At some point, termed *critical oxygen availability*, ER will become limited by and dependent on oxygen availability. At levels of oxygen availability below this point, an oxygen deficit exists, anaerobic metabolism and lactate production rise and metabolic acidosis occurs. Severe or extended periods of tissue oxygen deficit will result in damage to cellular function and structure with eventual cell death.

Table 7.1 Hemodynamic and oxygenation values

Variable	Formula	Normal Range
Hemodynamic		
Cardiac output	CO = HR × SV	
Cardiac index	CI = CO/BSA	3.5–5.5 L/min/m^2
Systemic vascular resistance index	SVRI = $\frac{79.9 \, (MAP - CVP)}{CI}$	800–1600 DYNE SEC/CM^5/M^2
Pulmonary vascular resistance index	PVRI = $\frac{79.9 \, (MPAP - PCWP)}{CI}$	80–240 DYNE SEC/CM^5/M^2
Oxygen transport		
Arterial oxygen content	Cao_2 = (Hb)(1.34)(%sat) + (PaO$_2$)(0.003)	17–20 ml/dl
Mixed venous oxygen content	Cvo_2 = (Hb)(1.34)(%sat) + (PvO$_2$)(0.003)	12–15 ml/dl
Oxygen content difference	A-vDO$_2$ = CaO$_2$ − CvO$_2$	3–5 ml/dl
Oxygen availability	O$_2$ avail = CaO$_2$ × CI × 10	550–650 ml/min/m^2
Oxygen uptake	VO$_2$ = CI × A-VDO$_2$ × 10	120–200 ml/min/m^2
Oxygen extraction ratio	$\frac{A-VDO_2}{CaO_2}$	0.15–0.29

HR = heart rate; BSA = body surface area; MAP = mean arterial blood pressure; MPAP = mean pulmonary arterial blood pressure; PCWP = pulmonary capillary wedge pressure; SV = stroke volume
Reprinted with permission of the publisher from Katz RW, Pollack MM, Weibley RE. Pulmonary artery catheterization in pediatric intensive care. Adv Pediatr 1983;30:169–190.

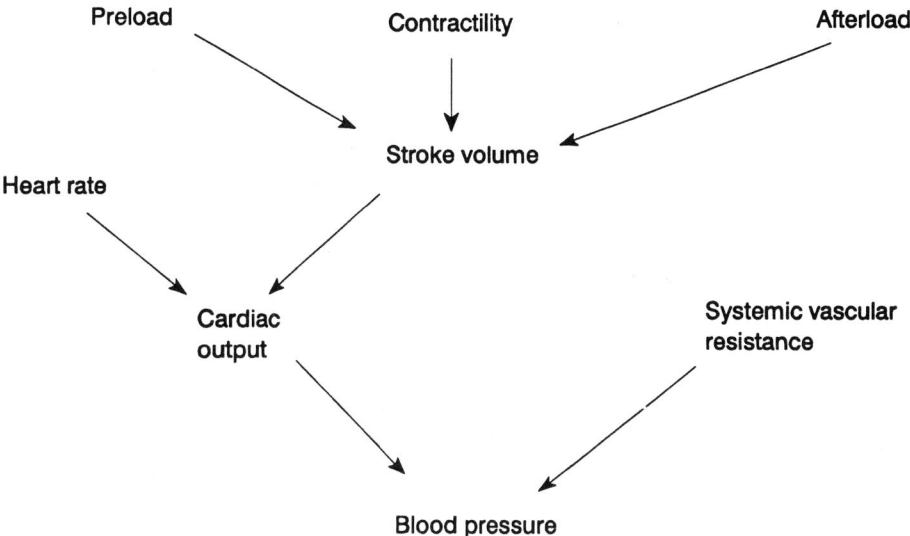

Figure 7.1 Interrelationship of the factors determining cardiac output and blood pressure. (Reprinted with permission of the publisher from Perkin RM, Levin DL. Shock. In Levin DL, Norriss, eds. Essentials of pediatric intensive care. St. Louis: Quality Medical Publishers, 1990.)

In many forms of shock, such as massive hemorrhage or pericardial tamponade, impaired oxygen availability is caused by impaired cardiovascular performance with low cardiac output. Cardiac output is a function of heart rate and the volume ejected per beat (stroke volume). Abnormalities of heart rate or rhythm such as bradycardia, extreme tachycardia, or dysrhythmias can produce shock. Stroke volume can be reduced by insufficient ventricular filling (inadequate preload), reduced cardiac contractility, or impeded ventricular emptying (increased afterload). Figure 7.1 depicts the interrelationship of factors determining cardiac output and blood pressure.

In some circumstances, such as sepsis or trauma, shock may occur with normal or increased cardiac output. Under these circumstances, oxygen and nutrient delivery may be inadequate for several reasons including increased demands for oxygen or nutrients, maldistribution of circulation at the organ or tissue level and failure of uptake or utilization of oxygen or nutrients at the cellular level.

Stages of Shock

Shock is not a single entity but rather a syndrome with progressive stages of severity: compensated, uncompensated, and irreversible. In compensated shock, intrinsic mechanisms restore and maintain vital organ function. This is achieved through a variety of neural, humoral, and cellular mechanisms. Compensatory mechanisms act to (1) preserve myocardial and cerebral blood flow at the expense of less vital organs such as skin, muscle, and splanchnic beds; (2) augment cardiac output through increased heart rate and contractility; and (3) restore circulating blood volume through vasoconstriction of capacitance vessels. Gross measures of cardiovascular homeostasis such as systemic arterial blood pressure, CI, heart rate, and peripheral perfusion may be normal or increased. Microcirculatory flow, however, is reduced and maldistributed. The recognition of shock during the compensated phase with institution of effective treatment allows for the best prognosis for recovery. When shock is primarily caused by cardiac dysfunction, intrinsic responses intended to augment perfusion often further depress function (Figure 7.2). As such in shock of primary cardiac etiology, a compensated phase is rarely seen.

In uncompensated shock, compensatory mechanisms become exhausted and may contribute to further propagation of the shock state. The function of vital organs such as the heart, lungs, kidneys, and brain begins to fail. The hallmark of uncompensated shock is the vasodilation of various vascular beds allowing pooling of blood with ensuing coagulation, platelet aggregation, release of mediators of vascular tone, vascular and cellular permeability, and chemotaxis. Cellular function deteriorates in both local and remote tissue beds. Measures of cardiovascular homeostasis such as systemic arterial blood pressure, heart rate, cardiac output, peripheral perfusion, and urine output are clearly abnormal during uncompensated shock. Survival remains possible during uncompensated shock; but the course is usually prolonged and commonly complicated by single or multiple organ dysfunction. Invariably hospital costs, duration of hospitalization, morbidity, and mortality are increased in patients who progress to uncompensated shock.

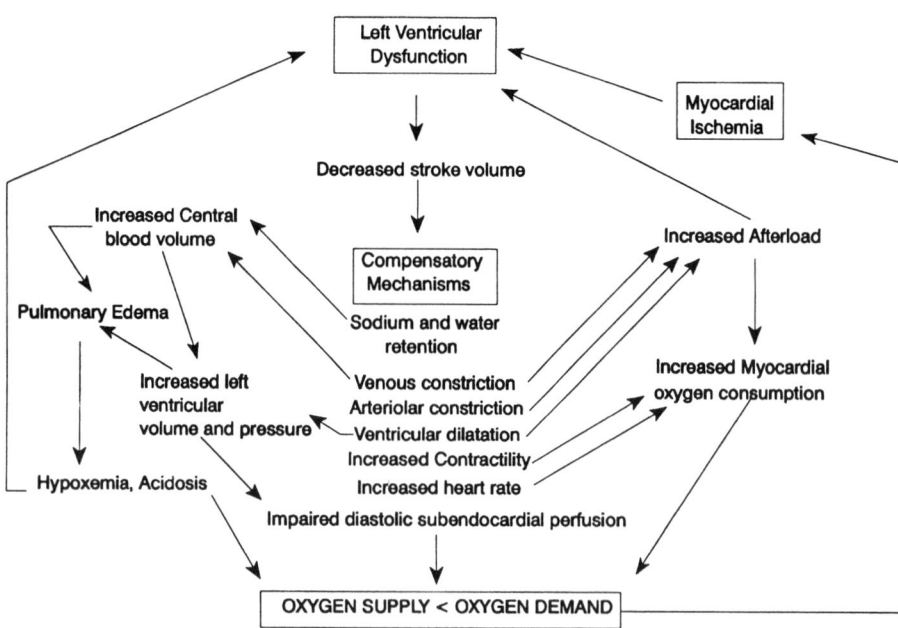

Figure 7.2 Self-perpetuating pathways in cardiogenic shock. (Reprinted with permission of the publisher from Perkin RM, Levin DL. Shock in the pediatric patient. J Pediatrics 1982;101(6):166.)

Irreversible shock signifies damage to vital organ systems of such magnitude that, despite therapeutic interventions, death eventually occurs. Measures of cardiovascular homeostasis may be ameliorated by therapy but this improvement is transitory.

DIAGNOSIS AND DIFFERENTIAL DIAGNOSIS
Classifications of Shock

The prototypical classification system for shock was proposed by Hinshaw and Cox in 1972. Their system uses four subclasses of shock: (1) hypovolemic (due to insufficient circulating volume), (2) cardiogenic (due to pump failure), (3) distributive (due to a defect in distribution of blood flow), and (4) obstructive (due to extracardiac obstruction to blood flow). Although useful, this classification system overly simplifies the issues concerning some forms of shock. For example, septic shock is classified under distributive shock. As the mechanisms underlying septic shock are coming to be understood, however, septic shock would be better categorized as a mixed class with components of hypovolemic, cardiogenic, and distributive shock contributing to the overall pathology. In addition, since obstructive shock causes decreased cardiac performance, many authors consider it a subset of cardiogenic shock. Table 7.2 shows many of the etiologies producing each classification of shock.

Hypovolemic Shock

Hypovolemic shock is the most common cause of circulatory failure in pediatric patients. Major categories include losses of water and electrolytes such as with gastroenteritis or diabetes mellitus, hemorrhage as after trauma or surgery, and plasma losses as with burns or so-called *third spacing* as occurs after intraabdominal surgery (Table 7.3). Losses may be external as with hemorrhage from a laceration or thoracostomy tube or may be more occult as with hemorrhage into the soft tissues after a long bone or pelvic fracture.

The unifying mechanism of hypovolemic shock is a loss of circulating blood volume (*preload*) that results in reduced ventricular filling with a consequent fall in cardiac output. Compensatory mechanisms, mediated predominantly through the sympathetic nervous system, act to restore perfusion to vital organs by vasoconstriction of less vital tissue beds.

During the compensated phase of hypovolemic shock, patients characteristically demonstrate tachycardia, cutaneous vasoconstriction with pale or mottled skin and a prolonged capillary refill time, and diminished pulse pressure demonstrable as thready pulses. Systemic arterial blood pressure is maintained during the compensated phase by elevation of systemic vascular resistance. If appropriate and sufficient restitution of circulating volume is provided during the compensated phase of hypovolemic shock, recovery is usually complete.

If adequate volume replacement is not provided, progression to uncompensated shock will occur. Uncompensated hypovolemic shock is characterized by profound vasoconstriction with ischemia to key organ systems, intravascular stagnation and

Table 7.2 Classification of shock

I. Hypovolemic
  A. Hemorrhagic
    1. Gastrointestinal causes
      a. Meckel's diverticulum
      b. Esophageal varicies
    2. Trauma
    3. Internal bleeding
      a. Blunt trauma
      b. Long bone or pelvic fractures
      c. Retroperitoneal bleeding (any cause)
  B. Nonhemorrhagic
    1. Gastrointestinal losses
      a. Vomiting
      b. Diarrhea
    2. Renal losses
      a. Excessive diuretic effect
      b. Osmotic diuresis (diabetes mellitus)
      c. Diabetes insipidus
II. Cardiogenic
  A. Failure of contractile mechanism
    1. Myocardial contusion
    2. Cardiomyopathy
    3. Myocardial "stunning"
  B. Impedance to ventricular outflow
    1. Intrinsic
      a. Aortic stenosis
      b. Interrupted aortic arch
      c. Coarctation of the aorta
	C. Impedance to ventricular filling
	    1. Intrinsic
	      a. Mitral stenosis
	      b. Atrial myxoma
	      c. Atrial thrombus
	    2. Extrinsic
	      a. Pericardial tamponade
	      b. Restrictive pericarditis
	      c. Tension pneumothorax
	  D. Valve failure
	    1. Acute mitral regurgitation
	    2. Acute aortic regurgitation
	  E. Dysrhythmia
	    1. Tachydysrythmias
	    2. Bradydysrhythmias
	  F. Myocardial rupture (trauma)
	III. Distributive
	  A. Sepsis
	  B. Toxic shock
	  C. Neurogenic
	  D. Anaphylaxis
	  E. Drug overdose
	  F. Trauma without hypovolemia
	  G. Hemorrhage shock and encephalopathy

Reprinted with permission of the publisher from Schuster DP, Lefrak SS. Shock in critical care. In Civetta JM, Taylor RW, and Kirby RR, eds. Critical care. Philadelphia: Lippincott, 1988;891.

Table 7.3 Causes of hypovolemic shock

Water and electrolyte loss	Hemorrhage
Diarrhea	Trauma
Vomiting	Surgery
Diabetes mellitus	Gastrointestinal bleeding
Diabetes insipidus	*Plasma losses*
Renal losses	Burns
Intestinal obstruction	Sepsis
Burns	Intestinal obstruction
	Peritonitis

Reprinted with permission of the publisher from Wetzel RC. Shock. In Rogers MC, ed. Textbook of pediatric intensive care. Baltimore: Williams & Wilkins, 1987;483.

pooling, and eventual damage to key organs such as the heart and the brain, leading to irreversible shock. Patients in the uncompensated phase of hypovolemic shock may be obtunded or comatose, oliguric or anuric, and hypotensive.

Cardiogenic Shock

Cardiogenic shock is defined as a hypoperfusion state in which the perfusion abnormality is due to primary cardiac dysfunction. Unlike adults, in whom coronary artery disease is common, primary cardiogenic shock is rare in children. All forms of shock as they progress into the uncompensated and irreversible stages, manifest cardiac dysfunction. Cardiogenic shock can be viewed as the final common pathway for all etiologies of shock.

Among the most common causes of primary cardiogenic shock in children is congenital heart disease. In several types of this disease, systemic blood flow depends on patency of the ductus arteriosus. These infants will present with cardiogenic shock on spontaneous ductal closure. Etiologies include hypoplastic left heart syndrome, critical aortic stenosis, interrupted aortic arch, and severe coarctation of the aorta. It may be difficult to distinguish these processes from the findings in shock due to neonatal sepsis. Another common cause of myocardial dysfunction associated with congenital heart disease is from myocardial injury during the postoperative period after repair of congenital heart lesions. Fortunately, the myocardium of the infant and child is surprisingly resistant to these insults and usually recovers except in especially severe or complex lesions.

Cardiogenic shock may occur as the consequence of a generalized hypoxic-ischemic insult. Etiologies include near-drowning, near-miss sudden infant death syndrome, and following cardiopulmonary arrest from other causes. Usually these patients also suffer severe brain injury because of hypoxia and ischemia. The myocardial effects can ordinarily be ameliorated, but death or severe disability in these patients is common because of their accompanying central nervous system (CNS) injury.

Other important etiologies of cardiogenic shock in children include dysryhythmias, drug intoxication, extrinsic inflow or outflow obstruction (tension pneumothorax or pneumopericardium, pericardial tamponade), metabolic disorders (hypoglycemia, cardiomyopathy), infectious disorders (constrictive pericarditis, myocarditis), and valvular disorders (regurgitant or obstructive).

Patients in cardiogenic shock rarely manifest a compensated phase in that compensatory mechanisms intended to support perfusion further impair cardiac output. These patients are as a rule tachycardic and hypotensive and have thready peripheral pulses and cold clammy skin. Further they may be mottled or cyanotic, have altered mentation, and are oliguric or anuric. Physical findings of hepatomegaly, jugular venous distension, and a gallop rhythm or findings such as cardiomegaly on chest radiograph, an increased central venous pressure or pulmonary artery wedge pressure may be helpful in differentiating cardiogenic shock from other varieties of shock.

Distributive Shock

Distributive shock results because of abnormal vascular tone producing a variable combination of venous pooling, physiologic shunting of vascular beds and increased vascular capacitance. Distributive shock, unlike other forms of shock, can occur in the face of normal or increased cardiac output. The various etiologies of distributive shock include anaphylaxis, neurogenic shock caused by cervical spinal trauma, drug overdose with an agent that causes vasodilation or vasomotor paralysis (barbiturates, antihypertensive agents, tricyclic antidepressants), and septic shock (Table 7.4). Septic shock, although historically included in the category of distributive shock, is more appropriately considered a mixed type of shock with components of hypovolemic, cardiogenic, and distributive shock. Patients with distributive shock are tachycardic and may have hypotension. They differ from patients with hypovolemic or cardiogenic shock in that during the early compensated phase they commonly have bounding pulses, wide pulse pressure, normal capillary refill time, warm distal extremities, and normal urine output. Findings also may include tachypnea, decreased systemic vascular resistance, low central venous pressure and pulmonary artery wedge pressure, and increased cardiac output. If not interrupted, later stages of septic shock are clinically similar to those in advanced hypovolemic or cardiogenic shock.

Patients with septic shock may be febrile or, especially in infants, hypothermic. They may have a leukocytosis with a preponderance of immature neutrophils or in severe cases may present with neutropenia. Hyperglycemia is common, and may occur, especially in young infants. In adults, septic shock is most commonly caused by gram-negative enteric bacteria. The offending organisms in children are more diverse and include both gram-positive and gram-negative bacteria, viruses, rickettsia, and protozoa (Table 7.5).

Table 7.4 Causes of distributive shock

Anaphylaxis	*Septic shock*
Antibiotics	Early phase
Vaccines	
Blood	*Drugs*
Local anesthetics	Barbiturates
Iodine contrast media	Phenothiazines
Insects	Tranquilizers
Foods	Antihypertensives
Neurologic Injury	
Head injury	
Spinal shock	

Reprinted with permission of the publisher from Wetzel RC. Shock. In Rogers MC. Textbook of pediatric intensive care. Baltimore: Williams & Wilkins, 1987;483.

Table 7.5 Common pathogens causing septic shock

Neonates	Children
Group B β-hemolytic streptococci	S. pneumoniae
Enterobacteriaceae	Neisseria meningitidis
Listeria monocytogenes	S. aureus
Staphylococcus aureus	
	Immunocompromised
Infants	Enterbacteriaceae
H. influenzae	S. aureus
Streptococcus pneumoniae	Psuedomonadaceae
S. aureus	Candida albicans

Reprinted with permission of the publisher from Wetzel RC. Shock. In Rogers MC, ed. Textbook of pediatric intensive care. Baltimore: Williams & Wilkins, 1987;483.

CLINICAL PRESENTATION
Effects of Shock on Organ Systems

Independent of etiology, shock is a process that affects all organ systems. The degree to which any particular organ system is affected will be a function of etiology, severity, and stage of shock.

Heart

Disturbed cardiac function may be the primary etiologic agent in shock as in children with congenital heart disease or cardiomyopathy. Under other circumstances, heart function may become disordered as a secondary manifestation of shock provoked by other mechanisms such as with trauma or sepsis. Secondary cardiac dysfunction can be broken down by the determinants of cardiac output noted earlier, specifically heart rate and rhythm, preload, contractility, and afterload.

Heart rate and stroke volume determine cardiac output. Young infants, especially neonates, have reduced amounts of myocardial contractile tissue and have very limited ability to increase cardiac output by increasing contractility. Therefore they are highly dependent on increased heart rate to improve cardiac output. As such, tachycardia is virtually always a manifestation of shock and represents a compensatory response. Excessive tachycardia, as may occur with extreme hypovolemia, hyperpyrexia, and high levels of either endogenous or administered catecholamines, is detrimental by reducing both diastolic ventricular filling time and coronary perfusion.

On occasion, especially in young infants subjected to hypoxic-ischemic injury to the myocardium or profound acidosis, *bradycardia* develops that dramatically embarrasses cardiac output. Atrial tachydysrhythmias can occur following myocardial injury or as a complication of pharmacological therapy (catecholamines, atropine). Ventricular tachydysrhythmias are rare but may occur in the face of severe disturbances of potassium or calcium concentrations, marked acid-base disturbance, hypoxic-ischemic injury, or direct myocardial traumatic injury, or drug overdose or from irritation caused by indwelling vascular catheters.

Preload is defined by the ventricular end-diastolic volume but can be estimated by the ventricular end-diastolic pressure. For the right ventricle, preload is estimated by the right ventricular diastolic pressure, right atrial pressure, or central venous pressure in decreasing order of accuracy. For the left ventricle, preload may be estimated by the left ventricular diastolic pressure or the left atrial pressure. In the absence of pathological intracardiac shunts or significant valvular pathology, the left ventricular preload may be estimated by the pulmonary artery wedge pressure, the pulmonary artery diastolic pressure, the right ventricular diastolic pressure, the right atrial pressure, or the central venous pressure in decreasing order of accuracy.

Preload is disturbed in all forms of shock. In hypovolemic shock, the primary disorder is a loss of intravascular volume with reduction in preload. In septic shock, anaphylaxis, or intoxication with a substance with vasodilatory properties, preload is reduced because vasodilation produces an expanded vascular space causing a relative hypovolemia. In primary cardiogenic shock, preload is commonly excessive due to the detrimental effects of renal compensatory efforts to augment cardiac output through reduced fluid excretion.

Diminished *myocardial contractility* causes shock with or without the presence of abnormalities of preload, afterload, or heart rate and rhythm. Decreased contractility may occur as a result of direct injury to the myocardium as in cardiomyopathy or myocarditis. Intracardiac surgery, such as for repair of congenital heart disease, especially procedures in which the ventricular muscle is incised, can result in decreased contractility. It may be diminished because of systemic consequences of shock that adversely affect myocardial performance including hypoxemia, lactic acidosis, myocardial ischemia, electrolyte abnormalities, and hypoglycemia and by the effects of endogenous circulating myocardial depressant agents (that is, myocardial depressant factor).

Afterload is the resistance against which the ventricle must eject its contents during systole. Systemic vascular resistance approximates afterload for the left ventricle as does pulmonary vascular resistance for the right ventricle (see Table 7.1). A few disease processes produce shock predominantly as a result of increased afterload. These include severe aortic stenosis and interrupted aortic arch anomalies that increase afterload of the left ventricle and pulmonary embolism, a rare cause of increased afterload of the right ventricle in children. Afterload is increased in all forms of shock except early phases of distributive and septic shock. This is especially true in primary cardiogenic shock as occurs with myocarditis and dilated cardiomyopathy.

Brain

Circulation to the CNS is protected during the compensated phase of shock. Despite this, significant clinical abnormalities are common, ranging from agitation to stupor or coma. The mechanisms involved may include disturbed microcirculatory flow, electrolyte and glucose abnormalities, and the release of both local and circulating factors with neurotransmitter properties. During uncompensated shock, cerebral blood flow may fall resulting in ischemic CNS damage. Ischemic brain injury may play a role in the development of irreversible shock.

Pulmonary

Early pulmonary manifestations of shock are tachypnea with hypocarbia and primary respiratory alkalosis. Later in the course of shock, tachypnea and hypocarbia persist as a compensatory response to metabolic acidosis from lactic acid accumulation. Eventually respiratory failure may occur primarily due to respiratory muscle fatigue consequent to inadequate supplies of oxygen and substrate to meet demands. Ventilatory demands may be increased due to altered pulmonary compliance secondary to interstitial and alveolar fluid accumulation. Fluid accumulation occurs because of capillary leak that commonly accompanies septic shock or from increased capillary hydrostatic pressure in left ventricular cardiogenic shock. Capillary leak and pulmonary hypertension are characteristics of the adult respiratory distress syndrome (ARDS), a potential complication of shock from any etiology but especially common following septic shock. Abnormalities of oxygen uptake within the lung are usually a consequence of intrapulmonary shunting caused by the development of pulmonary edema.

Kidneys

Through the renin-angiotensin system, the kidneys play a major role in the compensatory mechanisms of shock. The kidneys are also commonly damaged during shock. One of the most frequent causes of acute renal failure is hypoperfusion caused by shock states. Total renal blood flow is reduced during later stages of shock as the renal arteries are constricted, diverting blood flow to more vital organs such as the heart and brain. Oliguria is therefore caused by a combination of net decreased renal blood flow and increased tubular reabsorption.

Gastrointestinal Tract

Reduction of blood flow to the gastrointestinal (GI) tract is a major compensatory mechanism supporting systemic arterial blood pressure in shock. Several neural and humoral mechanisms are employed that result in vasoconstriction of the splanchnic vasculature. As a result, adverse consequences may result, including erosive gastritis, ischemic pancreatitis, and, perhaps most significantly, loss of the normal bacterial barrier function of the GI wall.

As a result of ischemia, GI bacterial flora and their products may translocate across the GI epithelium and into the portal circulation. These bacteria and bacterial products, particularly endotoxin, may be instrumental in the perpetuation of the shock state.

Liver

The liver is subject to ischemic injury during periods of reduced blood flow characteristic of shock. Ischemic hepatitis is typically marked by transient elevations in liver enzymes, particularly the serum transaminases, and moderate elevations in bilirubin.

Hematologic

Hemorrhagic shock with whole blood loss and subsequent mobilization of interstitial water results in decreases in hemoglobin and hematocrit proportional to losses. Shock from losses of body water or plasma, may result in variable degrees of hemoconcentration.

Coagulation

All forms of shock may include coagulation abnormalities. These abnormalities may take the form of mild elevations in prothrombin time (PT) and partial thromboplastin time (PTT) caused by hemodilution in hemorrhagic shock. Severe disseminated intravascular coagulation (DIC) with marked elevation in PT and PTT, thrombocytopenia, hypofibrinogenemia, and elevated circulating fibrin degradation products frequently accompany septic shock.

MANAGEMENT OF SHOCK
General Principles

It is important to emphasize that, since shock is progressive, management of the patient must be an ongoing process of evaluation, appropriate therapy, and reassessment of response to therapy. Repeated physical examinations concentrating on assessment of heart rate, blood pressure, peripheral perfusion (color and capillary refill time), respiratory pattern and effort, level of consciousness, and physical activity, as well as urine output, are the cornerstones in monitoring patients with shock. Many patients, especially those with hypovolemic shock from fluid and electrolyte losses, respond to initial therapy, obviating the need for more extensive monitoring techniques. Other patients, with later stages of shock or shock of other etiologies, will require more extensive monitoring techniques such as strict measurement of intake and output, arterial blood-gas measurement, monitoring of electrolytes and glucose, assessment of blood counts and coagulation profiles, continuous electrocardiographic monitoring, intra-arterial pressure monitoring, and central venous pressure monitoring.

For all forms of shock, simultaneous with or soon after initial stabilization, treatment of the underlying cause of shock must be initiated. Hemorrhage, internal or external, must be stopped with surgery performed if necessary. Septic shock will require broad spectrum antimicrobial therapy guided by the clinical presentation and the age of the patient (see Table 7.5) and may require drainage of a septic focus. Cardiogenic shock from congenital heart disease may require treatment with prostaglandin E_1 to open the ductus arteriosus pending surgical correction.

Cardiovascular Support

Support of the circulation is paramount in the treatment of shock. Central to shock therapy is the assurance of adequate flow of blood and delivery of oxygen to vital vascular beds such as the coronary, cerebral, and renal circulations. The cardiac output is dependent on heart rate, rhythm, and stroke volume; the latter is dependent on preload, contractility, and afterload. Therefore specific monitoring and therapy is presented for each of these factors.

Heart Rate and Rhythm

Patients with shock should have an initial assessment of heart rate and rhythm. All patients require repeated assessment of heart rate and most should have continuous electrocardiographic monitoring.

The most common finding will be sinus tachycardia. Marked tachycardia will embarrass cardiac output by restricting ventricular filling but usually will respond to fluid administration. Preload therapy is discussed in the next section. Occasionally patients will present with dysrrhythmias that limit cardiac output. Therapy of dysrhythmias should include evaluation and treatment for hypoxemia; acid base abnormalities; electrolyte disturbances, especially hypocalcemia, hyperkalemia, or hypokalemia; and hypoglycemia. Patients with an indwelling central venous catheter should have a chest radiograph done to check the position of the catheter tip. Occasionally, catheters become malpositioned with the tip lying in the right ventricle producing rhythm disturbances. Treatment may require drugs that modulate cardiac rhythm such as atropine or isoproterenol for bradycardia; digoxin, verapamil or adenosine for supraventricular tachycardia, and lidocaine or bretylium for ventricular tachydysrhythmias. On occasion, cardioversion or temporary pacemaker placement may be needed to achieve and maintain a stable perfusing rhythm.

Preload

Most forms of shock, with the exception of some types of cardiogenic shock, involve either an absolute or a relative hypovolemia that requires rapid therapy with intravascular volume expansion. Fluid administration should take the form of a rapid bolus of 10 to 20 ml/kg of fluid over ten minutes, followed by an evaluation of response. Further therapy should be guided by response and ongoing losses. In patients requiring fluid therapy in excess of 60 to 80 ml/kg, invasive monitoring should be strongly considered to guide subsequent therapy. The best choice of fluid for replacement in shock has been an area of ongoing debate in both the pediatric and critical care literature. The fluid options are listed in Table 7.6. A reasonable approach to fluid therapy is to use crystalloid in the form of 0.9 normal saline or lactated

80 | SYNOPSIS OF PEDIATRIC EMERGENCY CARE

Table 7.6 Intravenous fluids for volume resuscitation

Crystalloids
0.9% sodium chloride
Lactated Ringer's solution
Hypertonic sodium chloride

Colloids
5% human serum albumin in 0.9% sodium chloride
6% hydroxyethyl starch in 0.9% sodium chloride
5% plasma protein fraction in 0.9% sodium chloride
25% human serum albumin in 0.9% sodium chloride

Blood Products
Whole blood
Packed red blood cells
Fresh frozen plasma

Reprinted with permission of the publisher from Blummer JL. A practical guide to pediatric intensive care. 3d ed. St. Louis: Mosby Yearbook, 1990;71.

Ringer's solution for the first 40 to 80 ml/kg of replacement. If additional fluid restitution is required, consideration should be given to the type of fluid lost. If the cause of shock is hemorrhage, a transfusion of packed red blood cells may be necessary. With external losses of fluid and electrolytes, continued administration of crystalloid would be proper. If losses are of plasma, as in third spacing associated with septic shock, the use of colloid solutions such as five percent albumin, plasma protein fraction (Plasmanate) or hydroxyethyl starch (Hetastarch) may be suitable. There is no justification for the use of whole blood, plasma, cryoprecipitate or other transfusion subfractions such as platelets for the purpose of fluid resuscitation. The use of these blood components should be reserved for patients requiring correction of specific coagulation abnormalities.

End points for fluid resuscitation should be based on clinical response. The criteria for satisfactory volume resuscitation include a reduction in heart rate toward normal for age; improved cutaneous perfusion as measured by skin color, skin turgor, and capillary refill time of two seconds or less; improved renal perfusion as gauged by a urine output in excess of one ml/kg per hour, stable blood pressure appropriate for age, and normal mentation. In patients with ongoing internal or external losses or in whom cardiac function is not stable, repeated assessments will remain mandatory to assure that appropriate preload is sustained.

In patients with septic shock, cardiogenic shock, adult respiratory distress syndrome, or multiple organ system dysfunction, preload augmentation must be administered cautiously and should be guided by invasive monitoring. If cardiac filling pressures rise without either direct or indirect evidence of improved cardiac output, further volume administration will probably be detrimental, resulting in worse cardiac function and increased peripheral and pulmonary edema formation. Under these circumstances, augmentation of cardiac contractility using pharmacologic means is required.

Caution should be exercised in fluid resuscitation of patients with shock and concurrent CNS injury who are at risk for cerebral edema formation. Vigorous fluid therapy may correct shock only to have the patient succumb to cerebral herniation from increased intracranial pressure. In these patients, early inotropic support may be warranted to reduce total fluid requirements.

Contractility

The use of agents to augment contractility is necessary when volume resuscitation has been optimized and cardiovascular function remains inadequate. The choices for agents to improve contractility are shown in Table 7.7. The proper choice of agent depends on the clinical circumstance.

Patients with hypovolemic shock rarely require inotropic support. Patients with cardiogenic shock benefit from agents that improve contractility but do not increase systemic vascular resistance (*vasopressor effect*). Agents such as *dobutamine*, an analog of isoproterenol with potent inotropic effects with little effect on heart rate or systemic vascular resistance, may be ideal for such patients. *Amrinone*, a noncatecholamine agent whose mechanism of action involves inhibition of phosphodiesterase type III, is a moderately potent inotropic agent with some vasodilatory effects. Amrinone may be helpful in patients with cardiogenic shock who have increased systemic vascular resistance. Patients with cardiogenic shock who fail to respond to these agents may require the use of more potent agents such as epinephrine or norepinephrine. Although these drugs may be effective, they exact a heavy toll on the heart in the form of increased myocardial work and oxygen consumption. They also act to increase afterload through vasoconstriction. This effect further increases myocardial oxygen demand and may offset any improvement in contractility. Patients in cardiogenic shock with markedly increased afterload and those with atrioventricular valve regurgitation often benefit from the use of a combination of an inotropic agent with a systemic vasodilator (*afterload reducing agent*).

Patients with septic shock commonly will have cardiac dysfunction and low systemic vascular resistance. These patients benefit from agents with both inotropic and vasopressor actions. *Dopamine*, a precursor of norepinephrine, has complex dose-dependent cardiac and vascular effects. At low doses (1 to 3 μg/kg/min), dopamine acts as a vasodilator of the renal and mesenteric vasculature. At moderate doses (4 to 10 μg/kg/min), dopamine produces significant inotropic and chronotropic effects on the heart. At high doses (11 to 20 μg/kg/min), it has vasoconstrictive effects that increase systemic vascular resistance and arterial blood pressure. Dopamine is usually the initial drug of choice for septic shock. Patients who fail to respond to dopamine may require more potent vasoconstrictive agents such as epinephrine or norepinephrine to support circulation. When such agents are used, continuation of

Table 7.7 Commonly used cardiovascular drugs in shock syndromes

Drug	Dose (μg/kg/min)	Comment
Inotropic agents		
Norepinephrine (α-adrenergic)	0.05–1.0	Most frequently used for profound hypotension not responding to fluid or other inotropic drugs.
Epinephrine (α- and β-adrenergic)	0.05–1.0	Dose-related response; higher doses cause vasoconstriction. Useful in maintaining cardiac output and blood pressure in patients unresponsive to dopamine or dobutamine.
Isoproterenol (β-adrenergic)	0.05–0.5	Indicated in bradycardia unresponsive to atropine; as an inotrope if increase in heart rate is not excessive; may be helpful in reactive pulmonary hypertension.
Dopamine (α- and β-, and dopaminergic)	1–20	Cardiovascular effects are complex and dose-related; specific peripheral effects useful when low-dose infusion can restore cardiovascular stability and improve renal function.
Dobutamine (α- and β-adrenergic)	1–20	Racemic mixture whose overall activity is due to the sum of the individual stereoisomers; positive inotropic effect with minimal changes in heart rate or systemic vascular resistance.
Amrinone	1–10	Initial bolus infusion may be required. Limited data available in children.
Vasodilators		
Nitroprusside	0.05–8	Balanced arterial and venous dilator; may result in thiocyanate or cyanide toxicity.
Nitroglycerine	0.5–20	Venous dilator: dose not well established for infants and children.

Reprinted with permission of the publisher from Perkin RM, Levin DL. Shock. In Levin DL, Morriss, eds. Essentials of pediatric intensive care. St. Louis: Quality Medical Publishing, 1990.

dopamine in the low-dosage range will augment renal blood flow despite the vasoconstrictive effects of the other drugs.

Afterload

Patients with cardiogenic shock who manifest increased systemic vascular resistance or atrioventricular valve regurgitation, may benefit from the use of a systemic vasodilator. Caution must be taken when using vasodilators, especially in patients with low or normal blood pressure. Invasive cardiovascular monitoring, preferably using a Swan-Ganz catheter, is strongly advisable when the use of a vasodilator is contemplated.

The most commonly used drug is sodium nitroprusside. It has the benefit of a rapid onset of action and a short half-life, which facilitates titration. Sodium nitroprusside is a balanced vasodilator affecting arteriolar and venous capacitance vessels roughly equally. It should usually be used in combination with an inotropic agent such as dobutamine, dopamine, epinephrine, or norepinephrine. Nitroglycerine is a vasodilator whose effects are mostly on the venous capacitance vessels with less significant arteriolar effect. Nitroglycerine has the benefit of transcutaneous administration in more stable patients with congestive failure. As was noted earlier, amrinone afterload-reducing effects and may be helpful in the management of this patient subset.

Pulmonary

Virtually all patients with shock should receive oxygen supplementation. The adequacy of oxygen administration should be assessed using continuous pulse oximetry, arterial blood gases or both. Most patients with shock require endotracheal intubation and mechanical ventilation. Assisted ventilation is indicated in patients requiring an inspired oxygen concentration over 60 percent to achieve a PaO_2 of 60 mmHg or an oxygen saturation of 90 percent and in those demonstrating evidence of respiratory failure. Indications of respiratory failure include marked tachypnea, dyspnea, apnea, or a $PacO_2$ of 50 mmHg or greater. Patients with high oxygen requirements, rales on auscultation of the chest, and evidence of pulmonary edema on chest radiograph should receive increased positive end expiratory pressure (PEEP). Patients on mechanical ventilatory support usually will benefit from sedation using an infusion of a narcotic such as fentanyl (1 to 4 µg/kg/hr) with a benzodiazepine such as midazolam (3 to 5 µg/kg/min). Care must be exercised in giving sedatives and analgesics to hypotensive patients in that these drugs have vasodilatory effects. Some patients, especially those with ARDS, will require the use of neuromuscular paralysis with agents such as vecuronium or pancuronium.

Renal Support

Patients with shock should have a bladder drainage catheter (Foley catheter) placed for continuous monitoring of urine output. Blood urea nitrogen (BUN) and creatinine should be measured initially. Measurement should be repeated regularly for as long as shock or renal failure exist. Patients with oliguria or anuria, especially those with evidence of low cardiac output, may benefit from administration of a loop diuretic such as furosemide (1 to 2 mg/kg/dose). Low-dose dopamine may improve urine output because it acts to dilate the renal vasculature. Patients who develop acute renal failure may require dialysis (hemodialysis or peritoneal) or continuous arteriovenous hemofiltration (CAVH) to avoid fluid overload and to permit parenteral nutritional support.

Gastrointestinal Support

Patients with shock should have a nasogastric tube placed and applied at low intermittent suction. Measures should be taken to reduce the risk for gastrointestinal bleeding. Choices include the use of histamine blocking agents such as cimetidine or ranitidine or antacids administered through the nasogastric tube that act to prevent the production of gastric acid or to neutralize gastric acid respectively. There is evidence that the best method for reducing the risk of bleeding may be the use of sucralfate, a sulfated disaccharide-aluminum complex, that acts to protect the gastric mucosa from the effects of gastric acidity rather than by eliminating acid. This may be superior to the other methods because an acid milieu helps prevent growth of bacteria in the proximal bowel, the presence of which may promote bacterial translocation.

Hematologic Support

Shock patients should have a complete blood count (CBC) measured initially followed by repeated measurements until they are physiologically stable. Patients with hemorrhage and those receiving large amounts of asanguinous fluids should have CBCs measured more frequently. Ideally, to optimize oxygen availability, hemoglobin concentrations should be maintained at levels of 10 to 13 gm/dl. Concern about transmission of hepatitis or other viral agents may justify accepting lower hemoglobin concentrations in stable patients.

Coagulation Support

A coagulation profile, including a PT, a PTT, and a platelet count should be obtained initially on all patients with shock. If these are abnormal, the fibrinogen and fibrin degradation product concentrations should be measured, and the coagulation profile should be repeated at regular intervals until it is normal. Patients with isolated elevations of PT and PTT but with no evidence of bleeding may require no specific treatment. Patients who have active bleeding should receive fresh frozen plasma to replace clotting factors and vitamin K (1 mg/kg IV [intravenous]) to promote hepatic production of vitamin K-dependent clotting factors. Patients who have isolated thrombocytopenia should receive platelet transfusions if they are actively bleeding or if the platelet count falls below 20,000 per mm^3. Disseminated intravascular coagulation, as may occur particularly in septic shock, may require repeated administration of fresh frozen plasma, platelets and cryoprecipitate until the underlying cause is eliminated.

Experimental Therapies

A number of agents have been used in experimental models of shock and in clinical trials in humans. Corticosteroids have been used extensively, especially in septic shock. Their use should be discouraged since the results of a multicenter double blind clinical study in adults demonstrated no benefit to the use of steroids. In fact, mortality in the steroid-treated group was higher than it was in the placebo group. Naloxone, an opiate receptor antagonist, has shown promise in reversing hypotension in experimental models of shock. Results in human studies of naloxone are equivocal at best.

Perhaps the greatest promise lies in the use of passive immunotherapy for septic shock. In experimental models of shock, the administration of monoclonal antibodies to lipopolysaccharide (a component of endotoxin) dramatically reduces signs and symptoms of shock and improves survival. Similar findings have been made in studies of monoclonal antibodies to tumor necrosis factor, a cytokine involved in the expression and amplification of shock.

Further progress will require better understanding of cellular and biochemical effects of shock that result in cell injury and death, and better methods of assessment of regional oxygen availability and utilization will allow for more directed therapy.

SUGGESTED READING

1. Ayres SM. SCCM's new horizons on sepsis and septic shock. Crit Care Med 1985;13(10):846.
2. Bhatt-Mehta V, Nahata MC. Dopamine and dobutamine in pediatric therapy. Pharmacotherapy 1989;9:(5)303-314.
3. Blummer JL. A practical guide to pediatric intensive care, 3d ed. St. Louis: Mosby Yearbook, 1990;71.
4. Bonadio WA, Losek JD. Infants with myocarditis presenting with severe respiratory distress and shock. Pediatr Emerg Care 1987;3(2):110-113.
5. Braunwald E. Introduction—A symposium: Amrinone. Am J Cardiol 1985;56(3):1B-2B.
6. Bulkley GB, Oshima A, Bailey RW. Pathophysiology of hepatic ischemia in cardiogenic shock. Am J Surg 1986;151(1):87-97.
7. Cabal LA, Devaskar U, Siassi B, et al. Cardiogenic shock associated with perinatal asphyxia in preterm infants. J Pediatr 1980;96(4):705-710.
8. Crone RK. Acute circulatory failure in children. Pediatr Clin North Am 1980;27(3):525-538.
9. Demling RH. Colloid or crystalloid resuscitation in sepsis. In Sibbald WJ, Sprung CL, eds. New horizons in perspectives on sepsis and septic shock. Fullerton, Calif.: Society of Critical Care Medicine, 1986;275.
10. Desjars P, Pinaud M, Potel G, et al. A reappraisal of norepinephrine therapy in human septic shock. Crit Care Med 1987;15(2):134-137.
11. Driscoll AS, Gillette PC, McNamara DC. The use of dopamine in children. J Pediatr 1978;92(2):309-314.
12. Faden AI, Holaday JW. Opiate antagonists. A role in the treatment of hypervolemic shock. Science 1979;205(4403):317-318.
13. Friedman WF, George BL. Treatment of congestive heart failure by altering loading conditions of the heart. J Pediatr 1985;106(5):697-706.
14. Haupt MT. The use of crystalloidal and colloidal solutions for volume replacement in hypovolemic shock. Crit Rev Clin Lab Sci 1989;27(1):1-26.
15. Hinshaw LB, Cox BG. The fundamental mechanisms of shock. New York: Plenum, 1972;13.
16. Kallen RJ, Lonergan JM. Fluid resuscitation of acute hypovolemic hypoperfusion states in pediatrics. Pediatr Clin North Am 1990;37(2):287-294.
17. Katz RW, Pollack MM, Weibley RE. Pulmonary artery catheterization in pediatric intensive care. Adv Pediatr 1983;30:169-190.
18. Lees MH, King DH. Cardiogenic shock in the neonate. Pediatr Rev 1988;9:(8)258-266.

19. Luce JM. Pathogenesis and management of septic shock. Chest 1987;91(6):883–888.
20. Parker MM, Parrillo JE. Septic shock. Hemodynamics and pathogenesis. JAMA 1983;250(24):3324–3327.
21. Perkin RM, Levin DL. Shock. In Levin DL, Morriss, eds. Essentials of pediatric intensive care. St. Louis: Quality Medical Publishing, 1990.
22. Perkin RM, Levin DL. Shock in the pediatric patient. Part I. J Pediatr 1982;101(2):163–169.
23. Perkin RM, Levin DL. Shock in the pediatric patient. Part II. Therapy. J Pediatr 1982;101(3):319–332.
24. Perkin RM, Levin DL, Webb R, et al. Dobutamine: A hemodynamic evaluation in children with shock. J Pediatr 1982;100(b):977–983.
25. Pollock MM. Shock in infants and children. Emerg Med Clin North Am 1986;4(4):841–857.
26. Rackow EC, Falk JL, Fein IA, et al. Fluid resuscitation in circulatory shock: A comparison of cardiorespiratory effects of albumin, hetastarch, and saline solutions in patients with hypovolemic and septic shock. Crit Care Med 1983;11(11):839–850.
27. Scheinkestel CD, Tuxen DV, Cade JR, et al. Fluid management of shock in critically-ill patients. Med J Aust 1989;150(9):–510, 513–517.
28. Schuster DP, Lefrak SS. Shock. In Civetta JM, Taylor RW, Kirby RR, eds. Critical care. Philadelphia: Lippincott, 1988;891.
29. Shoemaker WC, Hauser CJ. Critique of crystalloid versus colloid therapy in shock and shock lung. Crit Care Med 1979;7(3):117–124.
30. Shoemaker WC. Pathophysiology and therapy of shock syndromes. In Shoemaker WC, Thompson WL, Holbrook PR, eds. Textbook of critical care. Philadelphia: Saunders, 1984;52.
31. Sprung CL, Schien RMH, Long WM: Controversies in the management of sepsis and septic shock. In Sibbald WL, Sprung CL, eds. Perspectives on sepsis and septic shock, new horizons. Fullerton, Calif.: Society of Critical Care Medicine, 1986;257.
32. Velanovich V. Crystalloid versus colloid fluid resuscitation: A meta-analysis of mortality. Surgery 1986;105(1):65–71.
33. Veterans Administration Systemic Sepsis Cooperative Study Group. Effect of high-dose glucocorticoid therapy on mortality in patients with clinical signs of systemic sepsis. N Engl J Med 1987;317(11):659–665.
34. Vincent JL, De Backer D. Initial management of circulatory shock as prevention of MSOF. Crit Care Clin 1989;5(2):369–378.
35. Weibley RE, Pimentel B, Ackerman NB. Hemorrhagic shock and encephalopathy syndrome of infants and children. Crit Care Med 1989;17(4):335–338.
36. Wetzel RC, Stiff JL, Rogers MC. Heart rate and rhythm as determinants of cardiac output. In Swedlow DB, Raphaely RC, eds. Cardiovascular problems in pediatric critical care. New York: Churchill Livingstone, 1986;257.
37. Wetzel RC. Shock. In Rogers MC, ed. Textbook of pediatric intensive care. Baltimore: Williams & Wilkins, 1987;483.
38. Witte MK, Hill JH, Blumer JL. Shock in the pediatric patient. Adv Pediatr 1987;34:139–173.
39. Zaritsky A, Chernow B. Use of catecholamines in pediatrics. J Pediatr 1984;105(3):341–350.
40. Zimmerman JJ, Dietrich KA. Current perspectives on septic shock. Pediatr Clin North Am 1987;34(1):131–163.

8

Dysrhythmias

Jagannath S. Surpure

Cardiac dysrrhythmias are uncommon in children because of low incidence of ischemic heart disease. Almost every type of dysrrhythmia recognized in adults, however, has been reported in the pediatric age group. There have been major advances in diagnosis and management. Rhythm disturbance constitutes an acute emergency if it compromises heart rate, and it has the potential for degenerating into a lethal rhythm. The most important component is the adverse influence on the cardiac output. Cardiac output is the product of stroke volume and heart rate. The fast rates compromise adequate diastolic filling/stroke volume and thus reduce cardiac output. The abnormally slow rates also cause inadequate cardiac output. The other conditions, such as asystole, ventricular fibrillation, and electromechanical (EMD) dissociation have no cardiac output. There is no measurable heart rate, therefore no stroke volume and cardiac output. Pediatric cardiac arrest or asystole is usually the end result of longstanding hypoxemia and acidosis secondary to respiratory compromise. Primary cardiac arrest is infrequent and is more often a result than it is a cause (Figure 8.1).

The common abnormal rhythms can be conveniently classified for therapeutic purposes based on heart rate (Table 8.1).

PATHOPHYSIOLOGY

The normal heart rate in children is related to age and is influenced by several physiologic and pathologic conditions. Therefore clinicians should be aware of wide variations in normal rates. The cardiac heart monitoring system can cause potential artifacts emphasizing the importance of clinical assessment and correlation before therapeutic interventions.

The electrocardiogram (EKG) graphically represents the sequence of myocardial depolarization. This depolarization activity begins at the sinoatrial (SA) node and advances to the atrioventricular (AV) node, ultimately progressing to the endocardium of both ventricles via the bundle of HIS. The ventricular depolarization is represented on EKG as QRS complex while repolarizaton as S-T segment and T wave. The mechanisms that produce fast rates include reentry and ectopic pacemakers. The reentry pathway is more common and may be present anywhere along the conduction system. Slow rates are due either to a slowing of the intrinsic pacemaker (sinus) or to a block in conduction system that may be complete or incomplete. Most slow rates in

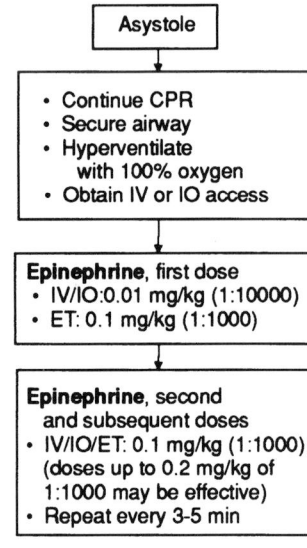

Figure 8.1 Asystole decision tree. (CPR = cardiopulmonary resuscitation, ET = endotracheal, IO = intraosseous, IV = intravenous) (Adapted with permission from Emergency Cardiac Case Committee and Subcommittee American Heart Association, Guidelines for cardiopulmonary resuscitation and emergency care: Pediatric advanced life support. JAMA 1992;268:2268–2275.

children are the result of hypoxia and acidosis and therefore are present during either cardiac prearrest or cardiac arrest situations.

Electromechanical dissociation (EMD) (Figure 8.2) is similar to asystole as there is no cardiac contraction and therefore no cardiac output. Even though the heart has electrical activity, it is ineffective in causing adequate muscle contractions. Ventricular fibrillation is rare in children. The myocardium has no effective contractions due to chaotic depolarization and repolarization.

CLINICAL ASSESSMENT

The patient may present with a variety of symptoms depending on age at presentation, including poor feeding, irritability, lethargy, pallor, dyspnea, sweating (evidence of congestive heart failure), syncope, dizziness, altered mental status (decreased cerebral blood flow), anginal pain (decreased coronary blood flow),

Table 8.1 Cardiac rhythm disturbances

Fast rates (tachyarrhythmias)	Sinus tachycardia (ST)
	Ventricular tachycardia (VT)
	Supraventricular tachycardia (SVT)
Slow rates (bradyarrhythmias)	Sinus bradycardia
	Atrioventricular blocks
Absent *or* disorganized	Asystole
	Ventricular fibrillation
	Electromechanical dissociation

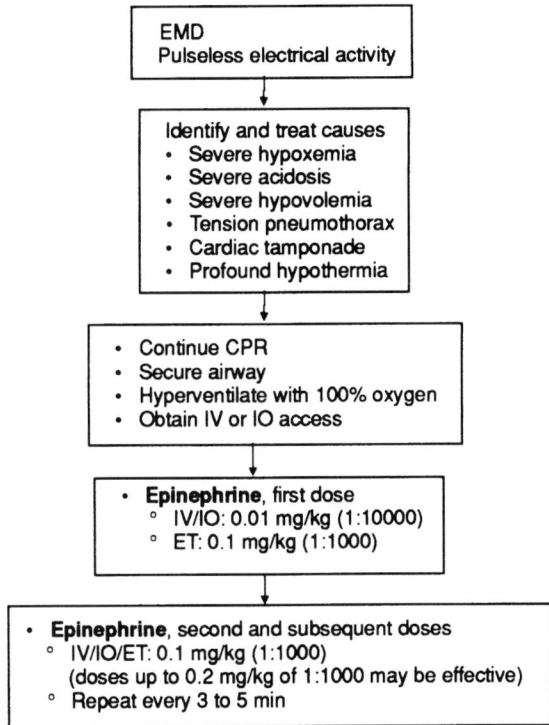

Figure 8.2 Algorithm 40 kg or less EMD. (Adapted with permission from Emergency Cardiac Case Committee and Subcommittee American Heart Association, Guidelines for cardiopulmonary resuscitation and emergency care: Pediatric advanced life support. JAMA 1992;268:2268–2275.

palpitation, or missed beats (perception of cardiac rhythm disturbance). A clinical assessment must include a careful history, thorough physical examination, prompt analysis of the EKG, and determination and monitoring of hemodynamic status.

The most common clinically significant cardiac rhythm disturbance in children is paroxysmal atrial tachycardia (PAT), also called SVT (Figure 8.3). Acute management is indicated when abnormal rhythm either compromises cardiac output or is unstable (Table 8.2), or when there is a potential for degeneration into a lethal, life-threatening rhythm disturbance such as ventricular fibrillation. The treatment may not be needed if the dysrrhythmia is stable and does not compromise cardiac output.

All unstable slow rates are treated the same way regardless of the specific diagnosis. Initial therapy consists of proper ventilation and oxygenation. Medications (atropine and sympathomimetic) may be required. All unstable fast rates require cardioversion regardless of the specific diagnosis. Sometimes it is difficult to distinguish the origin of the fast rate, whether it is ventricular or supraventricular. The wide fast rates are usually ventricular in origin and may require lidocaine. Ventricular fibrillation requires defibrillation and lidocaine.

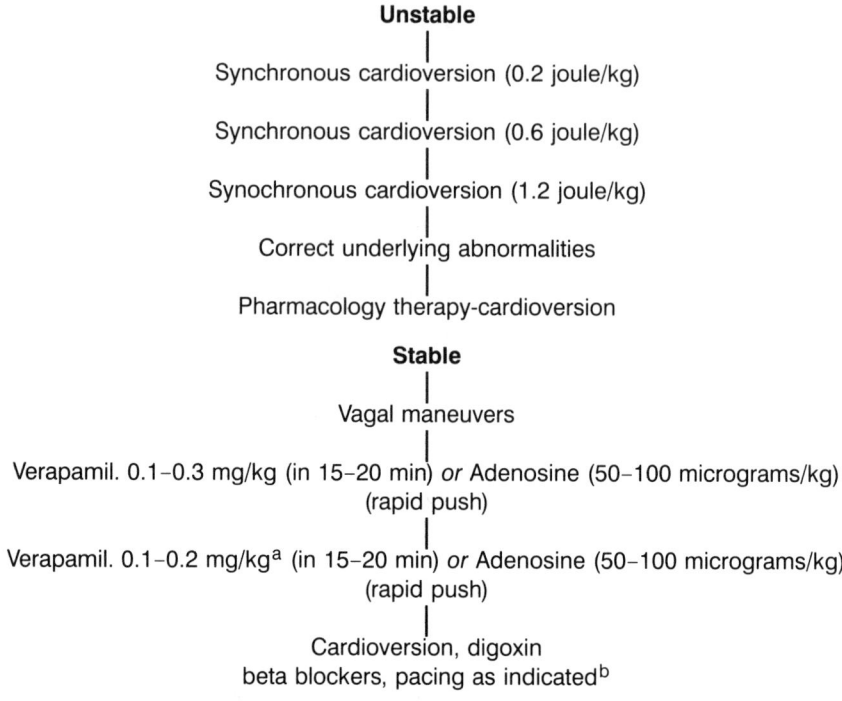

Figure 8.3 Algorithm 40 kg or less SVT. ([a]Note lesser second dose. [b]See text.)

SUPRAVENTRICULAR TACHYCARDIA

SVT or PAT is the most common type of rhythm disturbance in children with or without cardiac disease. Its prevalence in children is estimated as 1:25,000. Recently intracardiac electrophysiologic studies have resulted in better understanding of the mechanisms responsible for SVT. These mechanisms include reentry, enhanced automaticity, and triggered activity. Reentry is the most common form both in children and adults. The

Table 8.2 Unstable rhythms

Adolescent	Shock/collapse
	Chest pain—ischemia secondary to decreased perfusion of coronary arteries
	Congestive heart failure—resulting from decreased diastolic filling due to rapid heart rate
Child	Shock/collapse
	Congestive heart failure rare
Infant	Systolic blood pressure less than 60–70 mm/Hg
	Decreased peripheral perfusion
Newborn	Heart rate less than 80 per minute
	Blood pressure measurement difficult in newborn

accessory pathways are the basis for reentrant fast rhythms seen in the preexcitation syndromes of which Wolff-Parkinson-White (WPW) is the most common. The mechanisms for atrial flutter and fibrillation are either reentry, automaticity, or both.

Clinical Presentation

This varies with age, rate and duration of tachycardia, and associated structural heart disease. In infants the symptoms include irritability/lethargy, pallor, poor feeding, vomiting, cold and moist skin, duskiness, upper respiratory infection, and tachypnea. An infant who has had tachycardia lasting more than 24 hours usually presents with symptoms of congestive heart failure. Rarely an infant may present in cardiovascular collapse or as a near-miss sudden death. In older children, symptoms may be palpitation, dizziness, or syncope. About 20 percent of SVT in children has congenital heart disease and 20 to 50 percent has a concealed accessory bypass tract. Other causes include myocarditis, trauma, postcardiac surgery or catheterization, electrolyte imbalance, and digitalis toxicity.

The Electrocardiogram

The EKG shows rapid heart rate varying with age. In infants, it is approximately 240 beats/min, but it can be as high as 300 beats/min. The rhythm is usually regular; P waves may not be identifiable at higher rates. QRS duration is normal most (more than 90 percent) of the time. A rare QRS from aberrant conduction may be difficult to distinguish from ventricular tachycardia. If tachycardia is of longer duration, ST- and T-wave changes may be consistent with myocardial ischemia. In severely ill infants (sepsis, hypovolemia), it may be difficult to distinguish ST from SVT. In ST, the heart rate is usually less than 200 beats/min, and the rate may vary from beat to beat. Clinicians may be able to identify P waves on an EKG. The chest X-ray is usually normal; in SVT, however, the heart size may be enlarged. The EKG changes in WPW syndrome include short PR interval, a delta wave, and a wide QRS complex. In Lown-Ganong-Levine (LGL) syndrome, the EKG shows short PR interval and a normal or narrow QRS complex (Table 8.3).

Table 8.3 SVT—Differential diagnosis

Type	QRS Duration	Ventricular Rate/Rhythm	P Wave (II, III, AVF)
ST	Narrow	120–230/min variable	Urgent
SVT (AV nodal entry type)	Narrow	140–300/min regular	Inverted
Atrial fluter	Narrow	150–300/min variable	Saw-tooth pattern
Atrial fibrillation	Variable	150–300/min variable	Irregular

THERAPY

In most cases, immediate intervention is not required (Table 8.4) as the rhythm disturbance is usually well tolerated and the patient is hemodynamically stable. If this is so, a cardiac consult is obtained for pharmacologic intervention. SVT associated with hypotension or cardiovascular collapse, however, is a medical emergency and needs immediate intervention. In infants, it is also an emergency because exact duration of the problem is unknown. An EKG (12-lead) and a long rhythm strip should be obtained immediately. This may help in accurate diagnosis and with the etiology.

The use of a diving reflex (immersion of the infant's face in a basin of water at 5°C or ice bag application to the face for 10 to 20 seconds) can be effective. Vagal maneuvers, that is, carotid artery massage, are not usually effective in young children.

A clinician can digitalize the patient intravenously over 12 hours. The first dose of digoxin 10 microgram/kg is given slowly over 5 minutes followed by a second dose of 5 microgram/kg 6 hours later. The third and final dose (5 microgram/kg) is administered 6 hours later. Digoxin may take more than 2 hours to convert SVT. Propranolol (0.1 mg/kg IV [intravenous], maximum 5 mg) and verapamil have been effective and safe in adults. The dosage of verapamil is 0.1 to 0.2 mg/kg slow IV push to a maximum of 5 mg and may be repeated once in 30 minutes. Verapamil may cause apnea, bradycardia, and hypotension, and therefore it should be avoided, especially in infants less than one year of age, any child with hypotension and heart failure, or any patient receiving adrenergic antagonists. If verapamil is used, the blood pressure should be monitored closely. Recently intravenous adenosine (a short-acting purine nucleotide) has shown itself most effective (90 percent success rate) in both adults and children (adult dosage: 6–12 mg; children, 50 to 100 micrograms/kg). The advantages of adenosine include lack of adverse hemodynamic effects, safety when used with wide-ORS complex tachycardia, lack of interaction with other drugs, and a very short half-life (5 to 10

Table 8.4 Acute therapy of SVT in infants and children

Vagal maneuvers
Diving reflex
Unilateral carotid massage
Valsalva
Vomiting/gagging
Pharmacological*
Digoxin
Verapamil
Adenosine
Propanolol
Cardioversion
(0.5–2.0 joules/kg)

*See text for dosages.

seconds). In the presence of cardiovascular collapse, synchronized cardioversion (0.5 to 1.0 joules/kg) is used. Lidocaine bolus (1.0 mg/kg), prior to cardioversion, results in a higher success rate; infusion therapy with lidocaine 20 to 50 microgram/kg/min will assist in maintaining the rhythm. Bretylium may be used if lidocaine is successful. If the child is on digoxin or if digoxin toxicity is suspected, cardioversion should be tried with a lower dosage (0.5 joules), and the energy should be cautiously increased. If cardioversion needs to be repeated, the energy dosage is increased gradually to 2.0 joules/kg.

CONCLUSIONS

The stable patient does not require immediate therapy. The hemodynamically compromised or collapse patient, however, needs immediate intervention with attention to underlying etiology. The most common rhythm disturbance, SVT, is described in depth. The other rhythm disturbances, that is, asystole and EMD commonly secondary to respiratory arrest (hypoxia and acidosis) are described in depth in Chapter 1 (Cardiopulmonary Resuscitation).

SUGGESTED READING

1. Chameides L. Cardiac Rhythm Disturbances. American Heart Association/American Academy of Pediatrics. Pediatric Advanced Life Support Course textbook, 1988;61–67.
2. Deal BJ, Keane JF, Gillette PC, et al. Wolff-Parkinson-White syndrome and supraventricular tachycardia during infancy: Management and follow-up. J Am Coll Cardiol 1985;5:130–135.
3. Editorial Task Force. Dysrhythmias. American College of Emergency Physicians/American Academy of Pediatrics. Advanced Pediatric Life Support Course, 1989;45–57.
4. Garson A Jr. Supraventricular tachycardia. In Gillette PC, Garson A Jr., eds. Pediatric cardiac dysrhythmias, 1981;58:177–253.
5. Greco R, Musto B, Ariezo V, et al. Treatment of paroxysmal supraventricular tachycardia in infancy with digitalis, adenosine-5'-triphosphate, and verapamil: A comparative study. Circulation 1982;66:504–508.
6. Mehta AV. Supraventricular tachycardia in children: Diagnosis and management. Indian Journal of Pediatrics 1991;58:567–585.
7. Till J, Shinebourne EA, Rigby ML, et al. Efficacy and safety of adenosine in the treatment of supraventricular tachycardia in infants and children. Br Heart J 1989;62:204–211.

9

Congestive Heart Failure

Charles Cooper

Congestive heart failure in infants and children is a complex of symptoms originating from abnormal cardiac function. The symptoms may begin as barely perceptible to the parent; hence the children often present to the physician for medical care only after symptoms are far advanced.

In the young infant, congestive heart failure is most likely related to a structural defect of the heart. In the older child on the other hand, most often the congestive heart failure is secondary to an acquired illness or an acquired insult to the heart muscle itself.

A rapid determination that symptoms originate from abnormal cardiac function allows the prompt initiation of appropriate therapy.

Pathophysiology

As part of a broad classification of structural defects of the heart, a delineation can be made between obstruction to flow from the ventricular chamber (for example aortic stenosis) and defects associated with too much pulmonary blood flow as a result of a large left to right shunt (for example, large ventricular septal defect).

Congestive heart failure symptoms may further be divided into those originating in the right side of the heart (the pulmonary circuit) and those that are left-sided in origin (the systemic circuit). The failure represents dilatation and loss of ventricular function and thus the abnormalities of either pulmonary or systemic circulation.

Presenting symptoms of heart failure reflect a combination of changes in both preload and afterload. *Preload* refers to the volume of blood returning to the heart for circulation. *Afterload* refers to the maintained pressure against which the heart must empty the normal circulating volume of blood. Either part of this system can fail.

Generally obstructive lesions, an abnormal afterload to the heart, lead to deterioration of the musculature itself. Hypertrophied muscle initially is very efficient in its performance of work, but begins to contract poorly as it fails and becomes unable to overcome the increased afterload. Likewise the increase in dimension of the muscle itself may preclude adequate nutrition from the myocardial circulation and foster myocardial failure. As a result, residual volumes following emptying of the ventricle begin to increase, reflecting a stretching of the muscle fibers to a length that no longer behaves according to the Starling principle and fails to contract either sufficiently or vigorously. The cycle is set, resulting in increasing diastolic volumes and end diastolic pressures. Thus the muscle starts failing.

The left-sided failure results in the inability of the ventricle to pump an adequate volume for perfusion of vital organs against elevated pressure. This results in multiple organ failure with deterioration in respiratory, kidney, and neurologic functions. The poor tissue perfusion results in altered metabolism. Anaerobic metabolism causes the accumulation of acid products further aggravating the failing cardiac muscle and other vital organ functions. The resultant elevation of ventricular end-diastolic pressures leads to the inability of the left atrium to empty so that its pressure becomes elevated. This leads to the development of pulmonary venous hypertension, increasing abnormal respiratory symptoms, and eventual respiratory failure. The initial ability of the respiratory system to compensate for metabolic acidosis fails with the worsening of the pulmonary edema.

Right-sided obstruction behaves in a similar manner. The elevation of the right-sided end-diastolic pressure as a result of obstruction is reflected in decreased pulmonary blood flow. Increasing right atrial pressure results in systemic venous congestion causing edema of body organs and spaces.

Large volumes of blood delivered to the pulmonary circuit through a congenital defect causes a left-to-right shunt and an initial plethora to the pulmonary circulation. Mean pulmonary artery pressure is elevated, and pulmonary edema is present. Increasing retention of carbon dioxide with decreasing exchange for oxygen result in respiratory acidosis. The combination of hypoxia and acidosis will further insult the failing myocardium. The stretched myocardial fiber no longer contracts adequately according to the Starling mechanism, and low cardiac output ensues. Poor tissue perfusion leads to multiple organ failure and the institution of metabolic acidosis. Ultimately early symptoms of respiratory distress become frank symptoms of respiratory failure.

A unique group of patients, ranging in age from infancy to teenage, present with congestive heart failure secondary to rhythm disturbances. The rapid rhythm tachycardia results in inadequate cardiac output as well as inadequate myocardial perfusion. Symptoms reflect the failure of both ventricles. Rapid conversion by cardioversion or defibrillation to a normal rhythm is essential for returning heart function to normal.

Drugs and viral and bacterial illnesses, affecting other organs of the body, may also attack the heart muscle, the conduction system, or the even heart valves. As a result, there may be a combination of symptoms suggesting both right and left heart failure.

DIFFERENTIAL DIAGNOSIS

Infants and children may present in heart failure without a known history of congenital heart disease. Presentation to the physician and parent may also be confused with acute respiratory illness because the signs of respiratory distress mask the symptoms associated with congestive heart failure. Any afebrile illness associated with respiratory distress certainly should alert the physician to consider heart failure as the etiology for the respiratory symptoms.

Rarely an infant and child with nephritis and generalized edema may present mimicking congestive heart failure. Appropriate laboratory studies can help delineate the etiology quickly.

Rapid heart rates can be associated with many conditions and may not necessarily be abnormal rhythms. Treatment of the illness will cure the rapid heart rate. When in doubt, an electrocardiogram (EKG) can help clarify the presence or absence of an abnormal cardiac rhythm. Table 9.1 outlines abnormal assessments and physical findings and gives appropriate interventions.

Table 9.1 Differential diagnosis.

Assessment	Examination	Intervention
Respiration		
Tachypnea	Rapid rate Clear lung fields	Oxygen
Dyspnea	Rales and wheezes on auscultation	Lasix
Cyanosis	Rales, decreased breath sounds	Evaluate further; may need intubation and artificial ventilation

Continuing deterioration in any of these indicates need for intubation and artificial ventilation.

Respiratory arrest	No respiratory effort	CPR (cardiopulmonary resuscitation) Intubation and artificial ventilation
Circulation		
Heart rate	Auscultation of heart sounds Timing of rhythm Counting of rate	Medications Cardioversion Defibrillation (rare)
Central pulses	Palpation of quality to estimate Cardiac output	Inotropes
Peripheral pulses	Comparison of quality and strength to central pulses	Inotropes
Capillary refill (more than 3 seconds)	Determined in extremity as a measure of cardiac output and perfusion	Inotropes
Edema	Accumulation of tissue fluid as a result of decreased cardiac output	Lasix

LABORATORY EVALUATION

The laboratory evaluation for the patient with congestive heart failure is designed to help delineate the etiology and the initial steps of management.

A chest X-ray will reveal heart size, abnormal configuration, and pulmonary vascular pattern. Pulmonary pathology can also be ruled out as the etiology for the acute symptoms.

An EKG will rule out rhythm disturbances and chamber enlargement as etiology for the symptoms. In addition, the EKG serves as a baseline to further therapy.

A complete blood count (CBC) will reveal the absence of anemia and may help delineate infection as the etiology.

An electrolyte profile, including glucose and calcium, is to be determined. Electrolyte maintenance and replacement may be important in both the etiology as well as the treatment of the patient.

When possible blood-gas determination should be obtained. This is a particular problem with smaller infants and children. Warmed capillary beds may be the source for the blood sample when arterial sticks are neither feasible nor successful. A $PaCO_2$ of greater than 50 mmHg may indicate need for urgent intubation and ventilation.

Pulse oxymetry is useful in determining the success of peripheral oxygenation as well as a deterioration in the cardiac output. Poor cardiac perfusion will result in decreased readings.

Diagnostic studies, not part of the lifesaving management of the patient, are to be pursued when doing so is feasible. The patient who is not improving may require more sophisticated evaluation earlier in the course in order to determine the precise etiology and if possible the reason for limited improvement.

An echocardiogram is helpful in delineating structural abnormalities. It will be helpful in looking at and following myocardial function and is most diagnostic in the presence of a pericardial effusion.

Invasive cardiac catheterization with placement of the Swan Ganz cardiac output catheter may be necessary in order to monitor pulmonary artery pressures as well as cardiac output and vascular resistance during fluid management.

MANAGEMENT

Management of the patient with congestive heart failure requires frequent reevaluation and assessment of the patient to determine the need for further interventions. Rapid cardiopulmonary assessment as outlined in Table 9.2 is used to reassess the patient condition and progress of therapy frequently.

Cyanosis and respiratory distress not responsive to delivery of oxygen may warrant further intervention with intubation and ventilation. Deteriorating vital signs,

Table 9.2 Rapid cardiopulmonary assessment

Respiratory Assessment	Cardiovascular Assessment
Airway Patency	*Circulation*
Breathing	Heart rate
Rate	Blood pressure
Air entry	Peripheral pulses present/absent volume
Chest rise	Skin perfusion
Breath sounds	Capillary refill time
Stridor	Temperature
Wheezing	Color
Mechanics	Mottling
Retractions	CNS (central nervous system) perfusion
Grunting	Recognition of parents
Color	Reaction to pain
	Muscle tone
	Pupil size

Source: American Heart Assocciation. Textbook of pediatric advanced life support. Dallas: AA, American Academy of Pediatrics, 1990.

decreased saturations on oxymetry, and increasing work of ventilation are also indicators for further intervention.

Temperature control is an often neglected but important vital sign to follow. Body temperature in sick infants and children is frequently abnormally low and warrants frequent assessment to determine the need for warming procedures.

Heart rate may be rapid and is the body's response to maintaining an adequate cardiac output in the light of a failing myocardium. Digoxin in children remains the most used drug in the management of acute congestive heart failure. Apart from slowing heart rate, improved myocardial contractility increases cardiac output. In the patient with acute congestive heart failure, digoxin is given intravenously according to the following regimen:

Digitalizing dose:	40 micrograms/kg
Administration:	Only intravenously using the following dosage schedule
	½ dose initially
	¼ dose six to eight hours later depending on condition
	¼ dose six to eight hours after the second dose
Maintenance:	Approximately 12 hours after the last dose 10 micrograms/kg given as ½ dose every 12 hours

Diuretic therapy to remove fluid accumulation in the tissues, including the lung interstitial spaces, improves the patient significantly. The initial drug can be Lasix given as a dosage of 2mg/kg intravenously. The drug may be repeated every four to six hours. The close monitoring of electrolytes is essential. Bumex, a newer diuretic, is used frequently when the response to Lasix is less than expected. Sometimes alternating these two drugs produces the desired effect.

Maintenance fluids are usually given at approximately 60 percent of normal. In order to maintain an adequate output, an adequate stroke volume must be maintained. The patient in congestive heart failure may have a diuresis that decreases the preload. Therefore a delicate balance between fluid input and output must be maintained carefully, specifically during the frequent, large doses of diuretics use period.

Depending on the severity of the congestive heart failure, the use of inotropic agents and afterload-reducing agents (such as Dobutamine, Dopamine, Nipride, Inocor) might be indicated. These drugs are used as intravenous drips and require intensive management of the patient's vital signs, including urinary output and neurologic status.

The patient with rhythm disturbances precipitating congestive heart failure, that is, atrial or ventricular tachyarrythmias, require quick intervention with either cardioversion or defibrillation. An appropriate defibrillator with small enough joules should be available for the small infant and child. Recommended joules for cardioversion start at ¼ joule/kg. Recommended joules for defibrillation start at 2 joules/kg. Rarely the child or infant will require electrical pacing of the heart in order to maintain an adequate rhythm.

CONCLUSION

Congestive heart failure can cause mortality if an acute problem is not recognized and treated promptly. Since the symptom is merely part of a complex disease process, the patient will need to be admitted or transported to a facility that can delicately manage and diagnostically evaluate the care of these very sick infants and children.

SUGGESTED READING

1. Adams FH, Emmanouilides GC, Riemenschneider TA, eds. Heart disease in infants, children and adolescents. 4th ed. Baltimore: Williams & Wilkins, 1989;890-911.
2. American Heart Association. Textbook of pediatric advanced life support. Dallas: American Heart Association, American Academy of Pediatrics. 1990.
3. Carson A, Brickner JJ, McNamara, DG. The science and practice of pediatric cardiology congestive heart failure. 2007-2023. Lea & Febiger, 1990.
4. Schneeweiss A. Drug therapy in infants and children with cardiovascular diseases. Philadelphia: Lea & Febiger, 1986.

PART IV

Poisoning

10

Acute Pediatric Poisoning

David McCarty

Poisoning is a major medical problem of childhood, and therefore skill in diagnosis and emergency management is essential. In particular, acute intoxications must be immediately identified; prompt intervention may prevent illness or even death. The approach to emergency management of poisonings may be separated into three phases: (1) diagnosis; (2) assessment of severity; and (3) initial management.

Fortunately diagnosis is not usually a problem; most acute pediatric poisonings are witnessed or strongly suspected on presentation. Unsuspected poisoning may be very difficult to diagnose; physicians must keep intoxication in the differential diagnosis whenever a case is complex or confusing (Table 10.1), especially when life-threatening symptoms or multiple organ systems are involved.

Therapy should be rational and systematic but individualized; a "cookbook" approach is inappropriate. Assessment of severity is very important. Most poisonings are inconsequential, requiring only observation or minimal therapy, but some can be life threatening. In serious cases, supportive care takes precedence; if vital functions are sufficiently supported, most patients will recover. In other words, treat the patient, not the poison. Measures for decreasing absorption and/or increasing elimination of toxins are often helpful. Specific antidotes can be lifesaving when they are available. Reference sources (literature, consultant, poison information centers, and so forth) should be readily available and consulted routinely. Many poisons are encountered only rarely.

DEMOGRAPHICS

Most acute pediatric intoxications occur in defined subgroups. These groups differ in clinical presentation and potential for morbidity and mortality.

The largest group consists of children under five years of age, usually presenting with accidental ingestions. Substances ingested are usually therapeutic drugs, common household substances, or environmental agents such as plants. Fortunately, large amounts of the toxic agent are rarely ingested unless it has a pleasant taste or the toddler is fed by an older child. Serious effects are usually limited to agents with high intrinsic toxicity. Child abuse should be suspected in atypical cases.

A second group consists of patients of any age with iatrogenic toxicity. Exposures are usually relatively benign except for a few highly toxic drugs (for example,

Table 10.1 Clues to toxic etiology

Altered mental status	Metabolic acidosis
Cardiovascular compromise	Multisystem manifestations
Depressed or hostile patient	Seizures
Known substance abuser	Unexplained trauma (especially head)

theophylline, digitalis). It is important to keep in mind, however, that children often are treated with over-the-counter substances, home remedies, or folk medicines. Inquire about *all* treatment given, including over-the-counter and home remedies.

The last group consists of adolescents attempting suicide. Such intoxications are often difficult to manage. Large amounts of lethal substances may be ingested. History may be unavailable or unreliable. Patients may be uncooperative or actively resist therapy. Suicide gestures may prove lethal since the toxicity of readily available substances (for example, aspirin and acetaminophen) may not be appreciated. When dealing with suicide attempts, presume the worst.

DIAGNOSIS

If poisoning is definite or strongly suspected, the history (Table 10.2) can be focused to answer three questions: (1) What substance was involved? (2) How much was involved? (3) When did the exposure occur? Efforts should be made to obtain information from parents, siblings, or caretakers. The substance, in its original container, should be brought in for inspection. If it is not available, knowledge of its intended use may suggest its composition. Determining where the child was last seen and what medications or household or industrial products are in the home (particularly what substances or materials were used in the past 24 hours) may provide identification clues. When history is unavailable or inadequate, the clinician must presume a worst-case scenario.

Evaluation of severity begins with a brief physical exam (Table 10.3), first ensuring that the "ABCs" (airway, breathing, and circulation) are appropriately stabilized. Threats to life must be treated immediately. Once stability is assured,

Table 10.2 Important historical items in poisoning cases

For a known case:	
What substance was involved?	When did exposure occur?
How much was involved?	
For an unknown case:	
Activity of patient	Patient's appearance at scene
Chemicals/drugs in proximity	Sources of combustion products
Description of location	Suicide notes
Other victims	Unusual odors

Table 10.3 Physical examination

ABCs	Mental status
Vital signs	Eye changes (pupils, nystagmus)
Odors	Gag reflex
Secretions and excretions	Deep tendon reflexes
Autonomic activity	Skin and mucous membranes
Seizure activity	

findings helpful in determining or confirming the poison involved and in estimating severity of toxicity can be sought. Characteristic toxic syndromes (Table 10.4) known as *toxidromes* may be recognized (1). Preexisting medical illnesses should be assessed.

Reassessment at appropriate intervals is important; many toxins have a delayed onset of action. A period of observation is necessary for almost all toxic ingestions even if the initial examination is normal. For young children with seemingly benign ingestions, home observation is appropriate if the parents are reliable.

Laboratory evaluation may be helpful but has significant limitations. Simply detecting a drug on a "tox screen" does not mean that the substance detected is responsible for the patient's condition. Furthermore drug screening is not all inclusive; it is not possible to test for every potentially toxic substance. Laboratories vary in methods used and in technical expertise. Interpretation of results requires clinical correlation and judgement, and overreliance on drug screens should be avoided.

Appropriate use of the laboratory requires knowledge of specific tests to order, whether quantitative or qualitative results are needed, and what type of specimen (blood or urine) should be obtained. In general when the determination of the presence of a substance is the goal, urine screens are used since most substances have a much higher concentration in the urine than in the plasma. When determination of quantity is important, blood is preferred (6). Other specimens are of little value in the usual situation.

Some quantitative levels (Table 10.5) are essential for diagnosis and/or initial management of certain common and potentially serious intoxications. Other levels may be useful in confirming diagnosis or aiding management.

For serious poisonings, general laboratory tests are often needed. Serum electrolyte determinations allow calculation of the anion gap as well as of electrolyte disturbances. Arterial blood gases define respiratory and metabolic acid base status. Serum osmolarity allows detection of an "osmolar gap" (Table 10.6) and rough calculation of the concentration of osmotically active substances (sugars and alcohols). This is especially helpful when ethylene glycol or methanol levels are unavailable.

Table 10.4 Toxidromes

Anticholinergic	Psychedelic/hallucinogenic
Cholinergic	Sedative/hypnotic
Opiate	Sympathomimetic

Table 10.5 Important toxicologic assays

Toxin Levels Essential for Management	Toxin Assays Possibly Useful
Acetaminophen	Cannabinoids
Carboxyhemoglobin	Cocaine
Digoxin	Cyanide
Ethanol	Heavy metals
Ethylene glycol	Isopropyl alcohol
Iron/iron binding capacity	Lidocaine
Lithium	Opioids
Methanol	Phenytoin
Methemoglobin	Phencyclidine
Salicylates	Phenothiazines
Phenobarbital	Plasma and RBC cholinesterase
Theophylline	Sympathomimetics
	Tricyclic antidepressants

Abnormal hemoglobins (methemoglobin, carboxyhemoglobin) may produce a "saturation gap" (calculated arterial oxygen saturation minus the measured arterial saturation) (8). Finally, hepatic and renal function tests estimate capacity to metabolize toxins and/or to determine whether the toxin has damaged these organs.

Radiographic evaluation may be helpful in poisonings (Table 10.7). Abdominal X-rays may reveal heavy metals; chest X-rays show hydrocarbon pneumonitis; contrast studies detect concretions due to salicylates.

GENERAL THERAPEUTIC PRINCIPLES

Table 10.8 summarizes basic therapeutic measures involved in treatment of significant poisoning. Therapy may be classified as first aid, stabilization and support, or specific toxilogical.

First Aid

First aid measures may be useful if the patient is stable. For ocular or cutaneous exposures, contaminated clothing must be removed, solid material brushed off, and contaminated areas of the skin washed copiously with soap and water or with water alone if the contaminated area is the eyes. Parents should use gloves or other protective

Table 10.6 Calculation of osmolar gap

(Serum Na × 1.86) = BUN/2.8 + glu/18
Measured serum osm-calculated serum
Osm   = osmolar gap
Normal gap = 10 mOsm

Table 10.7 Toxic substances that are radio-opaque

Antihistamines	Heavy metals
Barium	Iodides
Calcium	Phenothiazines
Chloral hydrate	Potassium
Concretions*	Solvents (CCl$_4$, chloroform)
Drug-filled condoms	Tricyclic antidepressants
Enteric-coated preparations	

*Barbiturates, iron, glutethimide, meprobamate, salicylates, sustained-release theophylline.

measures. Dilution of ingested caustic agents with water or milk may be used in the *alert* patient but *not* if the child is drooling, having chest pain, or manifesting decreased mental status (9).

Other treatments must be mentioned to condemn their use. In particular, the so-called "universal antidote" (burnt toast, strong tea, and milk of magnesia), emesis induction by gagging, hypertonic saline, mustard water, soap suds, and mineral oil are ineffective and potentially dangerous. For significant exposures, the child should be transported to an appropriate medical facility via ambulance if necessary.

Stabilization and Support

Initial emergency department management should be directed to stabilizing the airway, breathing, and circulation. Appropriate basic and advanced life support measures should be instituted. Treatment with 100 percent oxygen should be given to all patients with significant toxicity, especially if carbon monoxide or cyanide toxicity is a possibility. Should the patient remain unable to protect the airway, endotracheal intubation should be performed. In general, loss of the gag reflex is an indication for intubation, but this may be difficult to determine. The most practical guide is that a poisoned, obtunded child who can be intubated without sedation or undue trauma *should* be intubated, unless the patient is comatose from a *rapidly* reversible cause (for example, opiate intoxication or hypoglycemia). Should significant patient resistance occur, the attempt may be terminated. Sedation should be avoided.

Table 10.8 Therapy of Intoxications

First aid measures	*Toxicologic therapies*
Removal from further exposure	Prevention of absorption
Decontamination	Enhancement of excretion
Transportation	Specific antidotes (if available)
Stabilization measures	Supportive therapy
ABCs	Preventive counseling
Seizure control	Psychiatric assessment (if patient is suicidal)
Dextrose, oxygen, naloxone, thiamine	

Respiratory distress that does not improve with use of the above measures should be carefully reevaluated for cardiopulmonary and toxicological causes. Should cardiopulmonary causes be ruled out, strong consideration must be given to the possibility of intoxication with a metabolic poison, especially if the venous blood is bright red (cyanide, CO) or chocolate-brown (methemoglobin). If these conditions are strongly suspected, immediate antidotal therapy may be lifesaving.

The next priority is circulatory adequacy. In general, hypotension from intoxication (if not due to hypoxia) is most commonly a result of loss of vascular tone with diminished peripheral resistance. Volume depletion may also play a role in producing hypotension due to toxin-associated diarrhea, vomiting, or diaphoresis. Lack of access to water (for example, from coma) or impaired thirst mechanisms may further reduce vascular volume. Myocardial depression may be seen with many overdoses, usually combined with peripheral vascular effects.

Initial treatment for toxin-induced hypotension consists of fluids and Trendelenburg positioning. Should fluid therapy fail, vasopressors may be necessary, using appropriate monitoring devices to guide therapy. Many toxins (notably tricyclic antidepressants) deplete norepinephrine stores in autonomic ganglia and blood vessels; thus indirect-acting agents such as dopamine and phenylephrine may be less effective than usual. Norepinephrine is the preferred vasopressor for such patients. Hypo- and hyperthermia may produce hypotension and can best be corrected with physical measures. If hypotension cannot be reversed by the previously mentioned therapy, inotropic agents such as epinephrine, dobutamine, calcium (for calcium channel blocker toxicity), and/or glucagon (especially for beta-blocker and calcium channel blocker effects) should be considered. Digitalis should be avoided.

Control of cardiac dysrhythmias, usually seen in adolescents with suicidal ingestions and in children who have ingested cardioactive drugs, is important in preserving circulation. Hypoxia must be corrected first if possible; if dysrhythmias persist, pharmacologic intervention and correction of electrolyte or metabolic factors are required. Hemodynamically significant bradycardias are treated with atropine, isoproterenol, or electrical pacing. Supraventricular tachydysrhythmias may be controlled with vagal maneuvers, adenosine, beta-blockers, alkalinization (for cyclic antidepressants), physostigmine (for severe anticholinergic toxicity), and (rarely) overdrive electrical pacing. Calcium channel blockers such as verapamil may cause dangerous hypotension, especially in infants, and are unproven in poisonings. Digitalis, cholinergic agents, and vasopressors should be avoided. Ventricular dysrhythmias may be controlled with lidocaine, phenytoin (especially for cyclic antidepressant- and digitalis-induced dysrhythmia), or alkalinization (cyclic antidepressants). Quinidine, procainamide, disopyramide, and bretylium should be avoided. Correction of hypomagnesemia may be very helpful, and magnesium may be a useful agent for ventricular dysrhythmia (especially for *torsades de pointes*, often drug-induced). A significant dysrhythmia occurring in the setting of digitalis intoxication is an indication for digitalis Fab (Fragment antigen-binding) fragments.

Hypertension, which may be life threatening in certain intoxications (sympathomimetics, MAO inhibitor interactions) is best controlled by alpha- and beta-blockade. Pure beta agents are theoretically hazardous since unopposed alpha effects may occur. Nitroprusside may also be used, and calcium channel blockers are theoretically attractive but unproven in this setting.

Seizures are common serious manifestations of intoxications, and toxic causes should always be considered when evaluating a seizure. Treatment is similar to that of status epilepticus from other causes. Phenytoin may not have its usual effectiveness when used for toxin-induced seizures, notably theophylline, cyclic antidepressants, and salicylates. Benzodiazepines and barbiturates tend to retain their efficacy, but some toxic seizures require general anesthesia. Alkali therapy should be given much more freely if the seizure was caused by cyclic antidepressants or salicylates; these agents penetrate the CNS (central nervous system) and myocardium much more readily in conditions of acidemia, increasing toxicity. Finally for refractory seizures, consider isoniazid-induced seizures, which may respond only to pyridoxine therapy.

Specific Toxicological Therapy

After the traditional ABCs, consider the "toxic ABCs." These measures should be considered standard in every potentially significant intoxication.

First are the routine antidotes—oxygen, glucose, naloxone, and thiamine. Hypoglycemia and hypoxia may be very difficult to diagnose clinically. Opiate overdose may not be associated with classic signs (for example, pinpoint pupils). Therefore for seizures, abnormal mental status, or focal neurologic deficits, use of these agents should be routinely considered. Thiamine is recommended to avoid precipitating Wernicke's encephalopathy by a glucose load. Significant adverse effects from these antidotes are rare, and they may be lifesaving.

Next gastric emptying by emesis or lavage and prevention of absorption by activated charcoal and cathartics must be considered. Endotracheal intubation prior to gastric emptying may be required to protect the obtunded patient's airway. Gastric emptying is controversial.

Ipecac-induced emesis has been used for many years and has been proven safe (when it is properly used) and consistently effective in producing emesis (though this does not necessarily equal effective toxin removal). Disadvantages of ipecac include delay in onset (15 to 30 minutes) of emesis, the possibility of aspiration should the patient seize or become comatose, variable efficacy, and the occasional occurrence of prolonged vomiting, which may interfere with activated charcoal or subsequent antidotal therapy.

Lavage, using a large-bore tube, is more consistent, rapid, and effective than is ipecac when emptying is delayed. Lavage is invasive and difficult to perform in an awake child. It should be performed, however, as soon as possible in ingestions involving significant amounts of potent toxins (for example, strychnine, camphor) even if the patient is awake, using sedation if necessary. To be effective, lavage must be carried out with a large-bore tube—30 to 40 French in adults, 16 to 28 French in children. A standard nasogastric tube is essentially useless except for very recent pure liquid ingestions or to administer ipecac and/or activated charcoal to a patient who is so uncooperative that standard lavage cannot be carried out.

Recent studies cast doubt on the usefulness of gastric emptying by either method. Some authorities now recommend using activated charcoal alone, but this is not yet universally accepted. In general, ipecac has no role in hospital management, though home use is likely to continue. Gastric lavage should be carried out in recent ingestions of substances that may produce life-threatening toxicity, especially those not well bound by activated charcoal (15).

Prevention of absorption is the next consideration. In contrast to gastric emptying, the value of activated charcoal is undisputed. Almost all toxic agents are adsorbed with the notable exceptions of small ions such as caustic agents, iron, lithium, and heavy metals. Hydrocarbons may also not be well adsorbed, but this is not clear. Activated charcoal is a very safe agent, especially when it is given as a single dose, and should be given routinely in almost all ingestions, except when emesis (occasionally produced by the agent) may be so detrimental as to outweigh its adsorptive effects as in hydrocarbon ingestion.

Cathartics are customarily added to the initial charcoal dose. An ionic cathartic (such as magnesium sulfate or citrate) or sorbitol should be given. In contrast to charcoal, multiple doses of cathartic are *never* indicated.

Recently a technique known as whole bowel irrigation has been advocated for certain ingestions, particularly for those in which activated charcoal is ineffective. This consists of the use of polyethylene glycolate solution or other agents resulting in an osmotic diarrhea, producing rapid gastrointestinal emptying without severe electrolyte loss. Although relatively new for pediatric use, the technique should be considered when charcoal is ineffective or when rapid gastrointestinal emptying is necessary (such as when sustained-release products are involved). Contraindications include ileus, obstruction, and gastrointestinal hemorrhage.

Antidotal therapy must be considered for certain ingestions. Such treatment is adjunctive, *not* a substitute for good supportive care. The most important antidotes currently available in the United States and their uses are listed in Table 10.9. A few antidotes for rapidly lethal toxins must be readily available; the physician should commit these to memory and be familiar with their use as there may be little time for consultation or review.

Next the feasibility and desirability of enhancing excretion should be considered. Most intoxication victims recover without such measures. Certain potent toxins, however (for example, lithium), require rapid excretion. Such methods work best for substances with small volumes of distribution, a mathematical concept that roughly equates to the substance's extracellular availability. For instance, cyclic antidepressants have a huge volume of distribution and are minimally affected by dialysis, while ethylene glycol, with a much smaller volume, is efficiently removed.

Methods available to enhance excretion include forced diuresis (rarely if ever helpful); alkaline diuresis; repeat-dose activated charcoal (*never with cathartic*); and

Table 10.9 Antidotes and their dosages

Drug/Toxin	Antidote	Antidote Dosage
Acetaminophen	N-Acetylcysteine	140 mg/kg orally (loading) 70 mg/kg every 4 hours, 17 doses (maintenance)
Anticholinergics	Physostigmine	Adult: 1 to 2 mg IV slowly Child: 0.5 mg or 0.02 mg/kg IV slowly
β-Adrenergic blockers	Glucagon	1 to 5 mg IV
Benzodiazepines	Flumazenil	0.2 to 0.3 mg
Bromide	Sodium chloride	
Carbamate insecticides	Atropine	2 to 4 mg IV as needed
Carbon monoxide (CO)	Oxygen	
Cyanide	Amyl nitrite perles Sodium nitrite	Adult: 300 mg Child: 10 mg/kg
	Sodium thiosulfate	Adult: 12.5 g IV Child: 1.5 mL/kg
Cardiac glycosides	Fragment, antigen-binding (Fab) antibody therapy	As necessary
Ethylene glycol	Ethyl alcohol	1 mL/kg of 95% solution, diluted (loading) 0.1 mL/kg/hour, diluted (maintenance)
Gyrimetra mushrooms	Pyridoxine	2 to 5 g IV slowly
Heavy metals	Dimercaprol (BAL) Penicillamine Disodium EDTA	
Isoniazid	Pyridoxine	2 to 5 g IV slowly
Iron	Deferoxamine	10 to 15 mg/kg/hour
Methanol	Ethyl alcohol	As for ethylene glycol
Narcotics	Naloxone	2 mg IV
Nitrites	Methylene blue	1 to 2 mg/kg of 1% solution
Organophosphates	Atropine Pralidoxime	1 to 2 mg IV as needed 1 g
Tricyclic antidepressants	Sodium bicarbonate	1 to 3 mEq/kg IV
Warfarin	Vitamin K_1	5 to 25 mg IV or IM

Reprinted with permission of the publisher from Bryson P. Comprehensive review in toxicology, 2d ed. Rockville, Md.: Aspen, 1989;11.

hemodialysis and hemoperfusion. Peritoneal dialysis is a poor substitute for hemodialysis. These methods are reserved for serious intoxications in hospitalized patients.

PATIENT DISPOSITION

The final decision in poison management is whether admission or transfer is required. Most toxins will manifest toxic effects within a six-hour period of observation. Some, however, will not (for example, acetaminophen), and it is imperative that it be reasonably certain that delayed effects will not occur. Other factors to consider are the accuracy of the history, the possibility of recurring exposure (for example, CO), reliability of follow-up, and availability of diagnostic and therapeutic services (for example, dialysis). Most importantly, adolescents who have attempted suicide (even as a "gesture") are at great risk for further, perhaps more successful, attempts and should have psychiatric evaluation. When in doubt, one must err on the side of admission. Should home discharge be feasible, counsel parents in prevention and first aid when such instruction is appropriate.

CONCLUSION

Intoxications represent a frequent serious problem for the pediatric emergency physician. Diagnosis requires skill in obtaining historical and physical findings to confirm suspected poisonings and a high level of suspicion for unsuspected ones. Determining the actual and potential level of severity of poisoning is crucial for determining treatment and disposition. Therapy begins with good supportive care. Use of antidotes and measures to decrease absorption and increase excretion are common with additional methods such as hemodialysis being used in serious cases. New concepts and therapies are being rapidly developed. Traditional methods are increasingly being questioned, and many older therapies and concepts are being dismissed. The field is rapidly evolving, and clinicians must strive to remain cognizant of current developments. For optimum results, scientific knowledge must be combined with good clinical skills.

REFERENCES

1. Bryson PD. Comprehensive review in toxicology, Rockville, Md.: Aspen, 1989.
2. Morenson HC, Greensher J. Pediatrics 1974;53:336–342.
3. Hansen HJ, Caudill SP, Boone J. Crisis in drug testing: Results of CDC study. JAMA 1985;253:2382–2387.
4. Inglefinger J, Isakson G, Shine D, et al. Reliability of the toxic screen in drug overdose. Clin Pharm Ther 1981;29:570–575.
5. Rockerbie RA, Campbell DJ. A random survey of drug screening proficiency. Clin Biochem 1977;10:138–139.
6. Helper B, Sutheimer C, Sunshine I. Role of toxicology lab in suspected ingestions. Pediat Clin North Am 1986;33:245–260.
7. Kellermann A, Fihn S, LoGefo J, et al. Utilization and yield of drug screening in the emergency department. Am J Emer Med 1988;6(1):14–20.

8. Goldfrank L, Flomenbaum N, Lewin N, et al. Goldfrank's toxicologic emergencies, East Norwalk, Conn.: Appleton and Lange, 1990.
9. Bayer M, Rumack B. Poisoning and overdose. Topics in emergency medicine, vol I. Rockville, Md.: Aspen, 1979;1–3.
10. Bayer M, Rumack B, Wanke L. Toxicologic emergencies. New York: Robert J. Brady Co., 1984.
11. Hall A, Rumack B, Karkal S. Increasing survival in acute cyanide poisoning. Emerg Med Rep 1988;9:17.
12. Slovis C. ED Management of unstable patients with status seizures. Emerg Med Rep 1989;10:9.
13. Delaney KA, Sauter D. Assessment and management of shock in the poisoned patient. Topics Emerg Med 1988;9(4):43–51.
14. Burton BT, Bayer MJ. Hazardous materials. Topics in Emergency Medicine, vol 7. Rockville, MD.: Aspen, 1985.
15. Hall A, Krenzelok E. Gastrointestinal decontamination: Sifting through supportive therapeutic options. Emer Med Rep 1991;12:19.
16. Barkin RM. Toxicologic emergencies. Pediatric Annals 1990;19(11):629–633.
17. Steinhart CM, Pearxon-Shaver AL. Poisoning. Critical Care Clinics 1989;4(4):845–872.
18. Tenenbein M. Whole bowel irrigation as a gastrointestinal decontamination procedure after acute poisoning. Medical Toxicology and Adverse Drug Experience 1988;3(2):77–84.

PART V

Trauma/Orthopedics

11

Acute Osteomyelitis and Septic Arthritis

William A. Herndon

Acute hematogenous septic arthritis and osteomyelitis can cause significant morbidity if they are not promptly diagnosed and properly managed. The character of these infections is changing (1). In the past, bone and joint infections in children have been responsible for significant mortality. The advent of antibiotics, the availability of newer diagnostic techniques, a better understanding of the pathophysiology of these infections, and advances in anesthetic and surgical management, however, have changed the course of these diseases. Despite these advances, diagnosis is often delayed. Outcome is directly related to time from onset of symptoms to institution of treatment. It is imperative that a high index of suspicion be present when a neonate, infant, or child presents with a limp, inability to bear weight, or refusal to use a limb.

Although they are sometimes present at the same time, this chapter will cover acute hematogenous osteomyelitis and acute hematogenous septic arthritis separately.

ACUTE HEMATOGENOUS OSTEOMYELITIS

Acute osteomyelitis is an infection of bone most often caused by the hematogenous spread of bacteria. It may occur in adults but is primarily seen in children. Osteomyelitis may also be caused by trauma or by penetrating wounds with subsequent direct inoculation of the bone by bacteria.

Fink and Nelson found the most common infecting organism in all age groups to be *Staphylococcus aureus* (2). Gram negative organisms, in addition to *Group A* and *Group B Streptococcus*, were predominant in neonates. *Haemophilus influenzae* was common in children up to the age of five, and *Streptococcus pneumoniae* and *Staphylococcus epidermidis* were present occasionally.

Pathophysiology

The most common site is the metaphyseal region of a long bone. An understanding of the pathophysiology of this condition requires knowledge of the vascular supply of this region. The nutrient vessel enters the diaphysis and branches to send small arterioles to the metaphysis. These vessels empty into venous lakes that in turn drain into the medullary cavity. In neonates, some of the arterioles cross the growth plate to supply the cartilaginous epiphysis. With time, the epiphysis develops its own blood supply and communication between the metaphysis and epiphysis is no longer present. This distinct separation of metaphyseal and epiphyseal circulation continues until closure of the physis.

Hobo demonstrated that bacteria injected into the osseous circulation caused infection in the metaphysis of a long bone (3). Some physicians hypothesize that two factors are responsible for this occurrence: (1) bacteria lodge in the sluggish venous lakes of the metaphysis and (2) reticuloendothelial cells are sparse in that area. After bacteria have become lodged in the region, an inflammatory response develops. Pus forms and may spread in several directions. Spread toward the medullary canal may occur but is readily walled off by the diaphysis. The direction of remaining spread depends to some extent on the age of the child. In neonates, pus may spread to the epiphysis via the blood vessels that cross the physis. In infants and children, pus spreads through the cortex and becomes subperiosteal. The periosteum in the child is thick and easily elevated by pus allowing spread along the shaft of the bone. Pus in the bone destroys the endosteal circulation, while the periosteal circulation to the bone is destroyed when the periosteum is elevated. The cortex becomes devascularized and forms a sequestrum. The well-vascularized perioseum lays down reactive new bone in an attempt to wall off the spreading infection and forms an involucrum.

Clinical Presentation

The most common complaint is pain. Neonates and infants usually will not use the involved extremity due to pain. The older child often will not use the extremity or, if the lower extremity is involved, will limp severely or refuse to bear weight. There may or may not be a history of trauma or of recent infection elsewhere in the body. It must be remembered that children fall every day, usually with very little sequelae. Often parents or the child may attribute symptoms to an injury. Recently evidence has been presented indicating that trauma may be causally related to the production of osteomyelitis (4). In addition, most animal models have required trauma to the bone to produce an infection reliably (5). Besides pain and refusal to use the limb, initial complaints may include fever, malaise, and decreased or absent appetite.

Pain, tenderness, erythema, and warmth over the metaphyseal region of a long bone indicates acute hematogenous osteomyelitis until proven otherwise. Swelling, erythema, and warmth are usually demonstrable in joints other than the hip. Fever is usually, but not always, present. Examination of the child must be careful, systematic, and above all gentle. In infants and young children, the first examiner often has the best chance at a reliable exam. Considerable patience is required. Very gentle joint range of motion should be performed and the metaphysis should be evaluated for tenderness. Careful, slow movement of the joint is usually tolerated with osteomyelitis, but not with septic arthritis.

Laboratory Evaluation

The diagnosis of early hematogenous osteomyelitis cannot be made with any single noninvasive test. The white blood cell count (WBC) is often, but not always, elevated. The erythrocyte sedimentation rate (ESR) is more consistently elevated but is not specific (4,6,7,8).

Radiographic bone changes (rarefaction, lysis, periosteal elevation) are not seen for 7 to 14 days after the onset of symptoms (Figure 11.1). Deep soft tissue swelling may be seen early and is good evidence of the presence of osteomyelitis. Comparison radiographs are helpful.

The technetium 99m bone scan is a sensitive test for the presence of osteomyelitis (9,10,11). It is not specific, however, and carries a significant incidence of false positives and negatives (12,13,14). Since the radioisotope localizes in areas of increased vascularity or new bone formation, a positive scan may be seen in fractures, tumors, and inflammatory processes. Unfortunately the bone scan has developed a reputation as the single best test for the diagnosis of osteomyelitis. In the right situations, it can be useful. It can be, and often is overused, however. Morrissy has indicated that the test is usually not required for diagnosis and adds nothing to the

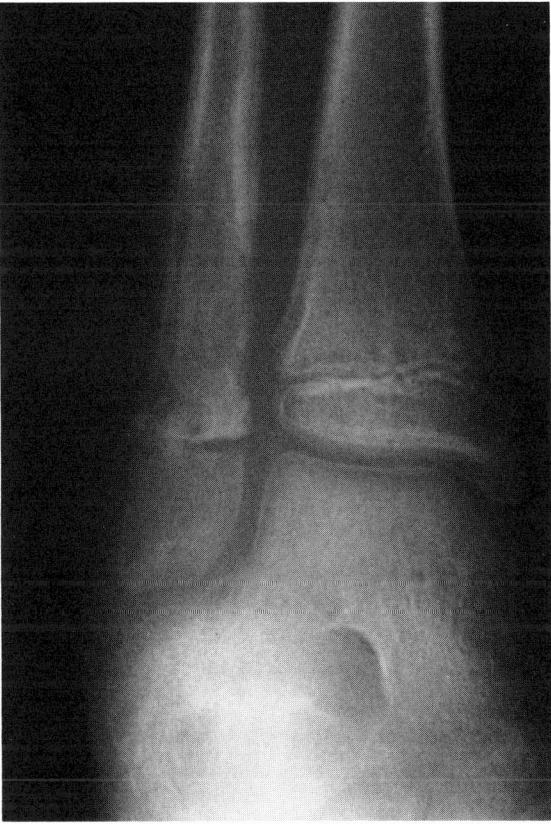

Figure 11.1 Advanced radiographic changes of acute hematogenous osteomyelitis of the distal fibula.

workup of a patient (4). There is no reason to get a bone scan when radiographic changes are present. The scan is often unreliable in neonates (12,13) and in the distal extremities (13,14). Nuclear imaging is most helpful in the diagnosis of axial skeletal infections and when multiple foci of infection are suspected. Gallium imaging has not been particularly useful.

An organism can be retrieved in from 60 to 80 percent of the cases of acute hematogenous osteomyelitis (1,2,4). Blood cultures should be done in all suspected cases and may be positive in 40 to 50 percent of cases.

The best way to retrieve an organism is by aspiration of the metaphysis. This not only confirms the presence of infection but also increases the chance of identifying the organism. Aspiration should be done before nuclear imaging. It does not interfere with later bone scanning and may make it unnecessary (15). Figure 11.2 demonstrates a logical workup for patients with suspected bone or joint infections.

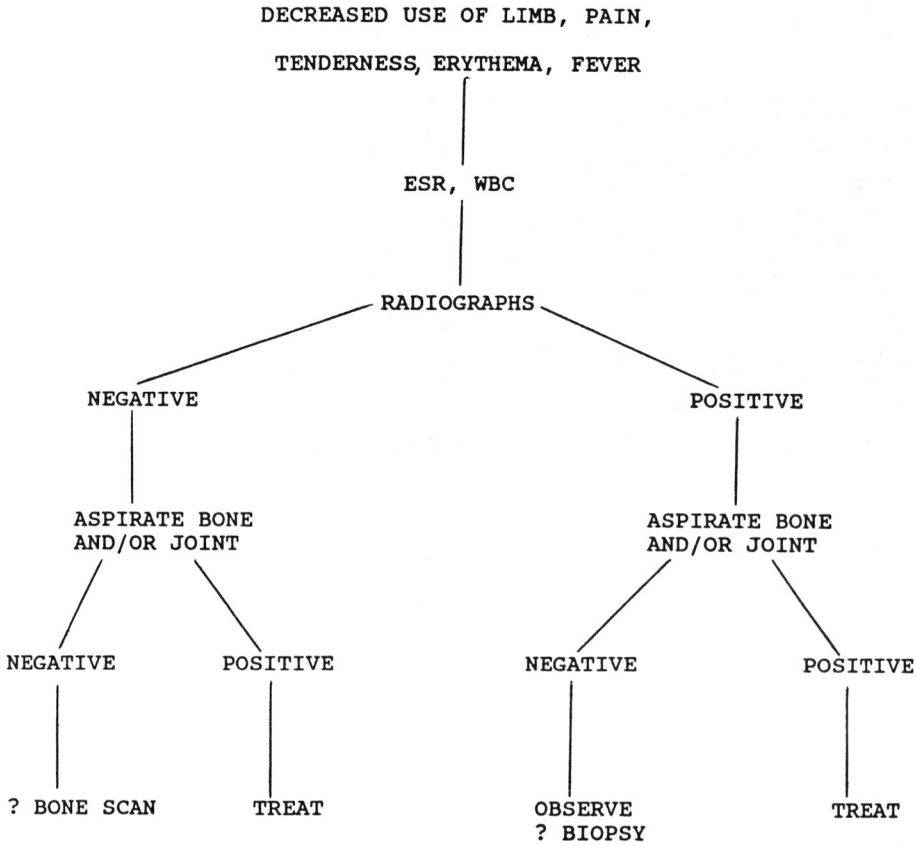

Figure 11.2 Suggested workup of suspected bone and joint infections in children.

Differential Diagnosis

The diagnosis of osteomyelitis is usually not difficult when a high index of suspicion is maintained. The presence of trauma may lead one away from the correct diagnosis. Clinically erythema and swelling may be attributed to cellulitis, which is usually caused by a penetrating wound or bite and which tends to be well localized and not associated with deep bone tenderness. As was stated previously, tenderness, swelling and erythema near the metaphyseal region of a long bone must be considered to be osteomyelitis until it is proven to be otherwise. Septic arthritis may be confused with osteomyelitis or may be present in addition to osteomyelitis.

Radiographically osteomyelitis is most often confused with a bone tumor or fracture. The clinical history and laboratory findings will usually be helpful, but in some instances, only a biopsy will establish the diagnosis when tumor is suspected.

Management

The proper management of bone and joint infections in children continues to be controversial. There is little disagreement, however, that outcome is improved with early diagnosis and rapid institution of treatment. Antibiotics are the mainstay of treatment for acute osteomyelitis. The place of surgery is more controversial.

Antibiotics alone are often sufficient for the treatment of acute osteomyelitis (2,5,6,16,17,18). This requires early institution of treatment with the right antibiotic. It is often necessary to begin antibiotic therapy before an organism has been identified. The choice of antibiotic depends on the age of the patient. Neonates require coverage against penicillin resistant *Staphylococcus aureus, Group B Streptococcus*, and enteric organisms. Initial therapy therefore usually consists of a penicillinase-resistant penicillin in combination with an aminoglycoside. More recently, cefotaxime alone has been used in this age group. In infants and older children, *Staphlococcus aureus* is responsible for at least eighty percent of all cases of osteomyelitis, and initial use of a penicillinase-resistant penicillin is recommended.

At present, there seems to be a general consensus that a short period of intravenous (IV) therapy can be followed by oral therapy. In general, oral therapy requires good initial response to intravenous therapy, identification of a specific organism, and patient compliance. The time of treatment required for adequate treatment has not been well documented. In the absence of good prospective studies, most authors use a course of six weeks of therapy (1,4,20,21).

Most authors agree that at least some form of surgical therapy is useful in certain cases of osteomyelitis (1,2,4,6,8,17,18,22). Indications for surgery include the demonstration of an abscess (from subperiosteal or bone aspiration) and unresponsiveness to medical therapy after two to three days. Figure 11.3 summarizes a recommended treatment protocol for acute osteomyelitis.

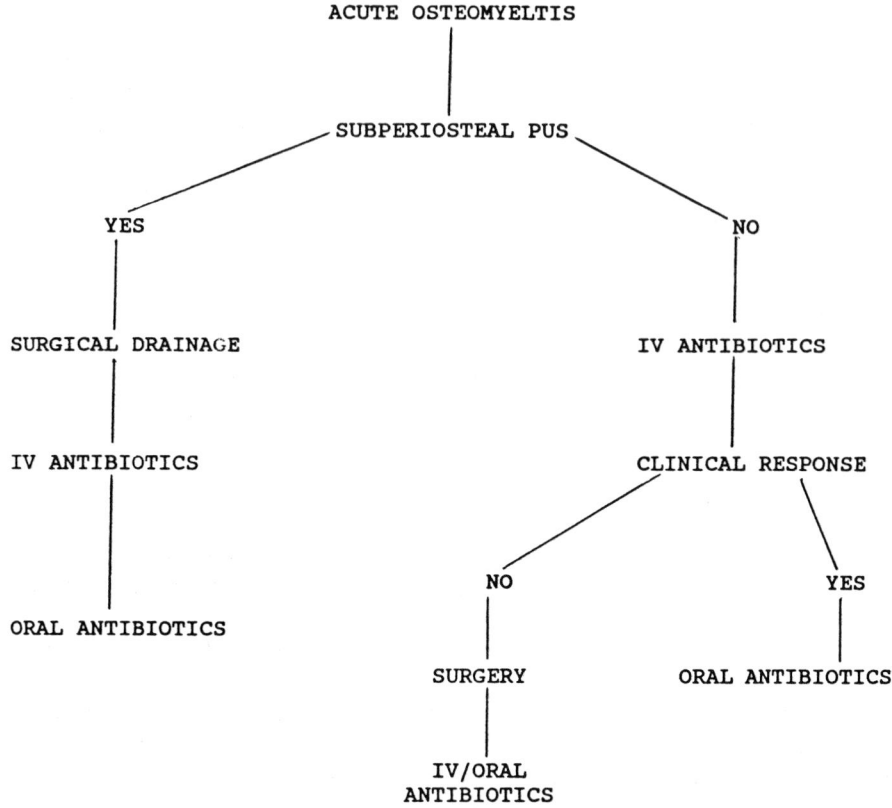

Figure 11.3 Suggested treatment protocol for acute hematogenous osteomyelitis.

ACUTE SEPTIC ARTHRITIS

Early diagnosis and early institution of treatment is even more important in cases of septic arthritis than in osteomyelitis since pus rapidly destroys joints. Infection may be established in one of three ways: (1) by hematogenous spread to the synovium, (2) by direct extension from an adjacent osteomyelitis, and (3) by direct traumatic introduction of bacteria into the joint. It most commonly involves the joints of the lower extremity, especially the knee and the hip (19). Spread from a focus of osteomyelitis occurs by two possible mechanisms depending on the age of the patient. In neonates, the infection spreads across the physis into the epiphysis (23). This explains the association of osteomyelitis with almost every case of neonatal septic arthritis (13). In infants and children, spread occurs directly from the bone into the joint space when the metaphysis is intra-articular (hip, shoulder, elbow).

Pathophysiology

After introduction of bacteria into the joint by either direct inoculation or hematogenous spread, bacteria are phagocytized by the synovium, and an intense inflammatory response occurs. The synovium produces an exudate of synovial fluid and white blood cells. Pus forms in the joint, and destructive enzymes released by the synovium, white cells, and some bacteria begin to destroy the cartilage matrix (24). The loss of ground substance changes the mechanical properties of the cartilage and the collagen becomes susceptible to mechanical destruction. As intra-articular pressure increases, further damage occurs. This is most pronounced in the hip where avascular necrosis can occur following tamponade of the retinacular vessels. It is important to remember that septic arthritis is initiated by bacterial invasion but that joint destruction is in most part caused by the body's response to the infection.

Clinical Presentation

Patients with acute septic arthritis present in a similar fashion to those with acute hematogenous osteomyelitis. Diagnosis in the neonate may be extremely difficult, and bone/joint infection may be identified as part of a sepsis workup. The neonate usually will not move the involved extremity (*pseudoparalysis*). The infant or child usually has extreme pain and tenderness and will not allow active or passive movement of the joint. Children will not bear weight if the lower extremity is affected. The hip joint, if it is involved, is held in flexion, abduction, and external rotation. Rotation of the joint will elicit crying from the child due to pain. More superficial joints are usually swollen, erythematous, and warm. Any joint motion causes pain and guarding. The patient appears ill and is irritable. Fever is usually, but not always, present (19).

Laboratory Evaluation

Morrey and associates found an elevated WBC in only a third of their patients but the ESR was significantly increased in most of the patients (25). Blood cultures may be positive in a third of cases.

Radiographs of the involved and contralateral uninvolved joint should be done but are not often helpful (26). Capsular distention or deep soft tissue swelling may by seen. Radiographs may be more helpful when the hip is involved since joint space widening can be seen early in the course of the disease (Figure 11.4).

Nuclear imaging is not useful. It characteristically demonstrates mild diffuse uptake of the isotope on both sides of the joint. Ultrasonography has recently shown promise in the diagnosis of septic joints (27). It requires experienced, trained personnel and may not be obtainable at all hours. If fluid is identified, aspiration is still required for diagnosis.

Suppurative arthritis is confirmed by joint aspiration. Failure to aspirate a suspected septic joint is inexcusable as it is easy, safe, and reliable. Fluid should be sent for gram stain, culture, and sensitivity and for a cell count. A WBC greater than

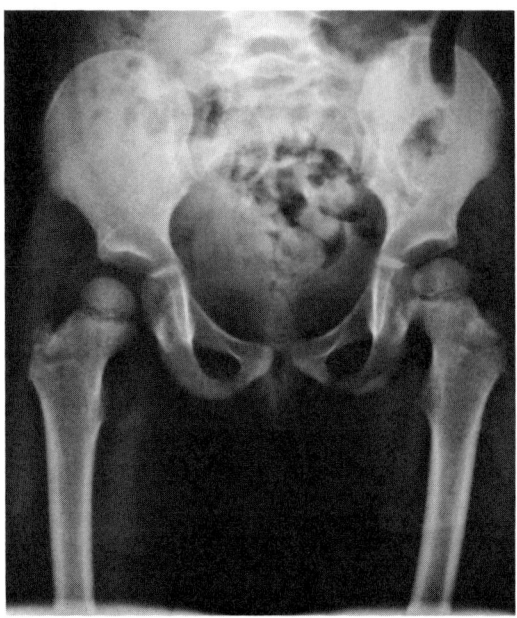

Figure 11.4 Widened joint space in a child with septic arthritis of the right hip.

50,000 is strongly suggestive of septic arthritis although inflammatory arthritis may also present with very high WBCs (28). Both septic arthritis and inflammatory arthritis have a predominance of polymorphonuclear leukocytes (greater than 75 percent). Any remaining fluid may be sent for protein and glucose determinations. In septic arthritis, the former should be elevated (greater than 2.5 percent gm) while the glucose level will be 40 to 50 mg/100 ml less than the serum value (drawn simultaneously).

Differential Diagnosis

The clinical presentation of the child with septic arthritis may be mimicked by several other conditions. Cellulitis and osteomyelitis may present in a similar fashion. Juvenile rheumatoid arthritis, acute rheumatic fever, transient synovitis, and even Legg-Perthes disease may present with a sensitive joint. Joint aspiration usually will readily differentiate septic arthritis from the other conditions.

Management

Treatment has two aims: (1) that the joint must be sterilized and (2) that products of the inflammatory response must be removed. Antibiotics easily cross the synovial barrier and reach sufficient concentration in the joint. Intra-articular antibiotics are not necessary. The method of removal of pus and debris from the joint is controversial.

As with osteomyelitis, adequate antibiotic management requires a short course of IV antibiotics followed by oral therapy (2,4,18,19,20). Optimal treatment times have not been well established. Jackson and Nelson have determined that minimum treatment times are three days for *N. gonorrhoeae*, two weeks for *Streptococcus* and *H. influenzae* and three weeks for *Staphlococcus aureus*, enteric bacilli, and Pseudomonas aeroginosa (19). In addition, helpful clinical guidelines include the initial response to antibiotics as well as the status of the ESR.

Treatment must often be initiated before an organism has been identified. Initial management depends therefore on patient age. Neonates are usually infected with enteric organisms, *S. aureus*, or *Group B Streptococcus* so that a course of either a penicillinase-resistant *penicillin* combined with an *aminoglycoside* or the use of *cefotaxime* alone is appropriate. In the age range from 6 to 24 months, both *S. aureus* and *H. influenzae* are common, and initial treatment needs to cover both organisms. Cefotaxime or cefuroxime cross the blood-joint barrier, and therefore both are effective against resistant strains of *S. aureus* and *H.influenzae*. Children older than five years are treated with a penicillinase-resistant penicillin. Of course after precise organism identification the antibiotic regimen should be changed when necessary.

The method of joint drainage possibly remains the most controversial issue in the treatment of bone and joint infections in children. Choices include multiple needle aspirations, open arthrotomy, and arthroscopy. Virtually all authors concur with immediate arthrotomy for the hip joint (29,30,31). Disagreement exists when treating joints other than the hip. The most important factor determining the outcome of septic arthritis is time from onset of symptoms to initiation of treatment (32). If treatment is begun less than five days after the onset of symptoms, a single aspiration accompanied by appropriate antibiotics will frequently lead to a good result. If the patient does not show a rapid clinical response or if fluid reaccumulates rapidly, drainage by arthrotomy or arthroscopy should be performed, and will ultimately produce a satisfactory result. Multiple needle aspirations are not recommended. They are painful and can further damage the joint. Early institution of treatment is more important than the method of drainage. The protocol (Figure 11.5) summarizes a recommended treatment regimen for acute septic arthritis of joints other than the hip.

CONCLUSIONS

The advent of antibiotics, newer diagnostic techniques, and perhaps the changing character of the infections has improved the outcome of the treatment of acute hematogenous osteomyelitis and acute septic arthritis. Mortality in the otherwise normal patient is virtually nonexistent today. Sequelae from the delayed diagnosis and improper treatment of these conditions, however, are still present. These include joint destruction, chronic osteomyelitis, and length and angular deformities of bone—each of which can be permanently disabling. A high index of suspicion combined with treatment based on the pathophysiology of the disease will lead to a satisfactory result in the majority

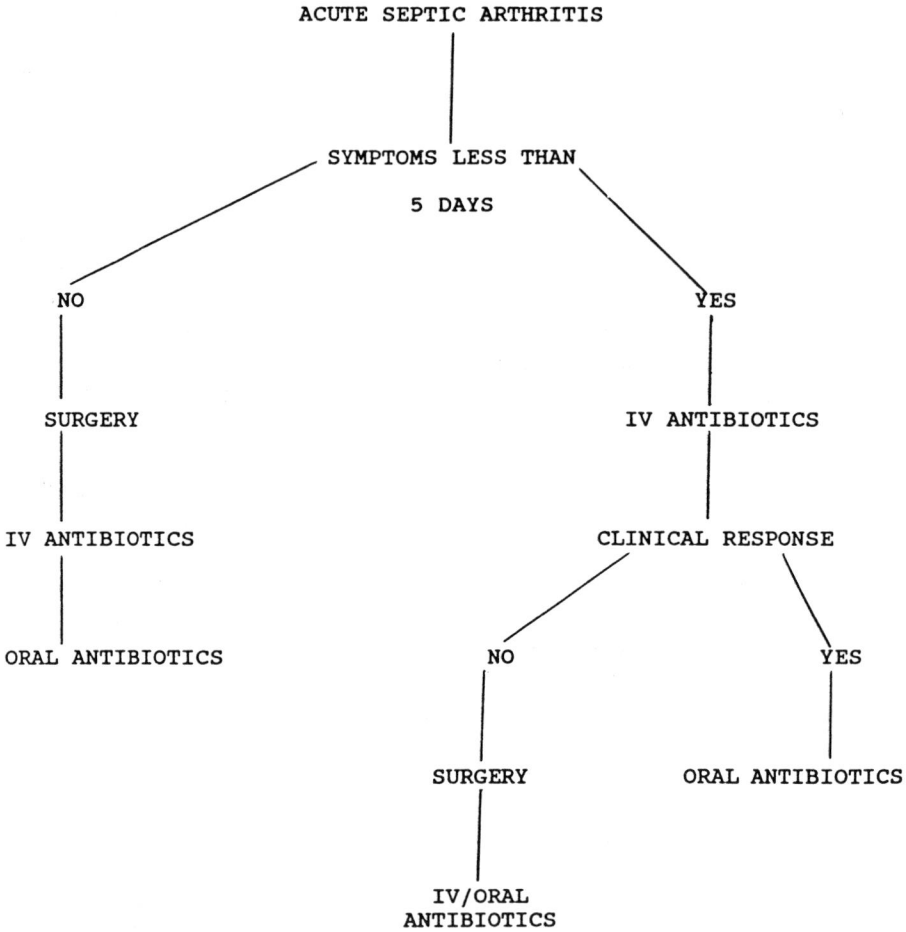

Figure 11.5 Suggested treatment protocol for acute hematogenous septic arthritis.

of cases. This approach recognizes that not all cases can be treated medically and that not all cases require surgery and emphasizes early diagnosis and rapid institution of treatment.

REFERENCES

1. Scott RJ, Christofersen MR, Robertson WW, et al. Acute osteomyelitis in children: A review of 116 cases. J Pediatr Orthop 1990;10:649–652.
2. Fink CW, Nelson JD. Septic arthritis and osteomyelitis in children. Clin Rheum Dis 1986;12:423–435.
3. Hobo T. Zur pathogenese der akuten haemotogenen osteomyelitis. Medicinalis Universitatis Imperialis in Kioto. Acta Scholae 1921;4:1–30.
4. Morrissy RT. Bone and joint sepsis in children. Instr course lect 1982;31:49–61.

5. Emslie KR, Nade S. Pathogenesis and treatment of acute hematogenous osteomyelitis: Evaluation of current views with reference to an animal model. Rev Inf Dis 1986;8:841–849.
6. LaMont RL, Anderson PA, Dajani AS, et al. Acute hematogenous osteomyelitis in children. J Ped Orthop 1987;7:579–583.
7. Morrey BF, Peterson JA. Hematogenous pyogenic osteomyelitis in children. Orthop Clin North Am 1975;6:935–951.
8. Vaughan PA, Newman NM, Rosman NA. Acute hematogenous osteomyelitis in children. J Ped Orthop 1987;7:652–655.
9. Duszynski DO, Kuhn JP, Afshani E, et al. Early radionuclide diagnosis of acute osteomyelitis. Radiology 1975;117:337–340.
10. Gelfand MJ, Silberstein EB. Radionuclide imaging. Use in diagnosis of osteomyelitis in children. JAMA 1977;237:245–257.
11. Howie DW, Savage JP, Wilson TG, et al. The technetium phosphate bone scan in the diagnosis of osteomyelitis in childhood. J Bone Joint Surg 1983;64-A:431–437.
12. Ash JM, Gilday DL. The futility of bone scanning in neonatal osteomyelitis: Concise communication. J Nucl Med 1980;21:417–420.
13. Herndon WA, Alexieva BT, Schwindt ML, et al. Nuclear imaging for musculoskeletal infections in children. J Ped Orthop 1985;5:343–347.
14. Sullivan JA, Vasileff T, Leonard JC. An evaluation of nuclear scanning in orthopaedic infections. J Ped Orthop 1981;1:73–79.
15. Canale ST, Harkness RM, Thomas PA, et al. Does aspiration of bones and joints affect results of later bone scanning? J Pediatr Orthop 1985;5:23–26.
16. Blockey NJ, Watson JT. Acute osteomyelitis in children. J Bone Joint Surg 1970;52B:77–87.
17. Cole WG, Dalziel RE, Leitl S. Treatment of acute osteomyelitis in childhood. J Bone Joint Surg 1982;64B:218–223.
18. Green NE, Edwards K. Bone and joint infections in children. Orthop Clin North Am 1987;18:555–576.
19. Jackson MA, Nelson JD. Etiology and medical management of acute suppurative bone and joint infections in pediatric patients. J Ped Orthop 1982;2:313–323.
20. Scoles PV, Aronoff SC. Current concepts review: Antimicrobial therapy of childhood skeletal infections. J Bone Joint Surg 1984;66A:1487–1492.
21. Waldvogel FA, Vasey H. Osteomyelitis: The past decade. N Engl J Med 1980;303:360–370.
22. Nade S. Acute haematogenous osteomyelitis in infancy and childhood. J Bone Joint Surg 1983;65-B:109–119.
23. Ogden JA, Lister G. The pathology of neonatal osteomyelitis. Pediatrics 1975;4:474–479.
24. Curtiss PH, Klein L. Destruction of articular cartilage in septic arthritis. J Bone Joint Surg 1963;45A:797–806.
25. Morrey BF, Bianco AJ, Rhodes KH. Septic arthritis in children. Orthop Clin North Am 1975;6:923–934.
26. Welkon CJ, Long SS, Fisher MC, et al. Pyogenic arthritis in infants and children: A review of 95 cases. Pediatr Infect Dis 1986;5:669–676.
27. Zieger MM, Dorr U, Schulz RD. Ultrasonography of hip joint effusions. Skeletal Radiol 1987;16:607–611.
28. Baldassare AR, Chang F, Zuckner J. Markedly raised synovial fluid leucocyte counts not associated with infectious arthritis in children. Ann Rheum Dis 1978;37:404–409.
29. Bynum DR, Nunley JA, Goldner JL, et al. Pyogenic arthritis: Emphasis on the need for surgical drainage of the infected joint. South Med J 1982;75:1232–1235.
30. Goldenberg DL, Brandt KD, Cohen AS, et al. Treatment of septic arthritis. Comparison of needle aspiration and surgery as initial modes of joint drainage. Arth Rheun 1975;18:83–90.
31. Howard JB, Highgenboten CL, Nelson JD. Residual effects of septic arthritis in infancy and childhood. JAMA 1976;236:932–935.
32. Herndon WA, Knauer S, Sullivan JA, et al. Management of septic arthritis in children. J Pediatr Orthop 1986;6:576–578.

12

Major Multiple Trauma

Douglas A. Boenning
Simon Cooper

Major trauma is defined as a severe, potentially life-threatening injury to one body system or serious multisystem injuries. Almost every child who sustains injuries of these types will require hospitalization for operative intervention, intensive care, or close observation. The physician in the emergency department should anticipate specific patterns of injuries associated with common mechanisms of trauma (for example, high-speed motor vehicle occupant, fall from significant height) and should be prepared to manage the child during the first hour in the hospital. This management includes assessing the extent of injuries, resuscitating the child in the trauma bay, intervening for abnormal vital signs or laboratory values, and developing a general plan for the patient's care after leaving the trauma room.

Children die from injuries more than from any other cause after the first year of life. In 1985, over 317,000 U.S. children 0 to 14 years were hospitalized for injuries. That same year almost 14,000,000 children sustained injuries that required medical attention or caused at least one day of restricted activity (10).

Because of the high annual incidence of childhood trauma, the emergency physician should be prepared to manage the severely injured child. Preparation also implies institutional readiness—a fully equipped location in the Emergency Department and a coordinated response team. No health care provider alone can adequately deliver care to the child with severe injuries. A team of individuals are necessary to perform various functions in the trauma room: manage the airway, establish vascular access, obtain blood specimens, monitor and record frequent vital signs, and intervene to stabilize the child. The other half of the support team outside the trauma room should include an individual to talk with family members in a quiet room, a radiology technologist, transport personnel, a security officer, and a nursing supervisor who controls traffic and functions as coordinator of communication with consultants, the operating room, and the central laboratory. At the Children's National Medical Center in Washington, D.C., 16 people respond to "trauma stats" with subsequent assessment and stabilization of most trauma patients within 15 minutes. In the general hospital setting where adult trauma assumes the larger role, the trauma team should practice occasional drills in response to different pediatric trauma scenarios.

PATTERNS OF INJURY

While each child is an individual, injury patterns repeat themselves. Some common injury mechanisms and their outcomes are:

1. Unrestrained occupant in a motor vehicle traveling over 25 mph
   a. Closed head injury
   b. Maxillofacial trauma
   c. Cervical spine injury
   d. Blunt trauma to chest and abdomen
2. Restrained occupant of a motor vehicle traveling over 40 mph
   a. Whiplash
   b. Abdominal lap-belt injuries (abdominal contents compressed against lumbosacral spine)
   c. Lumbar spine fractures or dislocations
3. Pedestrian or cyclist struck by motor vehicle traveling over 25 mph
   a. Lower extremity fractures (femur, tibia, and fibula fractures)
   b. Deep lacerations with significant blood loss
   c. If the child is thrown into the air: skull fracture, open or closed head injury, cervical spine injuries, blunt abdominal trauma.
   d. If the child is run over: blunt chest and abdominal trauma, rib fractures, pneumothorax and pelvic fractures.
4. Fall from height greater than 10 feet
   a. Central nervous system (CNS) trauma (skull fracture, spinal cord injuries)
   b. Long bone and foot fractures
   c. Blunt abdominal trauma including injuries to the liver, spleen or kidney
5. Penetrating trauma from stabbing or firearm injury
   a. Disrupted arterial or venous blood supply
   b. Perforated viscus
   c. Pneumothorax
6. Child abuse
   a. Fractures of the ribs, skull, long bones (spiral fractures and metaphyseal chip fractures)
   b. Ecchymoses, lacerations, sphincter tears
   c. Shaken baby syndrome (unresponsive child, seizures, full fontanelle, retinal hemorrhages, intracerebral bleed)

THE INJURY EVENT AND ACTIVATION OF RESPONSE

A serious injury event occurs involving a child. Witnesses activate the emergency medical service (EMS) system; paramedics arrive and begin a field assessment and stabilization (Table 12.1). Depending on the geographic locale, the child is transported to the medical center as a "scoop and run" or a well-packaged, immobilized patient with an intravenous (IV) line established. Ideally the hospital is alerted and

Table 12.1 Pediatric trauma score

Component	+2	+1	−1
Size	>20 kg	10–20 kg	<10 kg
Airway	Normal	Maintainable	Unmaintainable
Central nervous system	Awake	Obtunded	Comatose
Systolic blood pressure	>90 mmHg	90–50 mmHg	<50 mmHg
Open wounds	None	Minor	Major or penetrating
Skeletal	None	Closed fracture	Open/multiple fracture
Palpable pulse*	At wrist	At groin	Not palpable

*Used only if a proper sized blood pressure cuff is not available.
Adapted from McCarty DL, Surpure JS. Pediatric trauma: Initial evaluation and stabilization. Pediatric Annals 1990;19:584.

given an estimated time of arrival prior to the patient's appearance. The hospital physician in charge assesses the potential severity of the child's injuries and determines the level of institutional response. For example, in the child with relatively minor injuries and stable vital signs, no loss of consciousness, or an isolated injury such as a supracondylar fracture with good distal pulse, the trauma team is not required. In the more severely injured child, the trauma team is alerted. Institutional criteria vary on when to activate the trauma team. Some of the guidelines used at the Children's National Medical Center in Washington, D.C., are included in Table 12.2.

FIRST FIVE MINUTES IN THE HOSPITAL— PRIMARY SURVEY AND RESUSCITATION

When a child arrives in the trauma bay, multiple functions take place simultaneously. A paramedic provides a concise thirty-second report. The child is immobilized on a back-board with protection of the cervical spine by an appropriately-sized collar. The patient is disrobed and personnel apply cardiorespiratory monitor leads, a blood pressure cuff and pulse oximeter. Universal precautions are taken by everyone dealing with a bleeding child, handling blood specimens, or performing phlebotomy.

First, the examining physician looks at the entire child for 5 to 10 seconds to determine the overall extent of injuries, level of consciousness, and viability of the patient. Next the physician begins a systematic approach as described by the American College of Surgeons following the mnemonic "ABCDEFGH": Airway maintenance with C-spine control, breathing, circulation with control of hemorrhage, disability (neurologic status), exposure/extremities, Foley catheter, gastric tube, history (Figure 12.1).

The primary survey (ABCDE) rapidly identifies and intervenes for life-threatening conditions. The resuscitation phase begins almost immediately: providing supplemental oxygen, obtaining vascular access, administering volume-expanding

Table 12.2 Criteria for trauma stat

1. Mechanism of injury
   a. Unrestrained occupant at speeds of 25 mph or greater
   b. Restrained occupant at speeds of 40 mph or greater
   c. Hit by vehicle at speed of at least 20 mph
   d. Occupant ejected from vehicle
   e. Fall from height of 10 feet or greater
   f. Prolonged vehicle extrication of 20 minutes of more
   g. Dragged underneath vehicle or run over by vehicle wheels
   h. Any injury requiring helicopter evacuation from the scene
2. General location of injuries
   a. Shock following injuries
   b. Respiratory distress following injuries
   c. High suspicion of C-spine injury
   d. Uncontrolled traumatic hemorrhage
   e. Open fractures
   f. Severe maxillofacial injuries
   g. Unstable chest injuries
   h. Major pelvic injuries
   i. Blunt abdominal trauma with hypotension, rigidity, or significant tenderness
   j. Penetrating wound or crush injury to the head, neck, chest, abdomen, pelvis, or groin
   k. Neurological injuries producing prolonged loss of consciousness, altered mental status, posturing, seizures, lateralizing signs, or paralysis
   l. Major amputations
   m. Fracture of long bone in association with other injuries
   n. Two or more proximal long bone fractures
   o. Tracheal and laryngeal injuries
3. Physiological distress
   a. Patients with a Trauma score of 12 or less
   b. Patients with a Glasgow Coma Scale (GCS) score of 12 or less
   c. Patients with an Injury Severity score of 15 or greater
   d. Patients with a history of respiratory or cardiopulmonary arrest following injury

fluids, and eventually completing the mnemonic "FGH" (Foley catheter, gastric tube, and history). Following the primary survey and resuscitation phase, the secondary survey includes a more thorough physical examination.

Airway with Cervical Spine Control

Assess the patency of the oropharynx. A lusty cry is a welcome sound as it implies an unobstructed airway. Suction blood, saliva, or vomitus from the mouth and throat. The tongue often falls backwards obstructing the pharynx and glottis. A jaw thrust under the angles of the mandible pushes the tongue anterior, reduces noisy respirations, and unblocks the airway.

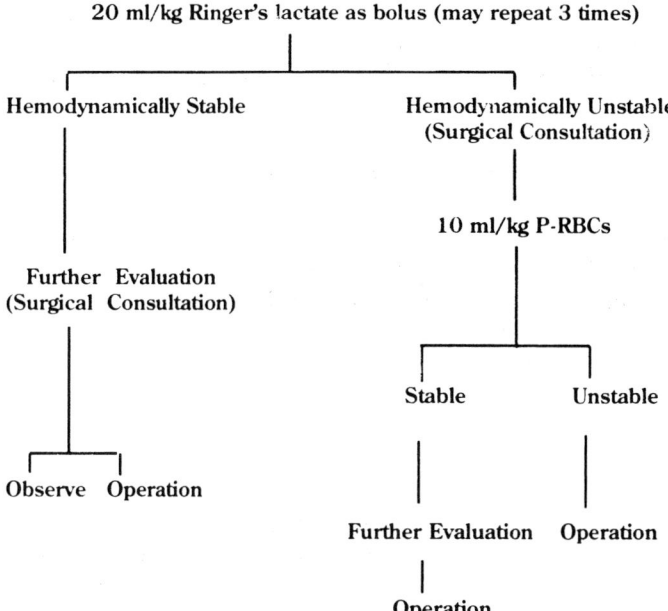

Figure 12.1 Resuscitation flow diagram for the stable and unstable pediatric patient. (Adapted from American College of Surgeons. Advanced trauma life support manual, 1989.)

If the child is already intubated, determine that a proper size endotracheal tube has been used, that it is inserted to a proper depth, and that it has minimal air leak. The endotracheal tube should be securely attached to the patient's face. Other children will require intubation based on indications discussed in the next section.

Breathing

Place 100 percent oxygen on the patient by either mask or nasal cannula. Inspect the chest for rate and regularity of breathing. Are there periods of apnea-bradypnea, periodic breathing, or Cheynes-Stokes respirations? Are chest excursions symmetric and sufficient to ventilate? Remember that infants are abdominal breathers. Auscultate air movement bilaterally noting asymmetry, decreased breath sounds, or lack of air movement. Suspect a pneumothorax when little or no air exchange is heard and there is poor chest wall movement, cyanosis, or hyperresonant percussion of the thorax. Agitation may be a sign of hypoxia. Hemothorax presents with decreased breath sounds and dullness to percussion. In the child with a suspected pneumothorax who is physiologically stable, obtain a stat chest radiograph. In the unstable patient, an emergent needle thoracentesis is performed in the fourth intercostal space at the anterior axillary line. Tube thoracostomy with continuous negative pressure is then required. If a hemothorax is suspected, make certain to establish IV access first then give adequate fluid volume prior to evacuating the chest. Any open chest wound must be covered with vaseline gauze to reestablish the integrity of the chest wall.

Patient respirations can be supported with a bag-valve mask and 100 percent oxygen. Intubation should be performed when a combination of airway, breathing, and neurologic factors are present. Any patient in uncompensated shock requires endotracheal intubation. Another common reason to intubate is ineffective respiration resulting from either mechanical or neurologic factors. Injuries or burns to the face, mouth, or neck often lead to edema and a compromised upper airway. Protecting the airway and lungs from gastric contents in the vomiting child is another indication for intubation. Intubate whenever optimum control of the airway is paramount such as in the paralyzed child (traumatically or pharmacologically) or in the child with increased intracranial pressure who requires hyperventilation. Rarely cricothyroidotomy is necessary in pediatric patients.

Circulation with Control of Bleeding

Apply pressure to any spurting or oozing wounds and maintain pressure on those areas. Assess circulation by looking at skin color and capillary refill, which should be two seconds or less. Listen to the heart to determine pulse rate, quality of heart sounds, or friction rubs. To assess the effectiveness of cardiac contractions, feel central and distal pulses on extremities.

Intravenous access is often not obtained in the field, especially in the infant or younger child. Vascular access should be obtained with the largest feasible catheter; success with a 24-gauge catheter, however, is far superior than no access at all. In infants, favored sites are antecubital fossa, saphenous, and dorsum of the hand. The external jugular vein is an alternative but is often inaccessible when the cervical spine has not been *cleared* radiologically. In the critically injured child, if percutaneous access cannot be obtained in a few minutes, consider an intraosseous route or vascular cut down. Intraosseous access is secured in the proximal tibia on the flat, medial portion two cm below the knee, aimed perpendicularly and away from the tibial growth plate. Use a bone marrow needle with stylet but remember that marrow is often not able to be aspirated, but the needle accepts manual pushes of fluid and medication. Later after volume resuscitation, the *usual* veins become more readily accessible by percutaneous attempts. A fractured leg precludes that extremity for intraosseous access. Cut-downs are best performed on saphenous or femoral veins.

Begin fluid resuscitation in the hypovolemic patient with Ringer's lactate solution at 20 cc/kg body weight. Remember that hypotension is a late sign of shock, and earlier signs (tachycardia, tachypnea, confusion, delayed capillary refill) require prompt management. If necessary, fluid boluses may be repeated three times and then whole blood (20 cc/kg) or packed cells (10 cc/kg) are administered (Figure 12.1).

Disability

Neurologic disability is briefly assessed. The level of consciousness can be categorized as *alert*, responsive to *voice*, responsive to *pain*, or unresponsive (AVPU). The Glasgow Coma Scale (GCS) (ranging from 3 to 15) scores the patient in three areas: best motor response, best verbal response, and eye opening (Table 12.3). A GCS score below 8 is predictive of serious head injury and poor outcome. In any unconscious child, the examiner should look for signs of increased intracranial pressure and of impending herniation. A more detailed neurologic evaluation can be conducted in the secondary survey.

Exposure/Extremities

The child should be completely disrobed to evaluate all regions of the body. Use trauma scissors to cut away clothing without disturbing the cervical spine or IV lines. This function should begin immediately on admission to the Trauma Room. Remember that children lose heat rapidly and need to be kept normothermic with heating lamps or warmed blankets. Extremities are examined for gross deformities, discoloration, swelling, amputations, and lacerations.

At this point the primary survey is complete. The resuscitation phase has begun. Vascular access has been established; monitoring equipment is in place; vital signs have been assessed more than once; blood specimens have been drawn; the airway has been stabilized; and the patient has been intubated if necessary. The FGH of the mnemonic is completed with Foley catheter, gastric tube, and history.

Table 12.3 Glasgow Coma Scale

Activity	Score	Infants (Best Response)	Children/Adults
Eye opening	4	Spontaneous	Spontaneous
	3	To speech or sound	To speech
	2	To painful stimuli	To pain
	1	None	None
Verbal	5	Appropriate words or sounds; social smile; fixes and follows	Oriented
	4	Cries but consolable	Confused
	3	Persistently irritable	Inappropriate words
	2	Restless/agitated	Incomprehensible words
	1	None	None
Motor	6	Spontaneous movement	Obeys commands
	5	Localizes to pain	Localizes pain
	4	Withdraws to pain	Withdraws to pain
	3	Abnormal flexion (decorticate)	Abnormal flexion (decorticate)
	2	Abnormal extension (decerebrate)	Abnormal extension (decereticate)
	1	None	None (flaccid)

Foley Catheter

Urine output is a good measure of adequate perfusion. In young children and unconscious victims, place a Foley catheter to monitor urine production (minimum 2cc/kg/hr) accurately. Gross hematuria or severe perineal ecchymoses preclude insertion of a catheter until urethral integrity can be established with an excretory urogram (IVP). Cooperative older children and adolescents may not require an indwelling bladder catheter.

Gastric Tube

A nasogastric tube should be inserted to decompress the stomach and reduce the volume of acidic fluid that could be aspirated. Bloody gastric contents are an early clue to serious abdominal injury. Use an orogastric tube if a cribriform plate fracture potentially exists.

History

Obtain additional history regarding allergies, medication, past illnesses and hospitalization, last meal, and events (mnemonic AMPLE) preceding the injury.

THE SECOND FIVE MINUTES—SECONDARY SURVEY

The secondary survey is a head-to-toe evaluation of the child. Special attention should be paid to the presence or absence of traumatic findings.

Head

Inspect the head for scalp lacerations that can bleed profusely. Is there any visible deformity or open defect? Palpate for asymmetry, depressions, defects, crepitus, and fontanelle size and tension. Large hematomas have raised edges and depressed centers, mimicking depressed skull fractures.

Eyes

Note the position of the eyelids and globes at rest along with any spontaneous movements. Determine if the globe has sustained a penetrating injury or subconjunctival hemorrhage and whether there is bleeding in the anterior chamber. A hyphema in a supine patient distributes around the limbus of the iris. Feel around the orbital rims for signs that indicate fracture such as tenderness, crepitus, or irregularity. Lid ptosis may be a preexisting condition or represent a cerebral hemispheric lesion. Spontaneous blinking indicates an intact pontine reticular formation. Provoked blinking from sound or light implies relevant sensory pathways are intact.

In the unconscious child, the eyes are a helpful gauge of CNS injury and its approximate location. Pupils should be symmetrical and reactive to bright light. Small pupils require close observation or magnification to detect reactivity. Some children have congenital anisocoria, which can explain unequal pupils in the patient without any obvious head trauma. A nonreactive, dilated pupil unilaterally raises the immediate concern of ipsilateral epidural (or subdural) bleeding requiring immediate intervention. If ipsilateral pupil dilation is associated with contralateral hemiplegia, lateral (uncal) herniation is occurring. Bilateral pupillary dilation is associated with central (tentorial) herniation, prolonged hypoxia, and brain death. Remember that some illicit drugs such as cocaine and amphetamine cause large nonreactive pupils as do pharmacologic agents such as atropine. Opiates, barbiturates, and psychotropics cause bilaterally small but reactive pupils.

An intact corneal reflex (lid closure, upward deviation of gaze) implies a normal brain stem from midbrain to lower pons. Oculocephalic (doll's eye) reflexes should never be tested until the cervical spine is deemed uninjured. Similarly oculovestibular reflexes (calorics) should not be performed if tympanic membranes are perforated. Finally the fundi should be examined for retinal hemorrhages, especially in an infant where a shaking injury is a possibility.

Ears

Look for bruising overlying the mastoid (Battle's sign), pathognomonic for basilar skull fracture (along with raccoon eyes or hemotympanum). Blood or gelatinous matter from the ear canals can be an ominous sign of CNS injury. Clear liquid in the ear canals can be spinal fluid or tears, most commonly the latter. Using an otoscope, examine the canal and tympanic membranes, noting perforations or hemotympanum. Hemotympanum has a subtle blue-purple hue rather than bright red. A red, injected tympanic membrane implies infection, a coincidental finding that may explain the presence of fever in many traumatized infants and preschool-aged children.

Nose and Mouth

Are cartilage and nasion aligned or misshapen? Is blood or cerebrospinal fluid (CSF) leaking from nostrils? Are nares patent? A septal hematoma will require evacuation.

The gums, lips, and tongue bleed readily and clot slowly. Attempt to determine the source of any blood loss from the oropharynx. Examine teeth for excess mobility, pain, crown fractures, and intrusions. Completely avulsed teeth can become foreign bodies in the mouth or airway. Disrupted orthodontic hardware in an adolescent may cause bleeding inside the lips as well as great anxiety to the patient and parents. A sublingual hematoma is associated with a midline mandibular fracture. Palpate the temporomandibular joint for tenderness and subluxation on movement.

Neck

If lateral cervical spine films do not rule out fracture, dislocation, compression, or subluxation, leave the collar in place. The radiograph should be reviewed by the treating physician and should expose the complete cervical spine and first thoracic vertebrae. If spinal cord injury without radiologic abnormality (SCIWORA) is suspected, leave the collar in place. Pseudosubluxation of C_2 on C_3 is a common finding in children. When the collar is removed, palpate the cervical spine for irregularities or pain. Often the sternocleidomastoid muscles are sore after a whiplash event. If discomfort cannot be isolated to the strap muscles only, replace the collar until more definitive studies can be performed, including open mouth views, swimmer's view, and/or computed tomography (CT).

Chest

An anteroposterior (AP) chest radiograph should be performed in all patients to detect bony injuries and pulmonary or cardiac problems. Palpate the length of both clavicles for deformity or crepitus often found in falls and sports injuries. Rib fractures may present with point tenderness but are unusual because the chest wall is so compliant in children. When rib fractures are present, large forces have impacted the thorax. In one study of blunt chest trauma, the presence of four or more rib fractures had a high correlation with mortality.

Heart

Reassess heart sounds. If the heart sounds muffle, neck veins distend, and pulsus paradoxus occurs (exaggerated drop in systolic blood pressure during inspiration), consider the possibility of cardiac tamponade. Tamponade is rare in children but should be considered when there has been a direct blow to the chest or any penetrating thoracic injury. Pericardiocentesis is performed with a plastic-sheathed needle entering subxyphoid and aiming toward the heart. A positive pericardiocentesis necessitates open thoracotomy.

Abdomen

Inspect the abdominal wall for distention and ecchymoses. A horizontal band of bruising can occur in the vehicle occupant wearing a lap belt and provides a clue to underlying injury. Similarly ecchymoses on the left or right upper quadrant can indicate spleen or liver lacerations respectively. Listen for the presence of bowel sounds. Palpate for tenderness in each quadrant and flanks. Push downward simultaneously on the anterior iliac spines to check the stability of the pelvic rim in addition to palpating the pubic ramus. Bladder injuries are commonly associated with pelvic fractures. Obtain a urine sample to determine whether hematuria is present; hematuria is defined as greater than ten red blood cells per high power field on microscopy.

Penetrating trauma to the abdomen with violation of the peritoneum will require exploration in the operating room.

Genitalia/Rectum

Look at the integrity of external genitalia. If bruising, swelling, or burns have affected the area, insert an indwelling Foley catheter before a urethral obstruction occurs. Perform a digital rectal examination for anal sphincter tone and detection of blood (obvious or occult) in the stool.

Extremities

Obtain AP radiographs of suspected limb fractures. Immobilize arms and legs with suspected fractures and determine the integrity of distal pulses. Absence of distal pulses should prompt a gentle attempt to realign the limb and an urgent arteriogram. A displaced femoral fracture presents with a painful swollen thigh that can hold a significant volume of blood. When a lower leg is broken, tibia and fibula are both commonly affected. If the patient was transported in traction or antishock trousers, use these devices for splinting and immobilization until definitive orthopedic care is rendered.

FURTHER DIAGNOSTIC STUDIES

In the trauma bay, the treating physician must determine which additional studies and consultations are necessary. All children deserve radiographs of lateral cervical spine, AP chest, and AP pelvis. Any limb deformity should also be radiographed. Additional plain films are indicated to evaluate the lumbosacral spine in children with lap belt injuries. Maxillofacial injuries can be delineated with plain radiographs.

In any child in whom vascular integrity has been compromised, consider contrast angiography. This modality is particularly helpful in penetrating injuries.

CT scans are important diagnostic studies that are invaluable in assessing head injuries and blunt abdominal trauma. Any child with a suspected skull fracture, loss of consciousness, or ongoing coma requires a CT scan of the head. With questionable findings on plain films, a CT can clarify issues surrounding the cervical spine.

Serious abdominal trauma occurs in one quarter of all multiply traumatized children. Peritoneal lavage, used more frequently in adult victims, has been supplanted by CT scans in children. While deep peritoneal lavage can be performed quickly in the trauma room, it is a nonspecific test, unable to pinpoint the origin of bleeding. (Any deep penetrating injury will require operative intervention no matter what.) The CT identifies specific organs injured and the extent of their damage. Many organ injuries such as liver lacerations and splenic hematomas are treated expectantly, and the CT provides a baseline assessment to which further studies can be compared. Indications for CT scans of the abdomen include: (1) localizing signs to the abdominal examination—abdominal pain, distention, absence of bowel sounds; (2) a hematuria of greater than 10 red blood cells per high power field (RBC/hpf) or blood in the stool; (3) an unconscious child with mechanism of injury consistent with abdominal trauma; (4) pelvic fracture; or (5) abused child with suspected abdominal injury.

The final role of the physician in the trauma bay is to coordinate consultations with subspecialists and help in reaching a decision regarding the hospital disposition of the patient. Invaluable consultants include all of the surgical subspecialties: orthopedics, neurosurgery, cardiothoracic surgery, urology, plastic surgery, ophthalmology, and oral surgery. Orthopedists are frequently needed in approximately one third of cases to provide definitive care of injured bones and joints following resuscitation and stabilization phases. Urgent orthopedic consultation is necessary with open fractures and loss of distal pulses resulting from fractures. The trauma physician should remember to administer tetanus toxoid and antibiotics to any child with an open fracture. When a neurosurgeon is required, it is often on a *stat* basis for such injuries as penetrating skull wound, depressed skull fracture, severe closed-head injury or spinal cord trauma. If the child demonstrates signs of increased intracranial pressure and impending herniation, the trauma physician must intervene immediately by elevating the head of the bed to 30°, intubating the patient, hyperventilating, and giving an osmotic diuretic to reduce brain swelling. If these temporizing measures do not work, the neurosurgeon may be required to reduce pressure with a burr hole prior to intervention in the operating room.

There are four general dispositions for the child who survives in the trauma room: operative intervention, intensive care unit (ICU), admission to a general ward or discharge home. The latter occurs infrequently and is generally not recommended. For the stable child with an isolated injury, a minimum of 24 hours of in-hospital observation is recommended. For the child with unstable vital signs following volume resuscitation, especially following a blood transfusion exceeding half the estimated blood volume, the child should be explored in the operating room to locate sites of hemorrhage and to control them. Open limb fractures, most depressed skull fractures, extensive lacerations and tendon injuries, orthopedic pinnings, and definitive thoracic and abdominal injury repair—all require transfer to the operating suite. The child who is stable following initial resuscitation in the trauma bay but who has sustained serious injuries with the potential for deterioration requires admission to an ICU with close nursing observation.

The "golden hour" begins at the time of injury, so it is important to transfer the seriously injured child to a regional trauma center promptly. A rapid response from a coordinated team of individuals assesses the extent of injuries, resuscitates the child, stabilizes vital signs, calls appropriate consultants, and arranges for the best hospital disposition of the child.

SUGGESTED READING

1. American College of Surgeons Committee on Trauma. Advanced Trauma Life Support Course for Physicians, Chicago, 1984.
2. Boenning DA, Taylor GA, Eichelberger MR. Role of computed tomography in evaluating abdominal injury of children. Emergency Pediatrics 1989;2:3–5.

3. Cooper A, Floyd T, Barlow B, et al. Major blunt abdominal trauma due to child abuse. J Trauma 1988;28:1483.
4. Eichelberger MR, Pratsch GL, eds. Pediatric trauma care. Rockville, Md.: Aspen, 1988.
5. Eichelberger, MR, Randolph JG. Progress in pediatric trauma world. J of Surg 1985;9:222.
6. Garcia VF, Gotschall CS, Eichelberger MR, et al. Rib fractures in children: A marker of severe trauma. J Trauma 1990;30:695.
7. Jaffe D. Wesson D. Emergency management of blunt trauma in children. N Engl J Med 1991;324:1477.
8. McCarty DL, Surpure JS. Pediatric trauma: Initial evaluation and stabilization. Pediatric Annals 1990;19:584.
9. Peclet MH, Newman KD, Eichelberger MR, et al. Patterns of injury in children. J Ped Surg 1990;25:85.
10. Rice DP, MacKenzie EJ and Associates. Cost of injury in the United States: A report to Congress. San Francisco; Institute for Health and Aging, University of California, and Baltimore: Injury Prevention Center, John Hopkins University, 1989.
11. Taylor GA, Eggli KD. Lap-belt injuries of the lumbar spine in children: A pitfall in CT diagnosis. Am J Radiology 1988;150:1355.
12. Young GM, Klein BL, Ochsenschlager DW, et al. The child with multiple injuries: Resuscitation priorities. Indian Journal of Pediatrics 1988;55:705.

13

Head Trauma

David J. Gower

Injury to the pediatric brain is common and ranges in severity from a minor bump on the head in an infant who falls to a teenager involved in motor vehicle accident with severe brain injury. Over one million children suffer from head injury each year, and one in ten adults have suffered head injury resulting in unconsciousness at some time during their childhood. Goldstein and Levin review some of the methodological errors inherent in the study of pediatric head trauma (1). These errors primarily involve improper or incomplete coding of charts that leads to an underestimation of the rate of injury. Perhaps the incidence of pediatric head trauma, particularly that associated with other types of injury, is far greater than is presently reported.

In all age groups, the rate of injury is greater for males than it is for females, but this difference is greatest for the adolescent. The mechanism of head injury varies depending on the age of the child. In patients under one year of age, automobile passenger-related trauma and falls around the home account for 87.8 percent of injuries. In the age group of five to nine years, pedestrian accidents become the most prominent mechanism of trauma, accounting for 39.3 percent of injuries. In the teenage years, the motor vehicle accident far outnumbers all other forms of injury and accounts for 51.8 percent of head traumas (1).

If persons at risk for head trauma could be identified from the general population, targeted preventive measures could be developed. To this end, researchers attempted to identify premorbid factors that would predict patients at risk for closed-head injury. While male gender, poor school performance, previous head trauma, low socioeconomic status, and living in congested areas have all been suggested as associated with an increased risk of head injury, there is no clear consensus with respect to these factors at the present time.

PATHOPHYSIOLOGY
Scalp Lacerations

Lacerations of the scalp are among the most common types of tissue injuries following trauma to the head. The scalp is a very vascular structure made up of five layers that include: *s*kin, sub*c*utaneous tissue, *a*poneurosis, *l*oose areolar tissue, and the *p*ericranium (SCALP). The large vessels that supply the scalp run just above the galea aponeurosis, and injury to this layer may result in significant blood loss. Debris from the accident site, as well as hair or clothing, may become entangled in the wound and should be removed meticulously prior to wound closure.

In rare instances, an injury to the scalp may lead to bleeding into the subgaleal space. The degree of trauma may be very minor or completely unrecognized by the patient. In one report, a child had her head against the window of a car that hit a bump and subsequently developed a doughy swelling of the scalp. The area of swelling associated with the subgaleal hematoma may be variable and is frequently associated with a headache. In general, time is the cure for these lesions, and no attempt to tap the fluid should be made since they frequently reaccumulate and, if infected, may lead to very serious complications (2).

Skull Fracture

In almost all cases, a simple fracture of the skull (Figure 13.1) will heal with time. This is because the edges of the fracture are naturally fixed into rigid approximation by the very nature of the skull itself and very little is necessary to promote the proper union of the bony edges. The significance of a skull fracture is as a marker of the amount of energy that was applied to the patient's head. A large amount of concentrated force is necessary to crack both tables of the skull, and one must be concerned about the amount of this energy that was transmitted to underlying structures. Thus the fracture may be an indication of a more severe injury to the brain.

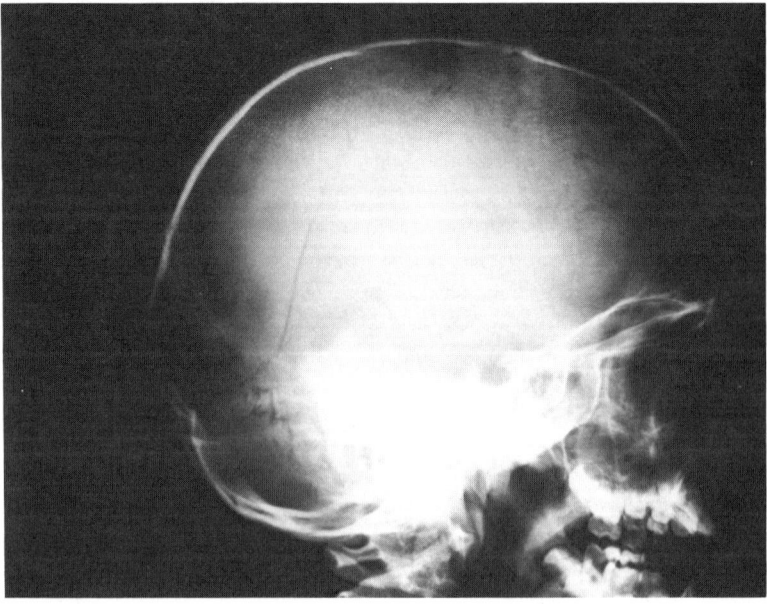

Figure 13.1 Photograph of a simple linear skull fracture.

In all skull fractures, the dura, which is closely approximated to the inner table of the skull, may be lacerated. In the older child, this will result in some collection of cerebrospinal fluid (CSF) under the galea, which will usually heal. In the child less than two years old, the dural laceration may result in herniation of the leptomeninges into the bony cleft. In this group of young children, the brain is growing at a very rapid rate, and the bony edges may not have time to heal properly before the leptomeningeal cyst pushes them apart. The growth and pulsation of the brain will lead to a growing skull fracture or leptomeningeal cyst. Repair of these cysts can be very difficult if they are left to grow to large size. The child less than two years old with a skull fracture should be closely followed to ensure that the fracture indeed closes as expected and does not progress to a growing cyst.

Depressed Skull Fracture

The depressed skull fracture (Figure 13.2) is quite a different entity from the simple skull fracture and more frequently requires surgical repair. Usually the injury is related to a focal area of force applied and may follow a hammer blow or a steering wheel across the forehead. The skin over the injury site may be open, closed, contused,

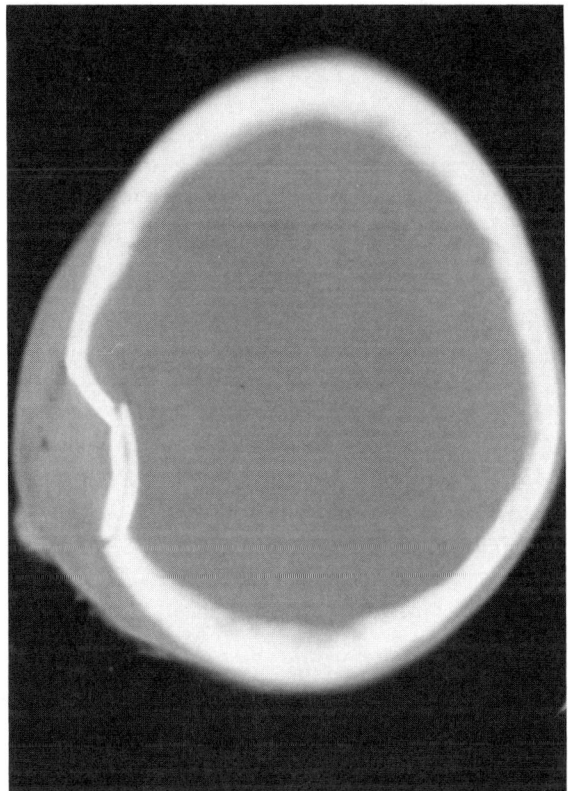

Figure 13.2 Compound depressed skull fracture caused by a hammer blow.

or absent. Brain may be present in the wound, or on rare occasions, severe cortical bleeding from a lacerated artery or vein may also be present. All depressed skull fractures should be evaluated by a surgical specialist to determine the extent of injury and the appropriateness of surgical decompression and repair. Minor depressions of the skull, less than bone skull thickness, may be observed since they will heal in a manner similar to a simple skull fracture. The more complicated injuries usually will require vigorous debridement and closure. In those injuries with exposed brain, the wound should be covered with a saline-soaked gauze to prevent drying of the brain prior to surgical repair.

In the very young child, the skull is more flexible, and the forces that would cause a fracture in an adult may only dimple the skull in the child. These injuries appear as a relatively large, smooth depression on the head. These injuries are surgically correctable in most cases, and the possibility of repair should be addressed.

Basilar Skull Fracture

Fractures of the skull through the base are not well seen on plain X-ray films but should always be considered in patients with head trauma. In these patients, the fracture almost always heals without surgical intervention except in the most severe cases. The factor that differentiates the basilar skull fracture from a fracture over the convexity of the brain is the associated structures that run through the base of the skull. Injury to the cranial nerves, vascular structures, or basilar dura may be disabling or in some cases fatal.

The carotid artery enters the base of the skull deep to the temporo-mandibular joint. The artery runs medially and emerges into the cavernous sinus. Approximately four to five cm of the artery is encased within the bone at the base of the skull, and a fracture across this bone may lacerate the artery. If this occurs, one of two things happens: (1) The blood will have nowhere to flow, and pressure on the artery will lead to a spontaneous thrombosis. (2) The other, and more likely, possibility is violent bleeding into the space of the middle ear and subsequent hemorrhage through the eardrum. Although uncommon, it is certainly not unheard of to have a traumatized patient die from bleeding through the ear. Usually this happens in a rapidly progressive injury that leaves little time for surgical control of the carotid at both ends.

All of the cranial nerves pass through the skull base and are at risk for injury from basilar skull fractures. Because of the anatomy of this region, some of the nerves are more commonly affected. A fracture through the anterior cranial fossa with injury to the olfactory apparatus will result in loss of the sense of smell. This is a far greater disability than one may consider at first. A large portion of the appreciation of taste is due to the sense of smell, and most people with total anosmia will complain of a loss of the taste of food.

Anterior fossa fractures may also lead to injury to the optic nerves or the nerves of ocular control passing through the superior orbital fissure. Probably the most commonly injured cranial nerves are the seventh, leading to a facial paralysis, and the eighth, leading to a sensorineural hearing loss. In the traumatized patient, the seventh nerve may also develop a delayed dysfunction, and therefore it is very important to document careful examination of facial movement. Injury to the lower cranial nerves, passing through the jugular or hypoglossal foramen, is relatively uncommon.

Fractures of bone usually lead to venous bleeding from the diploe. Basilar skull fractures are no exception to this rule, but the blood will pool in the subcutaneous tissues in very characteristic places. In the soft tissue behind the ear, the occurrence of blood accumulation and bruising is known as *battle sign* and accumulation in the periorbital region is known as *racoon sign*. Either of these signs should alert the clinician to the possibility of a basilar fracture and suggest the need for a careful cranial nerve examination as well as a computerized tomography (CT) scan with bone windowing.

Cerebrospinal Fluid Leak

At the base of the skull, the dura is applied tightly to the bony structure in a number of places. This relatively tight application of dura leaves it at risk for tear should a bony fracture occur. If the leptomeninges are torn, CSF may leak out through the fracture. Several pathways of CSF egress from the skull base are available. The fluid may leak into the air-containing sinuses and subsequently into the nasopharynx, resulting in rhinorrhea. Another major pathway of CSF flow is through the mastoid or floor of the middle fossa into the middle ear where it may pass through a ruptured tympanic membrane, producing otorrhea, or through the eustachian tube into the nasopharynx. In most cases, a CSF leak will stop within two weeks but should be watched carefully. The use of prophylactic antibiotics for this type of injury is controversial. On one side, advocates suggest that the bacterial flora is reduced by the use of such antibiotics and with it the risk of infection. Those opposed to antibiotic usage suggest that they encourage resistance without protection, and if a meningitis were to result from a CSF leak, the organism is more difficult to treat.

CSF leakage should be addressed and followed by a specialist who may elect to either drain CSF with a lumbar catheter or opt for surgical repair of the site of leakage.

Mass Lesions

The cranium is a closed space in which only a limited amount of volume may accumulate. The layers of the skull above the brain are the arachnoid, which contains the CSF, the dura, and the skull. Blood may accumulate in each of these areas, and the radiology and clinical syndromes are usually distinct.

The dura is loosely attached to the inner table of the skull. Blood accumulations must dissect the dura away from the skull in order to produce the characteristic lens shape seen on the CT scan associated with the epidural hematoma. Blood accumulation may be from venous sources as is the case with the skull fracture and bleeding from the diploe. The more characteristic source of blood causing the epidural hematoma is arterial. The middle meningeal artery runs within the structure of the temporal bone and in the first part of its course may be completely surrounded by bony investiture. Fracture of the bone across this bony canal will commonly lacerate the artery and cause a hematoma under pressure. This rapid accumulation of blood is the reason for the classical lucent period following head trauma prior to the onset of unconsciousness. In general, the relatively focal nature of the epidural and mechanism of injury leading to less diffuse brain trauma herald a better outcome than would be expected with other forms of hematoma accumulation.

If the small bridging vessels of the subdural space are torn, a subdural hematoma results. The plane of dissection for this blood is along a path of much less resistance than that for the epidural hematoma and leads to the characteristic crescent shape seen on the CT scan. In general, the outcome from a subdural hematoma is worse, perhaps because of associated brain trauma. The bleeding source, like in the epidural, may be either venous or arterial, and the clinical course will vary depending on the rapidity of mass lesion formation.

Bleeding may also occur within the parenchyma of the brain as seen in Figure 13.3. The classical areas to form posttraumatic hematomas are in the basal frontal lobes or in the temporal lobes. The reason for this characteristic location of these clots is unclear but may well be related to the surrounding bony structures. The frontal

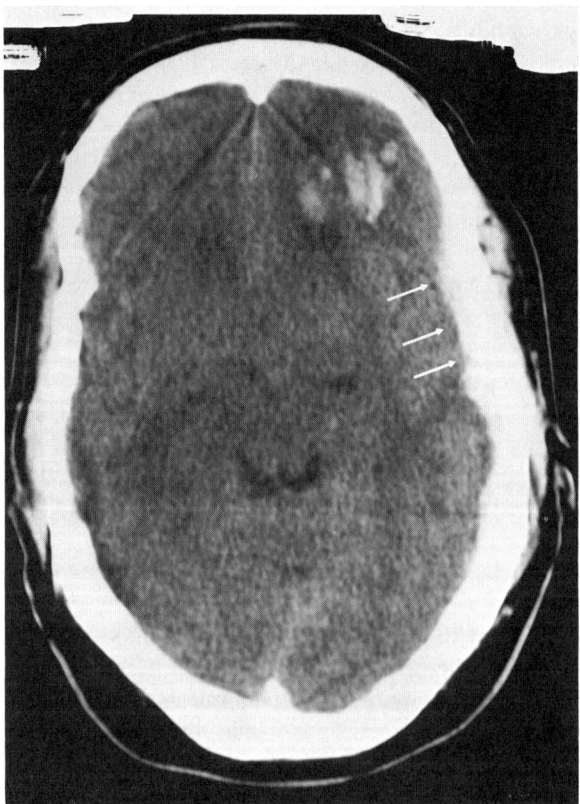

Figure 13.3 Small subdural hematoma (arrows) and associated intracerebral hematoma.

lobes sit on an irregular surface that may easily contuse them, and the temporal lobes sit within the confines of the middle fossa and have very little room for travel before encountering the bony edges. It is not uncommon in the traumatized brain to observe injury in one area of the brain with a similar injury directly across the head called a contra coup injury. Parenchymal bleeding may extend into the subarachnoid space or into the ventricles that may occasionally lead to acute hydrocephalus by obstruction of the outflow pathways and that therefore should be carefully watched.

Penetrating Trauma

Penetration of the layers of the brain and even of the brain itself by foreign material comes in all shapes and sizes, from the radio knob imbedded in the frontal lobes (Figure 13.4) to a piece of gravel just under the skull (Figure 13.5). Penetrating trauma should be dealt with as with any other form of head trauma. A CT scan is essential to determine the extent of injury and associated hematomas. In addition, an arteriogram may be indicated in some patients where major vascular structures are at risk by the missile as the laceration of the anterior portion of the superior sagittal sinus

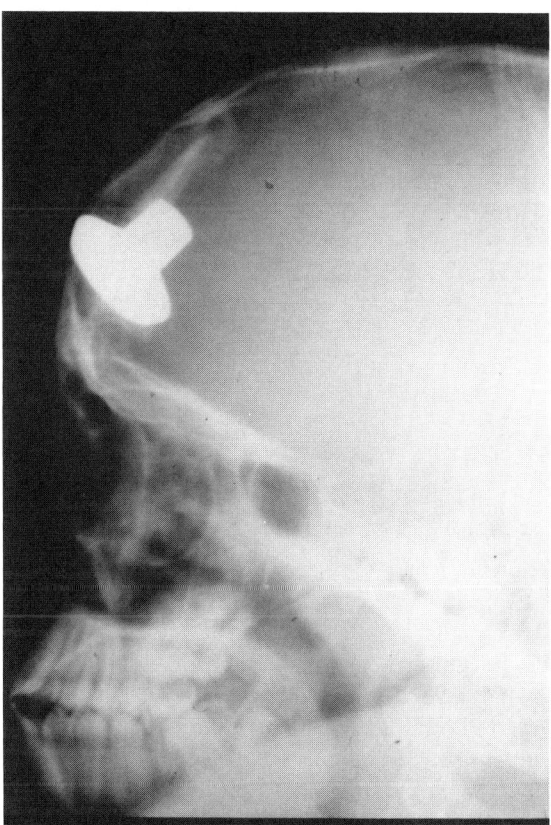

Figure 13.4 Photograph of a radio knob foreign body in the skull of a young child involved in a motor vehicle accident.

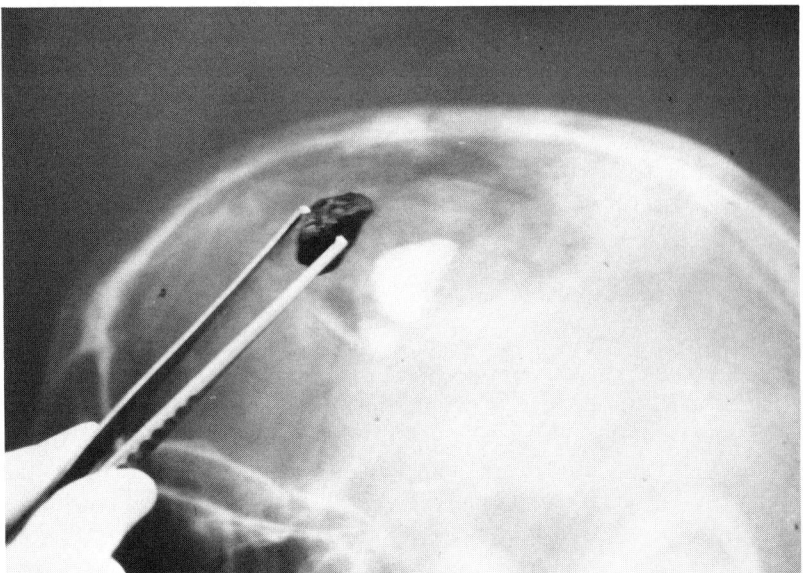

Figure 13.5 Photomicrograph of gravel removed from the skull of this child involved in a motorcycle accident.

in the patient seen in Figure 13.6. The foreign body should not be "pulled out" until adequate control of the injury site is available. In most cases, the missile should be removed only in the operating room with blood available for immediate transfusion. Even the most innocent looking thing sticking out of someone's head that beckons from across the room to "pull me out" should be avoided. Laceration of a major dural sinus may bleed profusely or allow air entry into this area, causing a major air embolism that could be more easily controlled in the operating room.

Concussion

The syndrome of concussion following impact injury to the head is poorly appreciated. Many patients are seen on a single visit and sent home after being found to be neurologically intact. Experimental studies have demonstrated disruption of axonal fibers following even relatively minor trauma. Many of the patients will develop headaches, concentration or memory problems, or dizziness that may persist for weeks or even several months. Imaging studies of the brain may show minor changes on magnetic resonance imaging (MRI) or be normal, yet some patients will experience problems with their jobs and other activities that require concentration. Reassurance and time are the only treatment, but alerting the patient to the possibility of a postconcussion syndrome and the need for follow-up is very important in avoiding problems that may develop.

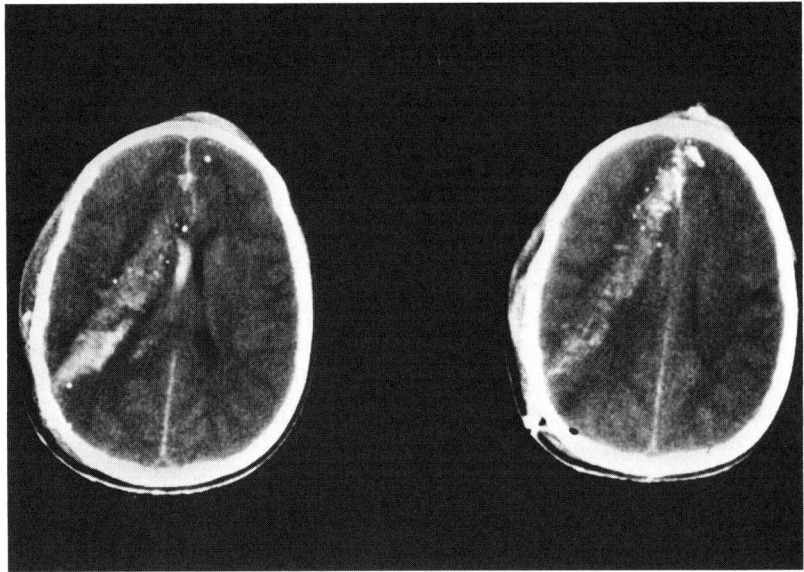

Figure 13.6 Gunshot wound in the head of this teenager with associated in-driven bone.

Closed-Head Trauma

The skull is a closed space that will only contain a constant volume of material. If mass is added to the intracranial contents, some natural compensation mechanisms will allow shifting of CSF into the vascular space and compression of the large venous structures. When mechanisms of compensation are exhausted and volume continues to be added to the intracranial compartment, the net effect will be an increase in pressure.

Cerebral perfusion depends on an adequate arterial pressure to force blood through the brain vasculature. An increase in the intracranial pressure above the mean arterial pressure will effectively stop the flow of blood into the brain and result in death of the tissue. In all cases, the cerebral perfusion must be protected, which can be most easily accomplished by maintaining intracranial pressure (ICP) below 20 mmHg.

The term *closed head trauma* implies an injury that does not penetrate the covering of the brain. The trauma may have been severe enough to cause intracerebral hemorrhage or subarachnoid bleeding, but the main pathophysiology of the injury is a concussive force. If energy is delivered to the CNS at these levels, areas of dysautoregulation of blood flow will develop. These areas will subsequently change their blood flow in response to the blood pressure and not in response to $PaCO_2$ and will subsequently produce mass by their enlarged vascular space. Control of the patient's blood pressure and intracranial pressure is essential in bringing about a good outcome. Early control of ICP may help reduce the amount of injury that the patient experiences.

CLINICAL PRESENTATION

The approach to the traumatized patient is summarized in the algorithm in Figure 13.7. The typical patient presents to the emergency department with a history of trauma and has an altered level of consciousness that alerts the clinician to the possibility of a head trauma. A variety of factors may contribute to the alteration of mentation and should be ruled out before the diagnosis of brain injury is made. In many traumatic situations, the patient may develop hypotension from a variety of causes that may be unrelated to a head injury. The basic ABCs (airway, breathing, circulation) of life support should be followed first to ensure adequate oxygenation of the blood and adequate blood pressure. The patient's body temperature may also effect the level of consciousness and should be taken into consideration (3,4).

Following the initial evaluation of the patient's status, the potential for toxic substances, most notably alcohol, causing an altered mental status should be considered as well as the serum glucose. These simple tests should be followed by more time-consuming toxicology screens. If these initial tests fail to demonstrate a reason for the patient's altered mental status, a diagnosis of head injury should be entertained.

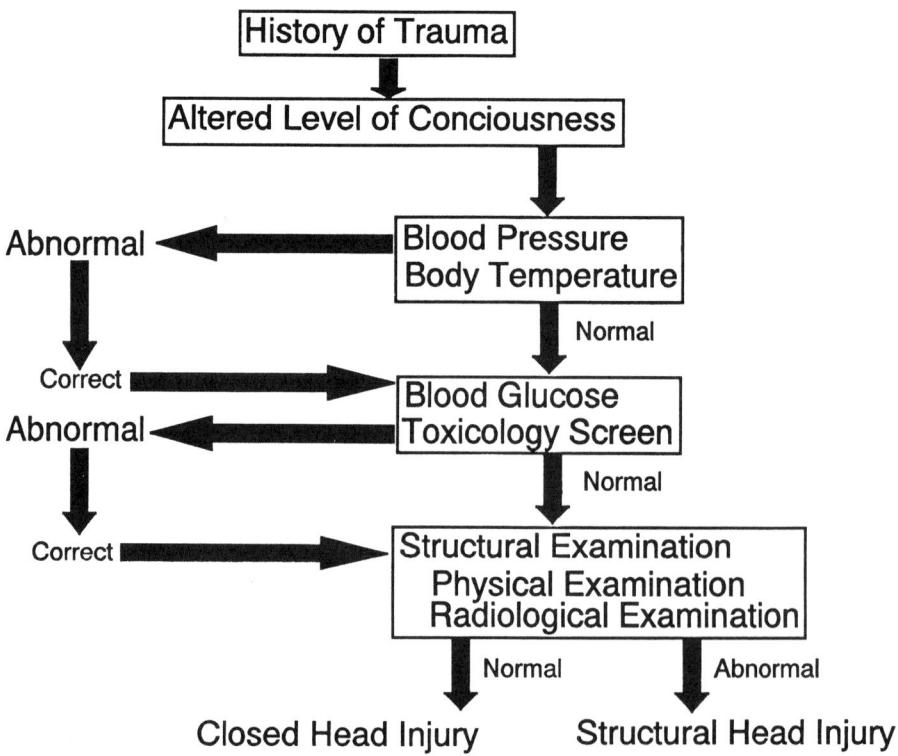

Figure 13.7 Algorithm for clinical presentation of the head-injured child.

HISTORY AND PHYSICAL

The history and physical are very important in the assessment of the patient with closed head trauma. The points of history that are most important are an assessment of the story that gives some idea of the amount of energy that the patient received during the trauma and how that energy was directed to various areas of the body. The initial response of the patient to the injury and at-the-scene reports of the patient's mental status are important in assessing the progression of the head trauma. If the patient was confused at the scene and is now normal, there is less reason for concern than there is with a patient in a reverse scenario. Detailed medical history is frequently unavailable during the initial assessment of the patient, and associated medical conditions such as insulin-dependant diabetes may not be known.

The physical examination should begin with a simple assessment of the ABCs of life support. During this assessment, some idea of the patient's mental status will be developed. A more formal assessment of the level of consciousness should follow using the Glasgow Coma Scale (GCS). Patients are felt to have a severe head injury if the GCS score is 8 or less. A minor head injury is felt to be a GCS score of 13 to 15. These classifications give some information about the intensity of therapy that will be required to treat the head injury and about the eventual outcome.

External examination of the patient may include an assessment of the cranial nerves to determine any dysfunction associated with a basilar skull fracture. The potential CSF leak or scalp laceration should be evaluated and ruled out.

Lacerations of the scalp are usually examined externally by palpation. This helps to find foreign bodies in the wound and to explore the possibility of a skull fracture. It is not uncommon that swelling of the pericranium may fool even the experienced examiner into thinking a fracture of the skull exists where none is present. CT scanning should be carried out on any patient with a suspicious wound to determine the integrity of the skull and the extent of injury to the underlying brain.

LABORATORY AND RADIOLOGY

Laboratory evaluation is essential to the evaluation of any patient who has undergone a major trauma. Blood counts and chemistries, arterial blood gasses and serum alcohol levels are done as mentioned above. In the brain-traumatized patient, routine clotting studies (PT [prothrombin time] and PTT [partial thromboplastin time]) should also be performed. When severe injury to the brain occurs, factors released into the blood will lead to a fulminant disseminated intravascular coagulopathy. This complication is a hallmark of a very bad outcome and indicates the degree of brain injury that may be present.

Computed axial tomography (CAT or CT for short) of the brain is the most important radiological evaluation to be performed. This test will help determine the presence of a surgically removable mass lesion or identify a patient with an injury more severe than clinical examination indicated and will require expectant observation. The use of contrast infusion dye in these patients is rarely indicated. The objective of the study is to identify intracranial blood, bone fragments, or foreign bodies—all of which will be high density on the study and not enhanced by contrast dye for up to 72 hours. The dye load from an infused CT scan is quite large and may compound renal injuries, particularly if the patient also received dye for renal examinations.

There is some controversy over the usefulness of plain skull films. The most important component of the radiological examination following trauma is the effect of the energy on the brain. This effect is imaged most effectively using CT scanning. The CT also has the advantage of imaging fractures at the base of the skull and depressed fractures better than can be seen on plain X-rays. For almost all types of head trauma, the CT scan provides more information than do plain skull films, but in limited instances (associated mandible or facial fractures) skull films may be indicated in addition to CT scanning.

The head is a relatively heavy object on a small flexible stalk. The patient with a serious head trauma should also have routine cervical spine X-rays to rule out associated injury. In the child with a relatively disproportionate head mass, associated injury to the cervical spine should always be suspected.

MANAGEMENT

In order to feel comfortable and perform adequately when presented with a patient with a severe head injury, it is important to have a clear scheme prepared to evaluate and treat a severe head trauma (5,6). The initial evaluation scheme for the patient with a traumatic coma has already been discussed in this chapter. The management scheme described in Figure 13.8. takes into account patients with a variety of both closed and open injuries.

A concise protocol for the control of intracranial pressure is a cornerstone to the development of a personal protocol for the management of trauma (7) (Figure 13.9). The most effective method of ICP control is through control of the patient's airway by the use of hyperventilation. Return of CO_2 to normal or reduction of CO_2 into a range of 25 to 30 mmHg will provide the greatest effect on the cerebral volume and subsequently on the ICP. In those patients where ICP control continues to be a problem, the use of an osmotic agent such as mannitol given intravenously (.75 to 1.0 g/kg) followed by a dose of furosemide (1.0 mg/Kg) will provide an effective next step in the control of ICP. The use of mannitol in a patient with inadequate control of the airway or in a patient who is hypoventilating is ineffective. Paralytic agents or narcotic analgesics administered to the patient following a thorough examination will increase the effectiveness of external ventilation efforts. The use of barbiturates in control of ICP may not be indicated in the acutely traumatized patient because of the adverse effects on the cardiovascular system and the resulting hypotension.

In some cases, neurological deterioration continues to occur despite adequate attempts to control ICP and may tempt one to drill exploratory holes to find the clot. There is little indication for exploratory burr holes in the emergency setting without adequate CT localization of a mass lesion. Surgical lesions are best dealt with in the operating room where adequate anesthesia is available to support the patient if a life-threatening event, in the form of hemorrhage or an air embolism, should occur.

Finally a CT scan of the head is a snapshot in time, and while the patient may be in the early evolution of a mass lesion at the time of the CT, that may not be

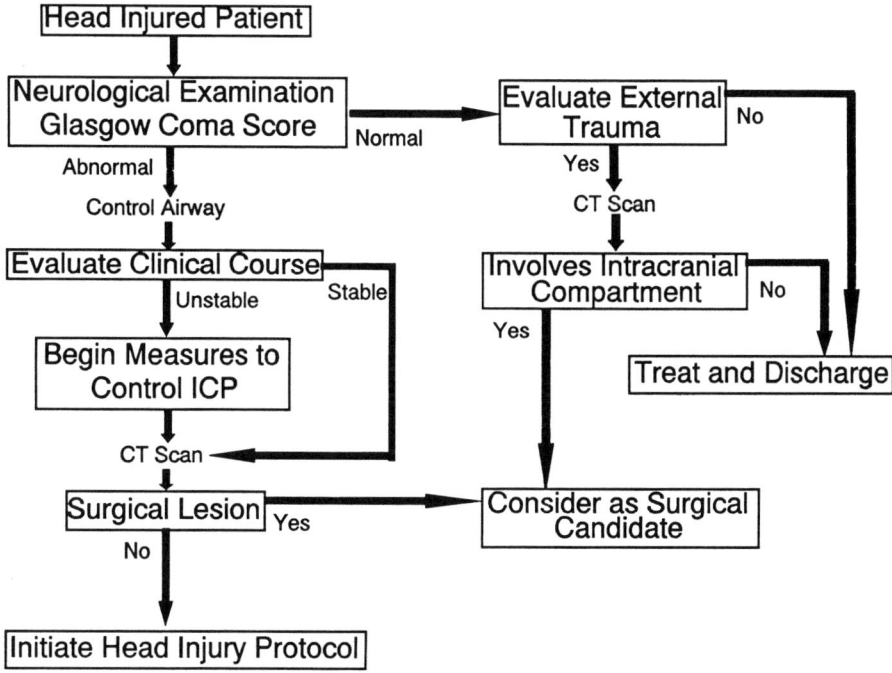

Figure 13.8 Algorithm for the management of the head-injured child.

adequately appreciated. If the patient continues to deteriorate or if focal lesions develop while the patient is undergoing evaluation for other injuries, one should not hesitate to repeat the CT scan to look for a change. Most commonly this scenario occurs when the patient is transferred to the hospital after obtaining a CT scan that is "normal" at another facility.

CONCLUSIONS

The process of handling head trauma in the traumatized child is constantly improving. Patient stabilization, transportation, and diagnostic capabilities have all contributed to better outcome (8). A thorough understanding and a plan in the mind of the pediatric emergency department physician in the form of "What would I do if

---

Elevate head of bed 30 percent to improve venous drainage
Control airway, hyperventilate to a $PaCO_2$ of 25 to 30 mmHg
Avoid circumfrensial taping of the endotracheal tube.
Restrict fluids to 75 percent maintenance

Osmotic agents, (mannitol .75 to 1.0 g/Kg IV [intravenous])
Sedation
Barbiturates

Figure 13.9 Steps for control of ICP.

a head-injured child presents at the doors right now?" is what has been summarized in this chapter as well as some points that may help in the assessment and treatment of the head-injured child.

REFERENCES

1. Goldstein FC, Levin HS. Epidemiology of pediatric closed head injury: Incidence, clinical characteristics, and risk factors. J Learning Disabilities 1987;20(9):518–525.
2. Kirkpatrick J, Gower DJ, Kelly DL Jr. et al. Subgaleal hematomas in children. Child Develop Ped Neurol 1986;28:506–514.
3. Sanford RA: Minor head injuries in children. Seminars in Neurology 1988;8(1):108–114.
4. Bullock R, Teasdale G. Head injuries. Br Med J 1990;300:1515–1518.
5. Pascucci RC. Head trauma in the child-review article. Intensive Care Medicine 1988;14:185–195.
6. Duncan CC, Ment LR. Head injury: Management in children. Conn Med 1988;52(6):331–334.
7. Gower DJ, Lee KS, McWhorter M. The role of subtemporal decompression in control of posttraumatic increased intracranial pressure. Neurosurgery 1988;23:417–423.
8. Bruce DA. Head injuries in the pediatric population. Curr Probl Pediatrics 1990;20(2):61–107.

14

Abdominal Trauma

E. Stevers Golladay
Dileep R. Vyas

Trauma is the leading cause of death in children aged 1 through 14 years. Blunt abdominal trauma occurs frequently and is second to head trauma as a cause of death in childhood accidents, but it is responsible for the majority of preventable deaths. Abdominal trauma is frequently associated with other injuries, and this combination tests the diagnostic and therapeutic skills of physicians. Although automobile accidents and auto-pedestrian accidents account for the majority of significant blunt abdominal trauma and falls account for most of the remainder, abused children may also present with major intra-abdominal injury (1). Child abuse should be suspected if the history is inconsistent with the injury. Penetrating injuries in general are becoming more common.

Appropriate triage, careful initial evaluation, rapid and appropriate diagnostic procedures, and vigorous management of immediate life-threatening conditions are essential to achieve the best results. Excluding immediate deaths in the field, mortality in multiply injured children with abdominal trauma approaches 7.5 percent (2).

PATHOPHYSIOLOGY

Proper evaluation and management of abdominal trauma in children requires knowledge of certain unique anatomic and physiologic characteristics of children. For instance, children have a relatively smaller anteroposterior abdominal diameter. The diaphragm inserts into the rib cage horizontally, providing a shallower, less spacious dome within which a comparatively large liver and spleen reside. The ribs, which are incompletely mineralized and more resilient than they are in adults, provide a less protective cage. The urinary bladder in young children is intraperitoneal and therefore ruptures more frequently. The close proximity of many vital organs in the child's small abdomen, a lesser amount of insulating fat and the relatively underdeveloped abdominal wall muscles also contribute to relatively more severe injuries per amount of force in children than in adults who experience blunt abdominal trauma. Children have diaphragmatic breathing. When the diaphragm is injured or irritated, ventilatory compromise results. Injury to the highly vascular organs such as the spleen, the liver, or blood vessels produces significant loss of blood. The hemorrhagic shock resulting from injury to intra-abdominal organs is the most serious and immediate threat to the child's life. Potentially life-threatening peritonitis and sepsis follow peritoneal contamination by ruptured hollow viscera.

INITIAL ASSESSMENT

The basic principles of initial assessment and resuscitation for a traumatized child remain the same as for an adult. The importance of appropriate management of the patient's airway, breathing, and circulation (ABCs) cannot be overemphasized. When profuse bleeding reduces circulating volume, the remaining blood must be fully oxygenated by administration of 100 percent oxygen and proper maintenance of ventilation. The cervical spine must be protected by a semirigid cervical collar until a cervical spine injury is properly excluded.

Exsanguinating intra-abdominal bleeding occurs without significant external evidence of injury. Hypovolemic shock is readily diagnosed when children present with signs of overt shock such as cold clammy skin, prolonged capillary refill, tachycardia, and hypotension, but if bleeding is slower, compensatory mechanisms of catecholamines and reflex vasoconstriction mask the signs of shock. These children may initially have tachycardia, irritability, or confusion but only when the compensatory mechanisms are overwhelmed by the continuous loss of blood, does profound shock occur. Overt or evolving shock is vigorously treated by replacement of lost intravascular volume with type-specific whole blood. Ringer's lactate or normal saline provide volume support until blood is available. As fluid may leak intra-abdominally, two large-caliber intravenous (IV) lines are established above the diaphragm and samples for laboratory analysis (Table 14.1) are obtained. Subclavian catheterization is fraught with undesirable complications in uncooperative children. If transcutaneous vascular access cannot be readily established, a venous cut-down is placed. A fluid bolus of 20 ml/kg should be administered over 5 to 10 minutes. The crystalloids (Ringer's lactate or normal saline) leak into the interstitial space rapidly. Three to four ml of crystalloid per ml of lost blood are necessary to restore intravascular volume. After several 20 ml/kg boluses of fluid, type O Rh-negative blood may be transfused if type-specific blood is unavailable. A pneumatic antishock garment (PASG) may be used to maintain circulation.

Once the ABCs have been addressed, monitors for heart rate, respiration, blood pressure, and oxygen saturation are placed. A nasogastric tube provides assessment of gastric content and decompresses the stomach. A Foley catheter decompresses the bladder, reveals the characteristics of its contents, and measures urinary output.

Table 14.1   Laboratory Studies for Abdominal Injury

CBC[a] blood type and crossmatch	Amylase, AST,[c] ALT,[d] arterial blood gas
Electrolytes—BUN[b]—blood sugar	Coagulation studies, urinalysis

[a]CBC = complete blood count
[b]BUN = blood urea nitrogen
[c]AST = serum aspartate aminotransferase
[d]ALT = serum alanine aminotransferase

Spontaneously voided urine is better for a microscopic examination, however. Normal prostatic position should be confirmed by a rectal examination prior to urinary catheter placement. If any question of urethral injury exists, a retrograde urethrogram should be obtained. Rectal examination assesses sphincter tone and provides for a guaiac examination.

Associated injuries are recognized, and changes from the initial presentation and the effects of resuscitative measures become evident by repeat assessment. Examination for respiratory pattern, abdominal girth, distention, abrasions, tenderness, rebound tenderness, rigidity or guarding, auscultation for bowel sound, or bruit is carefully performed. The rib cage and pelvis are compressed to establish the diagnosis of fracture. Multiple interval evaluations establish a pattern and alert the physician to subtle aberrations indicative of intra-abdominal injury. Children with intra-abdominal injuries, needing more than 40 ml/kg transfusion for stabilization, will usually need abdominal exploration.

DIAGNOSTIC PERITONEAL LAVAGE

Root and associates introduced diagnostic peritoneal lavage (DPL) in 1965 as an adjunct to clinical examination for the detection of intraperitoneal injury in patients with blunt abdominal trauma (3). Several subsequent studies have proven it to be a safe, rapid, and economical procedure. However, DPL is a nonspecific test that does not reveal the identity of the organ injured and may be falsely positive in approximately 5 percent of cases. Injuries to retroperitoneal structures such as the pancreas, the kidneys, and major vessels are not detected by DPL. False negatives occur with injuries to the urinary bladder, bowel, or diaphragm (4). It is best used as a screening procedure to detect free blood in the peritoneal cavity. DPL, even when it is strongly positive, does not mandate celiotomy in a hemodynamically stable patient but enhances the need for further evaluations. Positive DPL includes greater than 100,000 RBC/mm^3, greater than 500 WBC/mm^3, bacteria, vegetable fiber, and bile or amylase in excess of serum levels. Any of these may indicate the need for celiotomy.

COMPUTED TOMOGRAPHY

Computed tomography (CT) plays a major role in the evaluation of blunt abdominal trauma. It detects blood in the abdomen and identifies and precisely delineates the site of injury. The oral and IV contrast agents needed for optimal evaluation have some hazards, however. In addition in early pancreatic disruption or intestinal perforation, CT is not accurate. If it is immediately available and rapidly performed, CT is preferable to DPL for evaluation of blunt trauma.

INTRAVENOUS PYELOGRAPHY

IV pyelogram (IVP) identifies significant parenchymal disruption and potential renovascular injury. A single-shot IVP can be performed prior to abdominal exploration in unstable patients. CT, however, is more specific and as scan time decreases, the IVP will become less useful.

SPECIFIC INJURIES
Splenic Injuries

The spleen is one of two most commonly injured abdominal organs in victims of blunt abdominal trauma. Splenic trauma often occurs with little or no outward evidence of injury and may result from low energy impact. Rib fractures, pain from associated injuries, and the sensory loss from spinal cord trauma or altered mental status increase the difficulty of recognizing splenic rupture. A distended abdomen, tenderness in the left upper quadrant and referred left shoulder pain (Kehr's Sign), lower left-sided rib fractures, elevation of the left hemidiaphragm or a left pleural effusion often attend splenic injury. Plain abdominal radiographs can show the gastric air bubble shifted to the right because of compression from the splenic hematoma. Abdominal ultrasound may be used as a screening test for detecting splenic fractures. Emergency radionuclide scan can diagnose splenic and hepatic injuries and serve as a baseline as splenic healing progresses. CT is preferred because of the frequent association of other injuries (Figure 14.1). CT delineates splenic injury with high accuracy, and the degree of disruption noted aids in decision making.

Splenic injuries were treated by operation 15 years ago. Now the role of the spleen in the control of infection has lead physicians to attempt nonoperative management of splenic injury. That management consists of bed rest with intensive observation, IV fluids and judicious blood transfusion with frequent reevaluation by a physician experienced in dealing with multiply injured children. Operation for

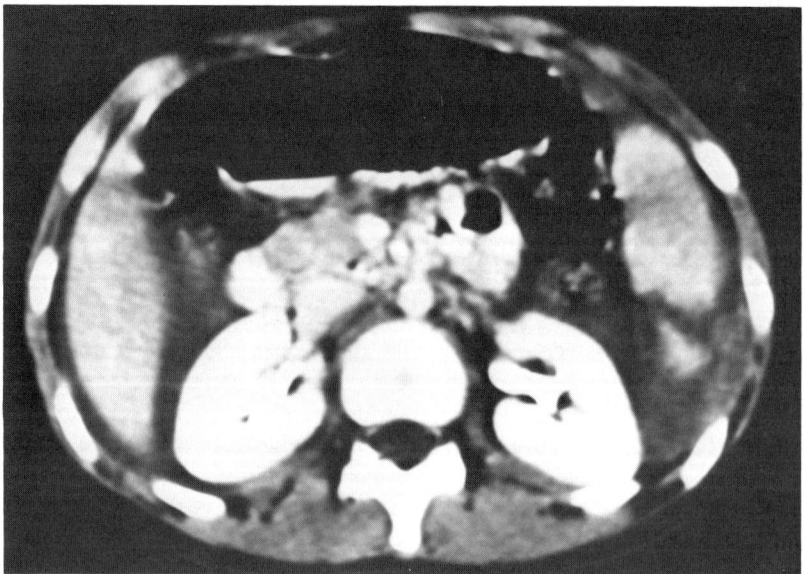

Figure 14.1 Contrast enhanced abdominal CT scan of a 12-year-old female, victim of motor vehicle accident, showing extensive splenic laceration with hemoperitoneum around the liver.

hemostasis is needed for children who fail to respond to resuscitation with blood loss replacement in excess of 40 percent of their calculated blood volume. Simple splenorraphy with omentoplasty and splenic autotransplantations are first considered (5). Splenectomy is only performed when alternatives are exhausted. The incidence of overwhelming postsplenectomy infection in splenectomized children may be lowered by autotransplantation of the spleen, appropriate vaccinations (pneumococcal and hemophilus influenza B), and the use of prophylactic antibiotics (penicillin).

Hepatic Injury

With routine use of CT for blunt abdominal trauma, it is clear that unsuspected hepatic injury is often present. The liver, the largest organ of the abdomen, is frequently the site of significant hemorrhage. Minor hepatic injuries are more common and frequently cause diagnostic and management problems. Right upper quadrant tenderness and abdominal distention may indicate hepatic injury but these signs are also commonly found in multiply injured and frightened children who cry and swallow large amounts of air. Minor elevations of liver enzymes detected in multiply injured children are not diagnostic of hepatic injury because of confusion with extrahepatic sources of those enzymes. Serum aspartate aminotransferase (AST) levels of more than 450 IU/L and a serum alanine aminotransferase (ALT) levels of more than 250 IU/L, in a recent retrospective review, were found to predict hepatic injury as correlated by CT (6). Liver enzymes above these levels should prompt further evaluations. CT, however, is the best diagnostic tool for detecting hepatic injury (Figure 14.2). Immediate operation is necessary to control major hemorrhage.

Children with stable injuries to the liver are admitted to the intensive care unit (ICU) and closely monitored while at bed rest and being given IV fluids. Extensive liver injuries can also be managed without operation. Hemobilia and hepatic abscess develop in two to six weeks in a small percentage of patients with hepatic injury. The overall mortality rate from liver trauma is about 4 percent (7).

Pancreatic Injury

Pancreatic injury usually occurs as a result of compression of the pancreas against the spinal column, which produces contusion or transection. Bicycle handlebar injuries, motor vehicle accidents, and child abuse account for most of the injuries to the pancreas. Pancreatic enzymes leak from disrupted ducts and produce a severe inflammatory response. Pancreatic injury usually presents with signs of pancreatitis such as abdominal pain, vomiting, fever, and epigastric tenderness. Amylase levels, often elevated following pancreatic trauma, may also be elevated in cases of injury to the salivary glands and are often normal even in severe pancreatic injury. Serial amylase levels are more helpful than a single measurement. Abdominal ultrasound and a contrast-enhanced CT will usually establish the diagnosis.

The initial management consists of rest, nasogastric suction, and administration of fluids. Pancreatitis pseudocyst, abscess, and fistula are complications that may require surgical intervention.

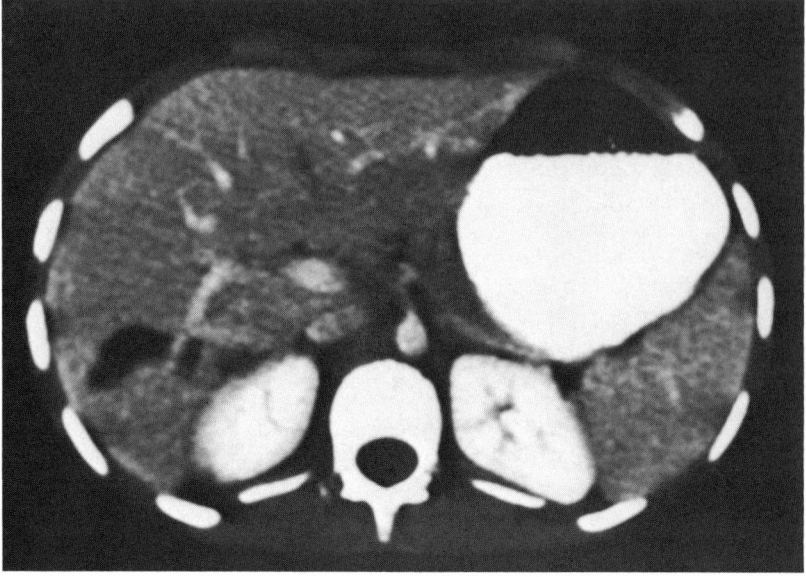

Figure 14.2 Abdominal CT scan of a 10-year-old female victim of motor vehicle accident showing hepatic laceration.

Intestinal Injuries

The incidence of hollow visceral injury in children with blunt abdominal trauma is less than 2 percent of pediatric trauma (7). Damage to the duodenum results from compression against the spinal column as in a bicycle handlebar injury. Increased use of seat restraints has decreased the overall morbidity and mortality from motor vehicle accidents. However, lap-belt use is associated with increased incidence of bowel and mesenteric injuries (8).

Duodenojejunal rupture and duodenal hematomas may also result from child abuse. Disruption of the intestinal integrity, avulsion of the gut from its mesenteric attachment, a submucosal hematoma, or a contusion may occur as a result of these forces. A large duodenal hematoma usually produces signs of high intestinal obstruction and mesenteric tears may cause significant intraperitoneal hemorrhage. Severe peritonitis and sepsis follow perforation of the intestinal tract. Abdominal pain, vomiting, and tenderness herald the onset of peritonitis. Free air under the diaphragm on an upright plain radiograph of the abdomen is diagnostic of intestinal perforation and mandates immediate surgical repair. Conservative management with rest, nasogastric suction, and parental nutrition are employed for less severe injury. The risk of infection in cases of intestinal perforation is high, dictating early and liberal use of antibiotics.

Renal Injuries

The kidneys are commonly injured by blunt abdominal trauma in children. Auto-pedestrian accident victims, automobile accident victims, and cyclists struck by motor vehicles frequently sustain renal injuries. Although the left kidney is more frequently injured, serious renal laceration is more often found on the right side (9). The signs and symptoms of renal injury are unreliable in diagnosing major renal trauma. Children with renal injuries may complain of flank pain. A renal mass, a flank hematoma, and tenderness of the costovertebral angle may be present. Gross hematuria usually occurs with major renal trauma. Major renal pedicle injuries, however, can present without hematuria (9).

IVP is the quickest, most readily available, and most cost effective means of evaluating suspected renal injury (10). A plain film followed in 10 minutes by one with contrast medium will define the presence or absence of functioning kidneys and the extent of injury. Unexpected congenital renal anomalies discovered during the evaluation, particularly ureteropelvic junction obstructions, are more common than is generally realized. Associated hepatic and splenic injuries make CT more useful as an investigating modality, and the extent of renal injury is better defined (Figure 14.3). The majority of blunt renal trauma consists of contusions and lacerations but renal pedicle injuries are found occasionally. The majority of children with blunt renal trauma are managed conservatively with bed rest, monitoring, and antibiotics. Operation for continuing blood loss, refractory shock, or renal pedicle injury is more unusual. Reconstruction of a pedicle injury must be done within 8 hours of injury for successful outcome (10). Acute renal failure, shock, urinary extravasation with or without urinary ascites, and abscess formation may complicate the management of renal injury. Hypertension, hydronephrosis, cyst, renal stone, renal atrophy, and renal intestinal fistula may manifest as late complications.

Ureteral Injury

Blunt ureteral damage is rare in children although disruption of the ureter at the ureteropelvic junction occurs, most often in young boys. Most ureteric injuries are caused by penetrating injury. Signs and symptoms of acute ureteric injury are few. A strong and forceful blow applied to the lumbar area or a penetrating wound that crosses the path of the ureter may warrant IVP. Diagnosis before scarring of ureteric tissue occurs is important for successful surgical repair (11).

Urinary Bladder Injury

Blunt trauma, usually motor-vehicle-related accidents, causes most pediatric bladder injuries. A penetrating object may rarely cause perforation of the bladder. The urinary bladder is intra-abdominal in children, and when it is full, it is vulnerable to rupture when sufficient force is applied. Approximately 7 percent of pelvic fractures are associated with vesical rupture (12). Both intraperitoneal and extraperitoneal

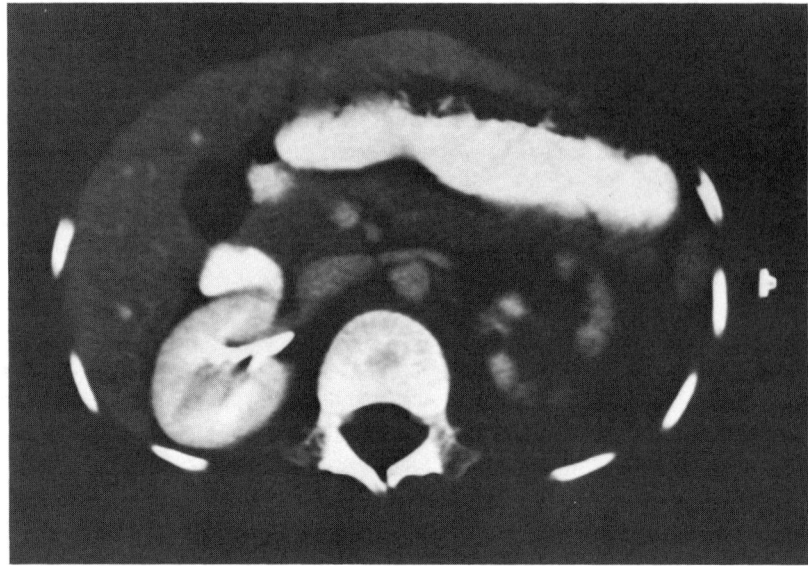

Figure 14.3 Abdominal CT scan of a 9-year-old male, who fell from a tree, showing lacerations of left kidney.

rupture can occur. The extravasation of blood and urine usually produces an abdominal mass and hematuria. Diagnosis is confirmed by IVP and cystogram. Before a retrograde cystogram is performed, however, urethral injury must be ruled out with a retrograde urethrogram.

Penetrating injuries and intraperitoneal injuries of the bladder are usually repaired and drained by suprapubic or transurethral catheter. Extraperitoneal bladder rupture is best diagnosed with contrast CT or a good cystogram (13). It is managed by continuous decompression by Foley catheter for 7 to 10 days.

Anorectal Injuries

Anorectal injuries in children usually result from sexual abuse. Although they are still uncommon, it appears that the incidence is rising. If the history of the event is not supported by the physical findings, sexual abuse is strongly suspected. A careful survey of victims of severe trauma includes examination for anorectal bleeding, anal sphincter tone, and position of prostate and for a perirectal mass. Sexually abused children may present with perianal petechiae or ecchymoses and may have rectal lacerations. With rectal perforation, serious infection develops within hours of injury and may present with fever, copious discharge, and erythema and edema of the anus and buttocks. Proctoscopic examination is necessary to study the extent of injury, and sedation or general anesthesia may be required for proper evaluation. Plain radiographs of the chest and abdomen will detect free air. If the possibility of sexual abuse exists, appropriate evidence and cultures for sexually transmitted disease must be collected. It is often necessary to admit these children to assess the possibility of evolving infection or the social dynamics of abuse. Immediate treatment usually depends on the extent of injury and varies from simple observation to operative repair. The incubation period for sexually transmitted disease is prolonged so these children must be followed up for an extended period to recognize the delayed presentation of venereal infections (14).

Miscellaneous Injuries

Injury to the abdominal aorta is very rare in children. The atherosclerotic changes common to the adult aorta increase the susceptibility to injury. The child lacks atherosclerotic changes, and the aorta is therefore less susceptible to rupture. Motor vehicle accidents or crush injuries account for most of the blunt injuries to the aorta. Gunshot wounds cause most of the penetrating injuries. Most victims die in the field. Survivors may show linear contusion of the abdominal wall; have a palpable mass; bruit; diminished or absent femoral pulses; and cold, cyanotic, and weak lower extremities (15). Abdominal ultrasound or aortography can confirm the diagnosis. The mortality is about 30 percent, mandating early surgical intervention.

Injury to the inferior vena cava is also very rare and is associated with high mortality (16). Profound exsanguinating shock is the rule rather than an exception. Retrohepatic caval tears with hepatic lacerations and many associated injuries are combined to yield a high mortality. Aggressive resuscitation and surgical intervention are necessary to reduce the likelihood of mortality.

Pelvic fractures are uncommon in children as the pediatric pelvis accommodates more energy without sustaining a fracture than is the case in adults. A pelvic fracture is usually the result of high-energy impact in children. More than 70 percent of pediatric pelvic fractures are a consequence of being struck by a motor vehicle (17). Injuries to multiple other organs usually occur. Retroperitoneal hematoma may be massive in children with pelvic fractures. Compression of the pelvic ring in the examiner's hands will usually prompt the diagnosis. Plain radiographs will demonstrate the presence of fractures although CT may be necessary to judge disruption of the sacroiliac joint. Lower urinary tract injuries frequently dictate the need for further diagnostic studies. A pelvic fracture does not require immediate intervention but the associated injuries or the excessive bleeding must be promptly treated (see Figure 14.4).

SPECIAL PROCEDURES: DIAGNOSTIC PERITONEAL LAVAGE

DPL is a procedure for detection of intraperitoneal blood, bile leak, and intestinal perforation. If celiotomy is indicated, DPL is not necessary. DPL should be avoided when there is morbid obesity, advanced cirrhosis, coagulapathy, advanced pregnancy or history of previous abdominal operation. CT, if it is readily available, is preferable to DPL in children. The procedure is performed under aseptic conditions

166 | SYNOPSIS OF PEDIATRIC EMERGENCY CARE

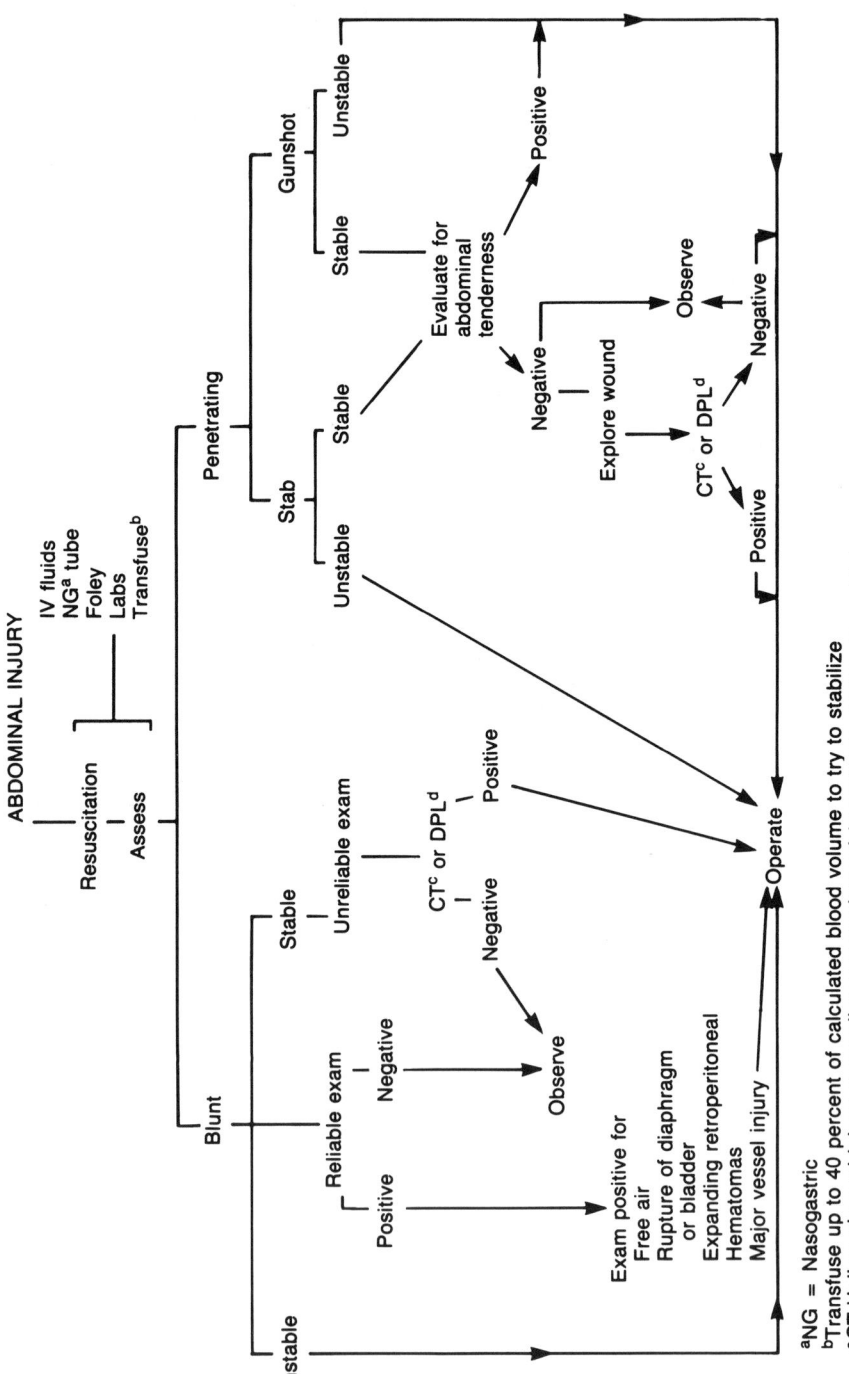

Figure 14.4 Algorithm

after the decompression of the urinary bladder and the stomach is accomplished. A small amount of local anesthetic is injected in the midline about one third the distance from the umbilicus to the symphysis pubis or in the umbilical ring. A small vertical incision (semicircular in the umbilicus) is carried through the skin and subcutaneous tissue to the fascia. A peritoneal dialysis catheter is advanced into the peritoneal cavity through a nick in the fascia and peritoneum. If blood flows from the catheter or is aspirated by syringe, the procedure is considered strongly positive. Otherwise 10 ml/kg (body weight) of warm Ringer's lactate or normal saline (up to 1 l) is instilled into the peritoneal cavity. Uniform distribution of fluid throughout the peritoneal cavity is accomplished by gentle agitation of the abdomen. The fluid is siphoned off into a container placed on the floor after 5 to 10 minutes (18).

REFERENCES

1. Cooper A, Thomas F, Barlow B, et al: Major blunt abdominal trauma due to child abuse. J Trauma 1988;28(10):1483–1487.
2. Zorlundemir U, Ergören Y, Yucesan S, et al. Mortality due to trauma in childhood. J Trauma 1988;28(s):669–671.
3. Root HD, Houser GW, McKinley CR, et al. Diagnostic peritoneal lavage. Surgery 1965;57:633–637.
4. Hawkins ML, Scofield WM, Carraway R, et al. Diagnostic peritoneal lavage in blunt trauma. Southern Med J 1988;81(3):293–296.
5. Büyükünal C, Danismend N, Yeker D, et al. Spleen saving procedures in pediatric splenic trauma. Br J Surg 1987;74(May):350–352.
6. Hennes HM, Smith DS, Schneider K, et al. Elevated liver transaminase levels in children with blunt abdominal trauma: A predictor of liver injury. Pediatrics 1990;86(1):87–90.
7. Oldham KT, Guice KS, Ryckman F, et al. Blunt liver injury in childhood: Evolution of therapy and current perspective. Surgery 1986;100(3):542–549.
8. Anderson PA, Rivera FP, Maier R, et al. The epidemiology of seat belt associated injuries. J Trauma 1991;31(1):60–67.
9. Quinlan DM, Gearhart JP. Blunt renal trauma in childhood. Features indicating severe injury. Br J Urol 1990;66:526–531.
10. Bass DH, Semple PL, Cywes S, et al. Investigations and management of blunt renal injuries in children: A review of 11 year's experience. J Pediatr Surg 1991;26(2):196–200.
11. Hoover DL, Bellinger MF. Genito urinary trauma. In Ehrich FE, Hildrich FJ, Tepas JJ III, eds. Pediatric emergency medicine. Rockville, Md.: Aspen, 1987.
12. Uehara DT, Eisner RF. Indications for retrograde cystouretrography trauma. Ann Emer Med 1986;15:3,270–275.
13. Corriere JN Jr, Sandler CM. Management of ruptured bladder. Seven years of experience with III cases. J Trauma 1986;26(9):830–833.
14. Finkel MA. Anogenital trauma in sexually abused children. Pediatrics 1989;84(2):317–322.
15. Reisman JD, Morgan AS. Analysis of 46 intra-abdominal aortic injuries from blunt trauma: Case reports and literature review. J Trauma 1990;30(10):1294–1297.
16. Wiencek RG Jr, Wilson RF. Inferior vena cava injuries—The challenge continues. Am Surg 1987;54:423–428.
17. Garvin KL, McCarthy RE, Barnes CL, et al. Pediatric pelvic ring fractures. J Pediatr Orthop 1990;10(5):577–582.
18. American college of surgeons, committee on trauma: Abdominal trauma. In Advance trauma life support program instructor manual. Chicago: ACS, 1988;111–130.

15

Thoracic Trauma

E. Stevers Golladay
Dileep R. Vyas

Thoracic injury is relatively less frequent in children than it is in adults; its incidence, however, appears to be rising (1). In children, these injuries are usually due to blunt trauma, but penetrating injury is becoming more common in preadolescents and teenagers (2,3). Mechanisms of injury follow a different pattern for various age groups. From birth to four years of age, child abuse and motor vehicle accidents predominate. In the 5- to 9-year-old age group, autopedestrian injuries are common and from 10 to 17 years of age, falls and bicycle injuries increase in frequency (4,5). In general, boys are at an increased risk.

The highly compliant chest wall of children allows for significant intrathoracic injuries to occur without ribs being fractured; thus this common indicator of severe injury in adults is not as useful in children (4). Associated injuries involving multiple organ systems increase the mortality of children with chest injuries (6). The mobility of the mediastinum in children dissipates force with a resultant lower incidence of injury to the airway and blood vessels, but conversely the faster mediastinal shift causes cardiovascular compromise more rapidly. The first few hours after injury yield the highest mortality, and therefore early diagnosis and therapy is essential (7).

INITIAL APPROACH

The initial priority to any child with a serious injury begins with the maintenance of a patent airway, adequate ventilation, and oxygenation. The cervical spine must be protected by a semirigid cervical collar until injury is excluded by adequate radiography. Patency of the airway can be maintained by displacing the mandible forward with a jaw thrust and by opening the mouth. Obstructing objects such as a foreign body or clot should be immediately removed. The airway must be suctioned free of blood and debris.

The adequacy of ventilation is assessed by the rate and the depth of respirations, activity of the accessory muscles, stridor, wheezing, grunting, cyanosis, and pallor. Administration of supplemental oxygen by face mask or nasal cannula or in conjunction with a bag-valve mask device is used when these signs are noted. The adequacy of oxygenation is judged initially by the color of the skin and mucosa and confirmed by pulse oximetry and blood-gas studies. Hypoxemia despite a patent airway and supplemental oxygen may herald severe pulmonary or cardiac injury such as pneumothorax, tension pneumothorax, hemothorax, or hemopneumothorax, cardiac contusion, pericardial tamponade, and vascular or septal rupture. Evacuation of the pleural or pericardial space with needle aspiration followed by the placement of a drainage tube is rewarded by improvement of status. Inadequate ventilation or oxygenation, rising oxygen requirements, rising $PaCO_2$, and falling PaO_2 dictate the need for intubation.

The adequacy of circulation must be assessed by mental status, heart rate, quality of the pulses, color and temperature of the skin, capillary refill, and blood pressure. Inadequate perfusion or shock causes further tissue hypoxia in children with chest injury. Loss of blood into the pleural space, abdomen, pelvis or thigh or an open wound can each exceed 40 percent of the blood volume and result in poor perfusion as can myocardial contusion and pericardial tamponade because of decreased cardiac output and hypotension (8).

Establishing two secured large-caliber intravenous (IV) lines is the next priority in any severely injured child. A type and crossmatch is obtained, and blood is sent to the laboratory for the investigations listed in Table 15.1 as soon as venous access becomes available. Intraosseous lines in infants and young children can be placed rapidly in the tibia or femur. Venous cut-down (saphenous, femoral, cephalic, or external jugular) provides reliable access early in the management of severe shock when percutaneous access is so difficult. Infusion of 20 ml/kg of Ringer's lactate over 5 to 10 minutes should be initiated after access is obtained to treat hypotension. A second bolus of 20 ml/kg over a similar period allows sufficient time for type-specific blood to be available for transfusion. Transfusion of O negative unmatched blood may be used prior to availability of type-specific blood (9). A detailed search for the extent of chest injury, other associated injuries, and the degree of physiologic derangement follows the management of ventilation and circulation. The child is exposed and examined completely. Catheters and monitors to record the heart rate, respiratory rate, electrocardiogram (EKG), blood pressure, urinary output, and pulse oximetry are then established. The stomach is decompressed with a nasogastric tube to prevent gaseous distention, subsequent vomiting, and possible gastropneumonic reflux in a patient with compromised ventilation. An orogastric tube is preferred if there is a nasal fracture or bleeding.

A child's surface area is larger in proportion to their body weight than is an adult's, and therefore children must be protected from hypothermia by warm blankets and overhead heaters.

Table 15.1 Laboratory Studies for Thoracic Injury

CBC[a] blood type and crossmatch	Arterial blood gas
Electrolytes—BUN[b]—blood sugar	Coagulation studies, urinalysis

[a]CBC = complete blood count
[b]BUN = blood urea nitrogen

A portable chest radiograph can be performed for unstable children although upright and lateral radiographs in the radiology department are preferred. Entrance and exit sites of penetrating wounds are marked. A 12-lead EKG should be obtained. Need for further studies such as esophagograms or aortogram is dictated by the signs attendant to abnormalities of these structures.

The following mnemonic may help memorize the initial approach.

Primary Survey/Resuscitation
A. Airway, "C" spine
B. Breathing
C. Circulation/hemorrhage control
D. Detailed examination (Data collection [vital signs, monitors, dextrostix])
E. Exposure, environmental control/(hypothermia, fever)
F. Foley
G. Gastric tube, blood gases

SPECIFIC INJURIES
Rib Fractures

The reported incidence of pediatric rib fractures in extensive trauma varies between 30 and 50 percent and implies that a significant fall, traffic accident, severe injury, or child abuse has occurred (1,4,6). Occupants as passengers in motor vehicles involved in accidents in older children and motor vehicle pedestrian accidents in younger children account for most pediatric rib fractures. Fractures of the first three ribs are often associated with bronchial, cardiac, or large-vessel injuries. The fractures of the lower three ribs are associated with hepatic and splenic injury (8). As the number of fractured ribs increases, so does the severity of injury and the extent of associated organ injuries thus increasing morbidity and mortality (10). Patients with rib fractures have localized pain on deep breathing, cough, or positional changes. The respiratory excursions may be diminished. A chest radiograph helps define the extent of injury. If pain is not controlled by analgesics, intercostal nerve block with a small volume of bupivacaine (0.25 percent) with epinephrine(1:200,000) is useful. As much as 1 ml/kg may be injected at the lower margin of the fractured rib and the ribs above and below the fracture level posterior to the fracture site (8,11).

Pneumothorax

Traumatic pneumothorax can follow penetrating or blunt injury and is usually associated with hemothorax. A small pneumothorax may be asymptomatic. A significant pneumothorax produces respiratory distress, tracheal shift, hyperresonance to percussion, and decreased breath sounds. Mediastinal shift, asymmetrical chest wall movement, tracheal shift, distended neck veins, and hyperresonance to percussion are signs of tension pneumothorax. Rapid respiratory deterioration of a mechanically ventilated patient with a well-placed endotracheal tube should arouse suspicion. Plain chest radiograph and lateral decubitus radiographs (with the suspected side upward) are diagnostic. Anterior second intercostal needle thoracostomy must be performed immediately if the child is severely stressed. A thoracostomy tube is placed posteriorly to evacuate the frequently present hemothorax better and aid in reexpansion of the collapsed lung. The thoracostomy tube allows evacuation of pneumothorax, hemothorax, and facilitates the re-expansion of the collapsed lung (8,11). Traumatic pneumothorax can yield as much as 15 percent mortality (6).

Open Chest

Open chest is an unusual injury in children with impailment on a fixed object as the most common cause. Penetrating injury to the thorax usually seals itself. If the penetrating object is large enough to leave a defect, a "sucking chest wound" may result. The pressure gradient between the thoracic cavity and the atmospheric pressure necessary for air exchange and venous return is destroyed, resulting in hypoxia and hypotension. If the chest wall hole is two thirds the diameter of trachea, air passes preferentially through the opening with respiration. The management of open pneumothorax requires its prompt closure with an occlusive dressing (a sterile towel or a gloved finger). This should be followed by a dressing with multiple layers of vaseline gauze extending at least five cm beyond the wound's edges. Securing the dressing with tapes on three sides with one side left open creates a flutter valve effect to prevent the development of tension pneumothorax. Definitive care requires placement of a chest tube through a separate wound followed by the surgical closure of the defect.

Hemothorax

Both blunt and penetrating injuries may result in hemothorax. Lacerations of the intercostal, internal mammary, and pulmonary vessels and occasionally rupture of a cardiac chamber or aorta are the causes of hemothorax. Parenchymal lacerations, because of the elastic recoil of lung tissue, low pulmonary artery pressure and the release of vasoactive substances, do not usually cause large-volume blood loss. Forty percent of the calculated blood volume may be lost into one hemithorax. A large hemothorax produces the compression of the ipsilateral lung, contralateral mediastinal shift, and shock. Tracheal shift to the contralateral side, dullness to percussion and decreased breath sounds are the usual signs. Upright chest or lateral decubitus chest radiographs show a collection of fluid in the costophrenic, cardiophrenic, or subpulmonic sites (Figure 15.1). Rapid infusion of fluid and blood is necessary to resuscitate the child. The vast majority of patients will require evacuation of blood by tube thoracostomy to provide effective air exchange, monitor ongoing loss and reduce the risk of fibrothorax (8). Traumatic hemothorax has a 2 percent incidence of empyema. Isolated traumatic hemothorax has low mortality, but for children with associated head and abdominal injury, the mortality rate approaches 70 percent.

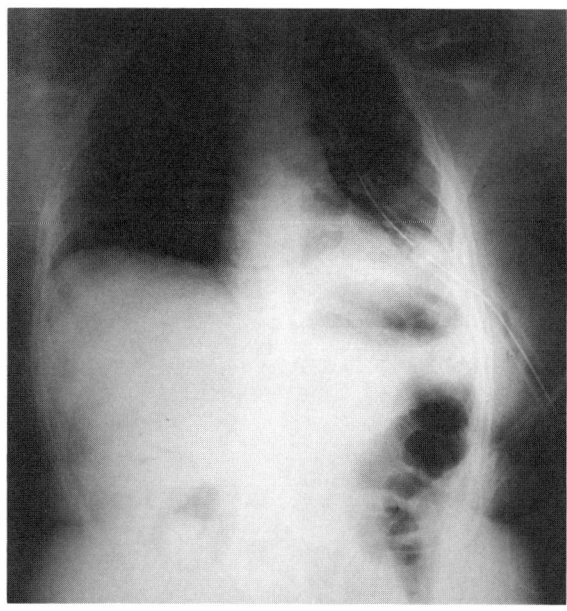

Figure 15.1 Chest radiograph of a 12-year-old female, victim of motor vehicle accident, showing left pleural effusion with a chest tube in place.

Pulmonary Contusion

The most common serious intrathoracic injury in children is pulmonary contusion. Pulmonary contusion, although associated with rib fracture or flail chest, often occurs without rib fractures (6). The lesion can be fairly localized or widely disseminated. The response of the lung to injury varies from minimal interstitial edema to rapid intra-alveolar extravasation of blood and fluid. Early institution of measures to limit interstitial pulmonary edema is important. These include judicious use of intravenous infusions, control of pain, and careful pulmonary toilet. Use of diuretics, bronchodilators, and prophylactic antibiotics should also be considered. Dyspnea, hemoptysis, dullness to percussion, wheezing, and crepitance develop with progression to respiratory failure. This mandates constant surveillance for hypoxemia and hypercarbia.

Chest radiographs may demonstrate peribronchial and/or perivascular infiltrate that can progress to consolidation (Figure 15.2). Arterial blood gases will establish the degree of respiratory compromise. Patients needing an FIO_2 of 0.4 to 0.5 by mask to maintain oxygen saturation will usually require endotracheal intubation and administration of positive end-expiratory pressure. Rapid institution of ventilatory support is critical in children with multiple contusions and multiple rib fractures and with those who require large-volume fluid resuscitation and those with deteriorating arterial blood gases. The arterial oxygen saturation should be maintained at about 90 percent. Pneumonia, fat embolism, and pulmonary embolism are common complications. The mortality varies with the severity of injury but may be as high as 70 percent when associated with other extra thoracic injuries.

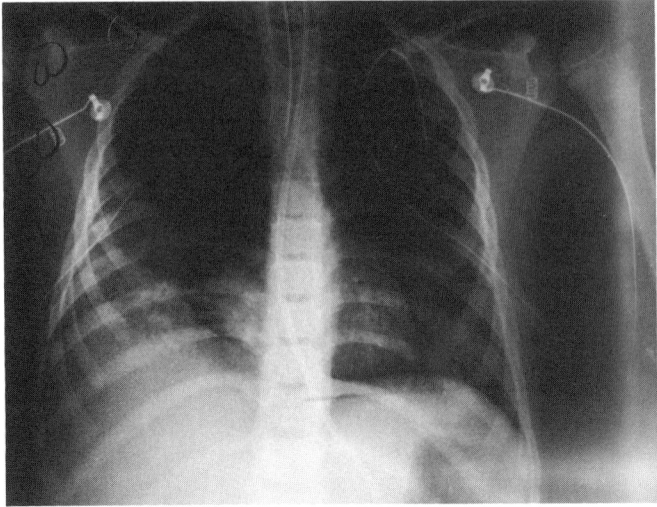

Figure 15.2 Portable chest radiograph of a 6-year-old male, victim of motor vehicle accident, showing right lower lung infiltrate compatible with pulmonary contusion.

Flail Chest

Although rib fractures are not unusual in childhood, the flail chest is rare. Lateral rib fractures and fractures of the sternum, pneumothorax, hemothorax, and pulmonary contusion are common associates of flail chest (8,12). Several contiguous ribs fractured at more than one point, may create a flail chest. Multiple rib fractures on chest radiograph do not constitute a flail chest. A section of chest wall must exhibit paradoxic motion during the respiratory cycle. Associated pneumothorax, hemothorax, or pulmonary contusion demand increased work of breathing, which increases paradoxic chest wall motion. Flail chest may not be apparent until the work of breathing is increased (13). In addition, chest wall muscle spasm may temporarily stabilize the flail, which becomes symptomatic as the muscles tire.

Initial therapy demands attention to ventilation and oxygenation. Not all patients with flail chests require endotracheal intubation and mechanical ventilation. The decision for such intervention depends on clinical and laboratory factors such as shock, hypoxia, hypercarbia, respiratory rate, associated head injury, and the necessity for general anesthesia for other injuries (12,14). Careful attention should be paid to fluid resuscitation. The lungs of a child with flail chest are very sensitive to fluid overload. Thus careful monitoring of pulmonary and cardiac function is necessary to optimize fluid administration (9). The treatment is primarily directed at pain control and the underlying pulmonary contusion. Pneumonia is a common complication (12,13). In children with two or more associated injuries, fractures of more than seven ribs, bilateral flail chest, and shock, the mortality can be as high as 95 percent. Late mortality is usually associated with pulmonary sepsis.

Tracheobronchial Disruption

Intrathoracic tracheobronchial injuries are rare. These injuries occur in a setting of high-energy impact and are usually associated with other injuries. Acute mortality is high. Timely diagnosis of these injuries is essential (15).

Three main mechanisms of injury are: (1) Sudden compression of the chest pulls the lungs apart, creating traction at the carina that results in a tear of the tracheobronchial tree. (2) A force applied while the glottis is closed causes high intrabronchial pressure that ruptures large bronchi. (3) Rapid deceleration generates shearing force at the areas of fixation such as the carina and causes rupture of the bronchus (16). Subcutaneous emphysema, dyspnea, hemoptysis, sternal tenderness, and positive *Hamman's sign* are common. Common radiographic findings include pneumothorax, pneumomediastinum, subcutaneous emphysema, accompanying fractures of clavicles and ribs, and pulmonary contusion. Bronchoscopy performed by an experienced person will confirm this diagnosis (17). The immediate treatment requires ventilatory support and a placement of a tube thoracostomy. The definitive treatment consists of primary suture of the lacerations. Overall mortality is approximately 30 percent (15,16).

Diaphragmatic Injury

Traumatic diaphragmatic injury is uncommon. Falls from heights and automobile accidents are the usual causes of blunt injury to the diaphragm. Gunshot wounds and stab wounds to the chest below the fourth intercostal space account for most of the penetrating injuries to the diaphragm and produce small holes with delayed presentations. Blunt trauma produces large radial tears. The gradient of peritoneal-pleural pressure facilitates the herniation of abdominal viscera into the chest, usually on the left side. Scaphoid abdomen, dullness to percussion on the chest, and the pathognomonic presence of bowel sounds in the chest establish the diagnosis.

Chest radiographs may show mediastinal shift, herniated viscera and elevation of the diaphragm or the presence of nasogastric tube in the intrathoracic stomach. Bowel contrast studies and positive contrast peritoneography may be helpful in difficult cases. If ventilatory support is necessary, bag-valve-mask ventilation should be avoided because insufflation produces further distention of the herniated gastrointestinal tract and causes further compromise of ventilation. Placement of a nasogastric tube helps to decompress a herniated stomach. Immediate surgical repair should be undertaken (8,9).

Chest pain or dyspnea in a child who has had blunt or penetrating trauma can signify a chronic diaphragmatic hernia and should warrant a chest radiograph. Chronic diaphragmatic hernias are better repaired by a thoracic approach. Acute diaphragmatic injury from blunt trauma has a 90 percent association with intra-abdominal injuries. Associated fractures of the lumbar spine are common.

Myocardial Concussion and Contusion

Cardiac concussion from blunt chest injury causes transient dysrhythmias and/or nonspecific ST-segment changes. There is no histopathologically identifiable lesion in this condition and the electrocardiographic abnormality is usually of no significance (18,19). Cardiac contusion results from forceful blunt injury that causes histopathologically identifiable lesions. The true incidence of myocardial injury after blunt injury is unknown. Signs and symptoms suggestive of myocardial contusion include precordial pain, diaphoresis, bruised precordium, tachycardia, low blood pressure, dyspnea, heart murmur, and precordial rub. Chest radiographs may demonstrate suggestive findings such as first rib or sternum fracture. Although many different tests suggest the diagnosis, there is no "gold standard" (20). Serial EKGs, serial creatinine phosphokinase isoenzyme (CK-MB) ratios, echocardiogram, pyrophosphate scan, multiple-gated acquisition (MUGA) cardiac scan and radionuclide angiograms are used to investigate cardiac function and perfusion (19–23). Common EKG abnormalities associated with myocardial contusion include ST-T wave changes and conduction abnormalities. Abnormalities of the other tests described here should enhance suspicion. Although most children will recover without serious problems, they should be admitted to a pediatric intensive care unit (ICU) and closely monitored as signs of pump failure, hemodynamic instability, or cardiac arrhythmia may arise and must be treated appropriately. The morbidity from myocardial contusion in hemodynamically stable patient without conduction abnormality is minimal.

Aortic Rupture

Aortic rupture is a common cause of death in automobile accidents in adults. Its occurrence in children is rare. It is usually caused by blunt injury such as a fall from a height of more than 20 feet or a pedestrian motor vehicle accident. The tear often occurs near the aortic isthmus, although some tears extend to involve the aortic arch or a cardiac chamber (24). Associated injuries are common, and immediate mortality is high. The survivors of aortic rupture have a contained hematoma or an intact adventitia. The child may complain of midscapular pain that radiates to the back and dyspnea and dysphagia are frequent. Hypertension in the upper extremity and hypotension in the lower extremities results from inadequate perfusion distal to the site of aortic rupture. Supraclavicular hematoma and deviation of trachea to the right can also be present. Obliteration of the aortic knob, widened mediastinum, fracture of the first or second rib, deviation of trachea, and/or esophagus (nasogastric tube) to the right on chest radiograph are suggestive of aortic rupture. A high index of suspicion, complimented by clinical and radiologic findings, will provoke aortography and lead to the correct diagnosis (24). Hypertension of the upper extremity, if present, may be controlled with the use of trimethophan (Arfonad) 0.1 mg/kg/min intravenously. Blood pressure should be continously monitored. Hemodynamic decompensation from blunt aortic injury is usually very rapid and massive, causing death from exsanguination. In a child with suspected blunt aortic trauma, immediate left anterolateral thoracotomy and repair may reduce the mortality. The mortality for patients who arrive alive in the emergency department is about 30 percent (8).

Hemopericardium

Hemopericardium can result from penetrating or blunt injury to the pericardial, epicardial, myocardial, or coronary vessels, intrapericardial great vessels, or cardiac chambers. Even a small amount of blood in the pericardial sac restricts cardiac activity and interferes with cardiac filling, producing cardiac tamponade. The presence of distended neck veins, low blood pressure, narrow pulse pressure, and distant heart sounds suggest the diagnosis. A decrease in systolic blood pressure in excess of 10 mmHg during inspiration, called *pulsus paradoxus*, is associated with pericardial tamponade. Widened cardiac shadow on chest radiograph, low voltage complexes on EKG, and peaked T-waves in the precordial leads with flat Ts laterally may also be present.

The initial management of hemopericardium consists of IV fluids to raise the central venous pressure followed by inotropic support of the blood pressure. Pericardiocentesis may temporarily relieve the symptoms, but open pericardiotomy must then be performed. Pericardial aspiration may not be diagnostic or therapeutic if there is clotted blood in the pericardial sac.

Esophageal Injury

Esophageal trauma can be caused by penetrating or blunt trauma. Blunt epigastric injury causes forceful ejection of gastric contents into the esophagus, significantly raising the intraluminal pressure that causes linear tears in the lower esophagus. Transmural rupture produces the leakage of gastric and esophageal content into the mediastinum, causing mediastinitis. Rupture from the mediastinum into the pleural space quickly follows, producing multifloral empyema.

The history of a severe blow to the lower sternum or epigastrium, pain or shock disproportionate to the severity of injury, fever, subcutaneous emphysema, pleural effusion, and the appearance of particulate matter or saliva in the chest tube drainage are suggestive or predictive of esophageal injury. Salivary amylase may be found in the chest tube drainage. Methylene blue, when it is swallowed, will also appear in the thoracotomy tube. The diagnosis may be confirmed by a water soluble contrast esophagogram. The initial treatment is directed toward drainage and the administration of fluid and antibiotics. The definitive treatment consists of the repair of the esophagus via thoracotomy (8).

The mortality of esophageal rupture is high when the diagnosis is delayed or the perforation of the esophagus is intra-abdominal.

Traumatic Asphyxia

Traumatic asphyxia occurs when the chest is flattened between a compressant force and a hard surface during maintenance of a closed glottis. It is most typically seen after an automobile passes over a child's chest. The resilient chest wall of a child allows compression of the heart, the lungs, and the great vessels to occur without rib or sternal fractures. A sudden, sharp rise in the intrathoracic pressure causes the pressures in the supraclavicular vessels and the head and neck capillary pressures to rise. The classic feature of traumatic asphyxia is a supraclavicular cyanosis of the neck and the face and a V-shaped distribution of the cyanosis in the posterior intrascapular area. Other frequently associated clinical features include petechiae of the head and neck, subconjunctival hemorrhage, epistaxis, hemoptysis, hematemesis, blurred vision, mental dullness, and hyperpyrexia. Cardiac injury and pulmonary contusion may also be associated. Peripheral or spinal paralysis occurs rarely. The treatment is largely supportive and consists of elevation of the head of the bed, oxygen supplementation, and fluid limitation. Associated injuries may dictate more invasive procedures to maintain homeostasis and are largely responsible for the associated morbidity and mortality. More than 90 percent of the cases, however, recover completely without specific treatment.

SPECIAL PROCEDURES
Tube Thoracostomy

Emergency tube thoracostomy may be necessary to drain air, fluid, or both from the pleural cavity and help reexpand the lung. The usual site for the placement of a chest tube is the fifth intercostal space anterior to the midaxillary line on the affected side (Figure 15.3). The diameter of the selected tube should approximate the width of the intercostal space through which it is to be placed. A wide area of skin around the placement site is antiseptically prepared and draped. The proposed incision site, usually the skin overlying the seventh rib in the midaxillary line, is infiltrated with local anesthetic. A 1 to 3 cm skin incision is used to develop a craniad posterior tunnel. The pleural space is entered through the fifth intercostal space. The chest tube is directed by a hemostat through the tunnel so that the tip of the tube is located at the posterior third intercostal space. The tube is connected to an underwater seal or suction at negative 10 to 20 cm water pressure. The tube is secured to the skin with nonabsorbable sutures. A chest X-ray verifies the tube position, adequacy of pleural space drainage, and the reexpansion of the lung. It may also reveal previously unrecognized lung pathology.

Pericardiocentesis

Pericardiocentesis is used for aspiration of cardiac tamponade. It is best done in the operating room with continuous EKG monitoring. The xiphisternal area is antiseptically prepared and draped. A long large-caliber over-the-needle cannula is inserted in the left xiphocostal angle and advanced toward the left shoulder at a 30

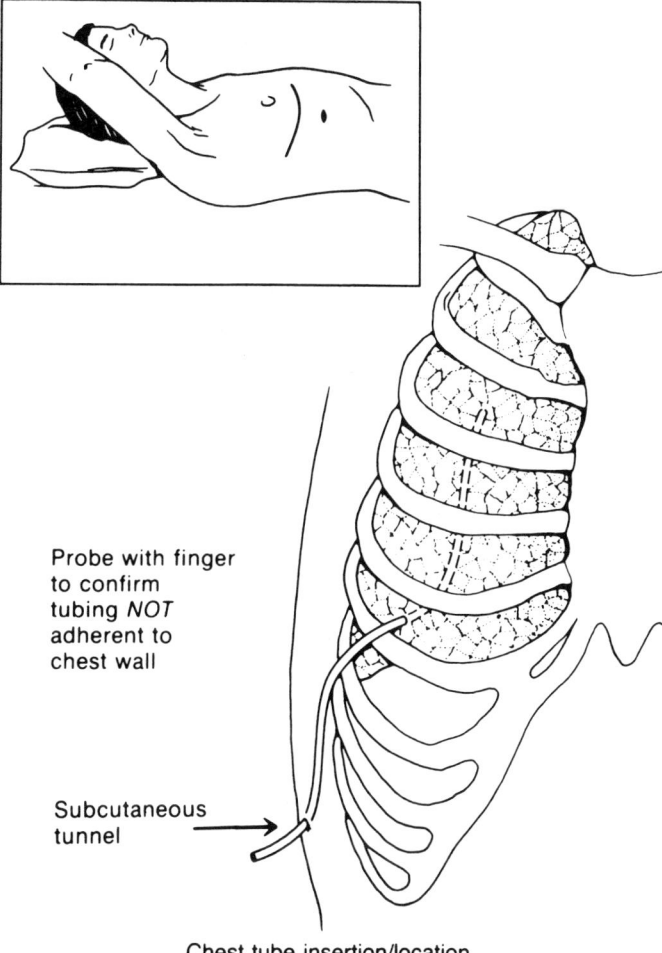

Chest tube insertion/location

Figure 15.3 Placement of tube thoracostomy. (Reprinted from Ehrlich FE, Heldrich FJ, Tepas JJ. Pediatric emergency medicine. Rockville, Md.: Aspen, 1987;73, with permission from Aspen Publishers, Inc. © 1987.)

to 45 degree angle to the plane of the body (Figure 15.4). A 20 ml syringe maintains a small negative pressure as the needle is advanced. When the needle tip penetrates the pericardial sac, blood will appear in the syringe. If the needle is advanced into the myocardium, an injury pattern (ST-T changes or QRS widening) will appear on the EKG monitor. The needle should be withdrawn slightly if an injury pattern appears. Once the needle tip is in the pericardial space, the cannula is advanced into the pericardial sac, and the needle is withdrawn. The cannula is connected to a syringe and stopcock, and the pericardial space is drained.

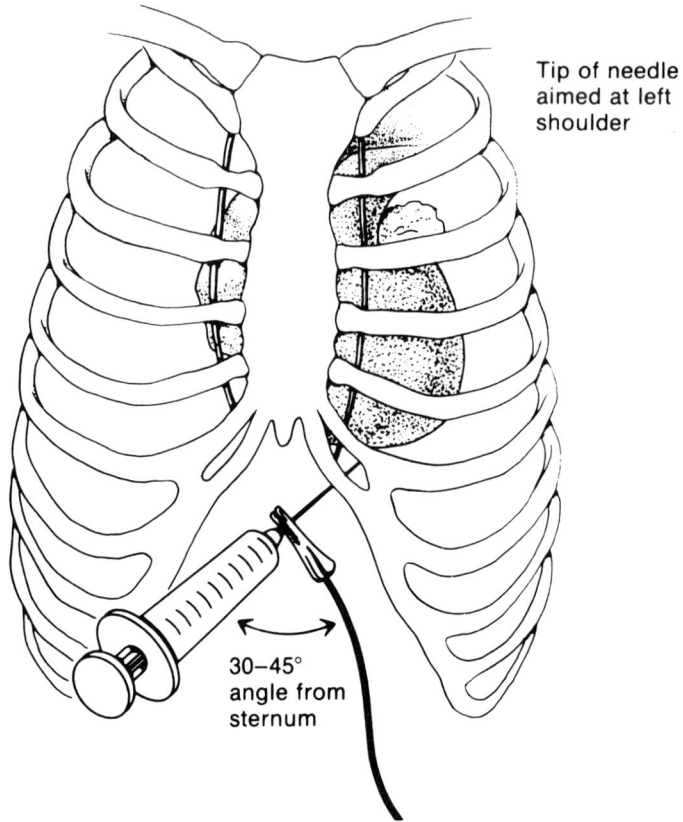

Figure 15.4 Location and technique of pericardiocentesis. (Reprinted from Ehrlich FE, Heldrich FJ, Tepas JJ. Pediatric emergency medicine. Rockville, Md.: Aspen, 1987;73, with permission of Aspen Publishers, Inc., © 1987.)

REFERENCES

1. Haller JA, Little AG, Shermeta DW. Thoracic trauma in children. Pediatr 1984;74:813–819.
2. Barlow B, Niemirska M, Gandhi RP. Ten years experience with pediatric gunshot wounds. J Pediatr Surg 1982;17:927–932.
3. Barlow B, Niemirska M, Gandhi RP. Stab wounds in children. J Pediatr Surg 1983;18:926–929.
4. Nakayama DK, Ramenofsky ML, Rowe MI. Chest injuries in children. Ann Surg 1989;209:676–681.
5. Pecklet MH, Newman KD, Eichelberger MR, et al. Patterns of injury in children. J Pediatr Surg 1990;25:85–91.
6. Pecklet MH, Newman KD, Eichelberger MR, et al. Thoracic trauma in children: An indication of increased mortality. J Pediatr Surg 1990;25:961–966.
7. Thomas ARL, Anderson I. Pediatric trauma: Secondary survey. BMJ Sept 1, 1990;433–437.
8. Golladay EG. Injuries to the heart and chest in children. Mount Kisco, N.Y.: Futura, 1983.

9. American College of Surgeons, Committee on Trauma. Thoracic trauma. In Advance trauma life support program instructor's manual. Chicago, 1988;89–110.
10. Garcia VF, Gotschall CS, Eichelberger MR, et al. Rib fractures in children: A marker of severe trauma. J Trauma 1990;30:695–700.
11. Golladay ES. Thoracic injuries. In Ehrlich FE, Hildrich FJ, Tepas JJ, III. Pediatric emergency medicine. Rockville, Md.: Aspen, 1987;69–83.
12. Freedland M, Wilson RF, Bender JG, et al. The management of flail chest injury: Factors affecting outcome. J Trauma 1990;30:1460–1468.
13. Landercaper J, Coghill TH, Strutt P. Delayed diagnosis of flail chest. Crit Care Med 1990;18:611–613.
14. Trinkle JK, Richardson JD, Franz JL, et al. Management of flail chest without mechanical ventilation. Ann Thorac Surg 1975;19:355–362.
15. Jones WG, Mavrondis C, Richardson JD, et al. Management of tracheobronchial disruption resulting from blunt trauma. Surgery. 1984;95:319–323.
16. Kirsh MM, Orringer MB, Behrendt DM, et al. Management of tracheobronchial disruption secondary to non-penetrating trauma. Ann Thorac Surg 1976;22:93–101.
17. Baumgartner F, Sheppard B, deVirgilio C, et al. Tracheal and main bronchial disruptions after blunt chest trauma: Presentation and management. Ann Thorac Surg 1990;50:569–574.
18. Doty BD, Anderson AE, Rose RF, et al. Cardiac trauma: Clinical and experimental co-relations of myocardial contusion. Ann Surg 1974;180:452–460.
19. Tellez DW, Hardin WD Jr, Takahashi M, et al. Blunt cardiac injury in children. J Pediatr Surg 1987;22:1123–1128.
20. Wisner DH, Reed WH, Riddick RS. Suspected myocardial contusion: Triage and indications for monitoring. Ann Surg 1990;212:82–86.
21. Golladay ES, Donahou JS, Heller JA. Special problems of cardiac injuries in infants and children. J Trauma 1979;19:526–531.
22. Ildstad ST, Tollernd DJ, Weiss RG, et al. Cardiac contusion in pediatric patients with blunt thoracic trauma. J Pediatr Surg 1990;25:287–289.
23. Langer JC, Winthrop AL, Wesson DE, et al. Diagnosis and incidence of cardiac injury in children with blunt thoracic trauma. J Ped Surgery 1989;24:1091–1094.
24. Clark DE, Zeiger MA, Wallace KL, et al. Blunt aortic trauma: Signs of high risk. J Trauma 1990;30:701–705.

PART VI

Central Nervous System

16

Spine Injuries

Curtis Gruel

Fortunately, injuries to the spine and spinal cord are rare in children. They deserve serious attention, however, for several reasons. If they are not recognized and treated appropriately, they can have devastating consequences, including paralysis, deformity, and pain. Also they are not easy to recognize, particularly because of the numerous normal radiographic appearances of the child's spine that may resemble fracture or instability. Finally these injuries may assume different patterns and require different treatment than do their adult counterparts.

The true incidence of pediatric spinal injury is not known. It has been estimated that 2.5 to 3.3 percent of all spinal injuries occur in children. The incidence is usually reported to be higher in males, and it increases with age, probably due to vehicular trauma, sports activities, and other risk-taking behaviors. Cervical spine birth trauma should be considered in a newborn with decreased tone, a nonprogressive neurologic deficit, and a negative history of a familial neurologic disorder. During ages 3 to 5 years, falls from heights, motor vehicle accidents, and child abuse are the most common causes. From 6 to 15 years, they are usually the result of motor vehicle accidents and sports injuries. The number of spine injuries in children that result in spinal cord injury (SCI) is also unknown. Paraplegia is three times more common than quadriplegia. The importance of SCI in producing paralysis is obvious.

Another sequela of SCI in children is spinal deformity. This is most common in younger children, with higher levels of injury, with spasticity, or when a laminectomy has been performed. Children with simple fractures and no SCI tend to remodel, and deformity is seldom progressive.

PATHOPHYSIOLOGY

Injuries to the spine and spinal cord in small children may assume different patterns and behave differently than they do in adults. This may be explained by some basic anatomical and physiological differences between children and adults. First the cartilaginous plates in the child's spine are still growing. This explains certain injury patterns peculiar to children since the growth plates constitute an area of mechanical

---

The author would like to thank Doctors Theresa Stacy and Timothy Tytle for their help in locating figures for this manuscript.

weakness in a motion segment; also injury to the plate or further growth in the presence of paralysis or spasticity can lead to progressive deformity. On the other hand, the child's spine has some ability to remodel after simple fractures. Second the child's spine has more inherent ligamentous laxity than does the adult spine, accounting for the fact that SCI can occur without fracture or dislocation. Third the child's head is proportionately larger than is the adult's thus imparting more energy to the spine. This also requires different positioning in the child to achieve reduction of cervical spine injuries. Fourth, the facet joints are oriented more horizontally in the child, allowing more motion normally, especially in the cervical spine. Most cervical spine injuries in children occur at the upper end, as opposed to adult injuries, which often occur in the lower cervical spine. By around ages 8 to 10, the child's spine has achieved nearly adult proportions, and the injury patterns more closely resemble those seen in adults. The last difference between children and adults is fortunate in that children have a greater potential to recover from SCI.

It is possible for children to sustain SCI without a visible fracture on plain radiographs, linear tomograms, or computed tomography (CT). This is known as spinal cord injury without radiographic abnormality (SCIWORA). The SCI may be complete or incomplete. The incidence of SCIWORA among all SCIs in children is reported to be between 5 and 67 percent. The most popular theory to explain this phenomenon centers around the greater elasticity of the immature spine, which allows it to elongate more than the spinal cord before disruption occurs. The proportionately larger head-to-body size ratio and the relatively poorly developed neck musculature explain why the injury is more common in the younger age groups and in the upper cervical spine. The onset of paralysis may be delayed, or the paralysis may be precipitated or exacerbated by a second episode of trauma. The injury may be recognized by myelography or magnetic resonance imaging (MRI). Somatosensory evoked potentials (SSEP) may be useful in the presence of concomitant head injury or as a baseline.

CLINICAL PRESENTATION

Injury to the spine and spinal cord should be immediately suspected in any child who has sustained multiple trauma, especially from a motor vehicle accident (Figure 16.1). This is especially true if a head injury has occurred. Lacerations, abrasions, or contusions around the head and neck should alert one to the possibility of cervical spine injury and may serve as valuable clues as to the mechanism of injury. In the unconscious patient, a diligent search must be made to rule out injury to the spinal column and to assess the status of the spinal cord. Radiographs of the entire spine should be obtained. The motor and sensory levels and the presence or absence of reflexes should be determined (to serve as a baseline). The spine should be protected by log rolling and positioning with such devices as sandbags or soft collars. Anyone complaining of neck or back pain following injury should be evaluated. Similarly any complaint of numbness or weakness, even if it is transient, should be taken seriously. Some patients with an injury to the upper cervical spine (such as an odontoid fracture) will complain of numbness or paresthesias in the occipital nerve distribution. Any

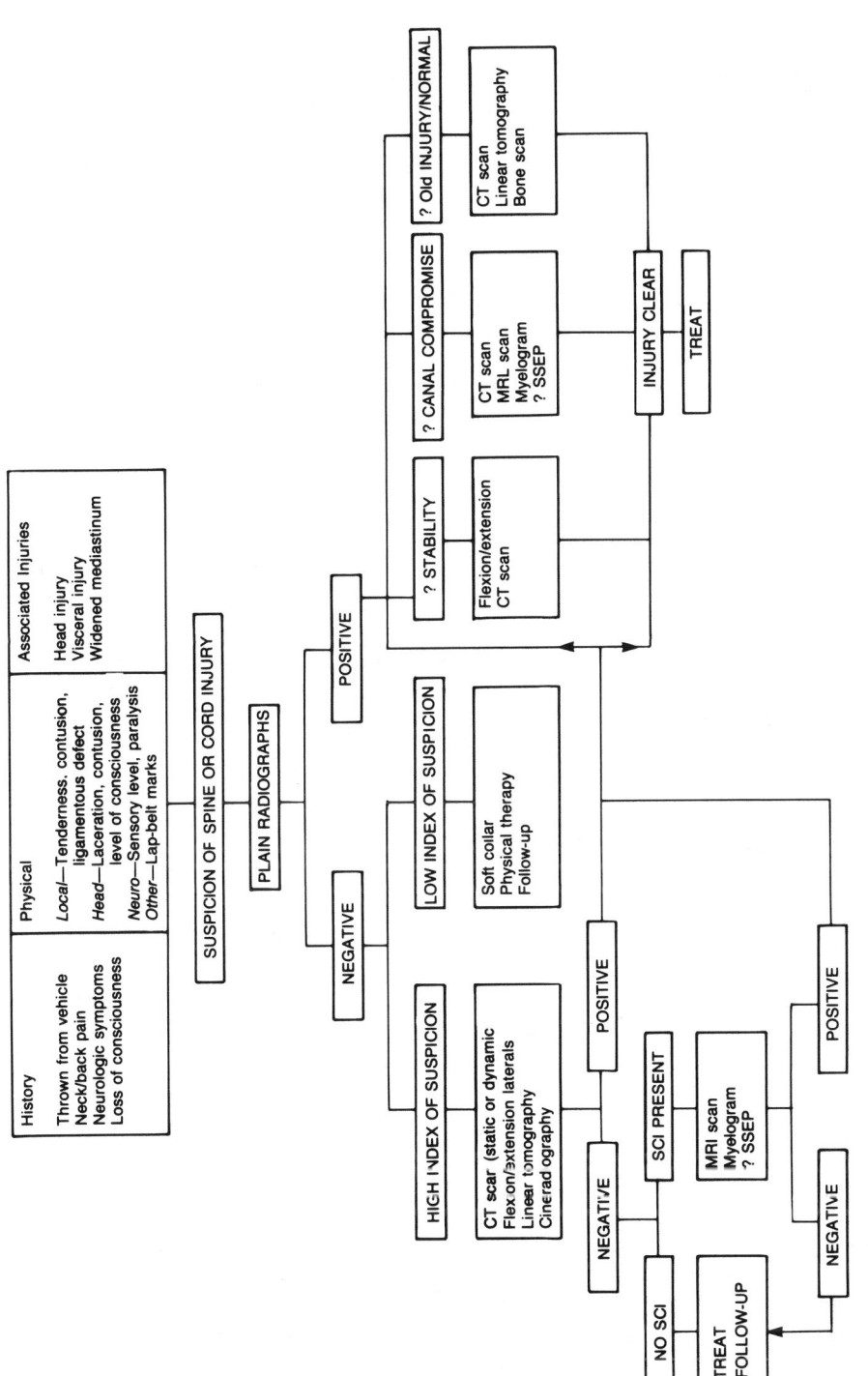

Figure 16.1 Clinical presentation of spine and spinal cord injuries in children.

patient with significant visceral injury from blunt trauma should be suspected of spinal injury. A widened mediastinum may be the first indication of a thoracic spine injury and is thought to result from bleeding at the fracture site. Occasionally a child will present with torticollis following a minor injury. This is especially common following an upper respiratory infection and is often due to atlantoaxial rotatory fixation (AARF). The laboratory evaluation will be considered further later.

DIFFERENTIAL DIAGNOSIS
Normal Findings

The most frequent source of confusion in the evaluation of spinal injuries in children is the rather common occurrence of normal findings or variations that may resemble fractures or instability. It is necessary to have some familiarity with these to avoid confusion that can result in overtreatment.

Growth Centers

There are numerous secondary ossification centers in the immature spine. These can resemble fractures, but can usually be recognized by their positions, by their smooth sclerotic margins, and by the absence of soft tissue swelling. Most vertebrae form from three ossification centers, one in the centrum and one in each neural arch. The arches usually fuse in the midline posteriorly by age two to four years and are seldom a source of confusion (Figure 16.2a). There is also a cartilaginous line between the neural arch and its junction with the central ossification center on each side. These are known as the neurocentral synchondroses and are usually closed by three to six years of age. They can be mistaken for fractures of the neural arch. The ring apophyses form during adolescence, disappearing by skeletal maturity, and appear as small points of ossification at the superior and inferior ends of the vertebral bodies (Figure 16.2b). They are seldom mistaken for fractures but may themselves be subject to injury during adolescence. There is a horizontally oriented growth plate at the base of the dens, which is contiguous laterally with the neurocentral synchondroses. This usually disappears by five to seven years of age. Most fractures of the odontoid in children occur through this growth plate (Figure 16.2c).

Pseudosubluxation

Between 19 and 40 percent of normal children under age eight will demonstrate up to 4 mm of anterior movement of the second cervical vertebra on the third during flexion and extension radiographs. This may also occur at the segment between the third and fourth vertebrae. It is believed to be the result of the normal horizontal orientation of the facet joints and the greater ligamentous laxity present in this age group. It may be recognized by the absence of soft tissue swelling and by the fact that the posterior elements align, even in the position of apparent subluxation (Figure 16.2d). The retropharyngeal space in a child should be no more than 7 mm, and the retrotracheal space should be no more than 14 mm although both can be affected by crying, position changes, and the amount of adenoid tissue present.

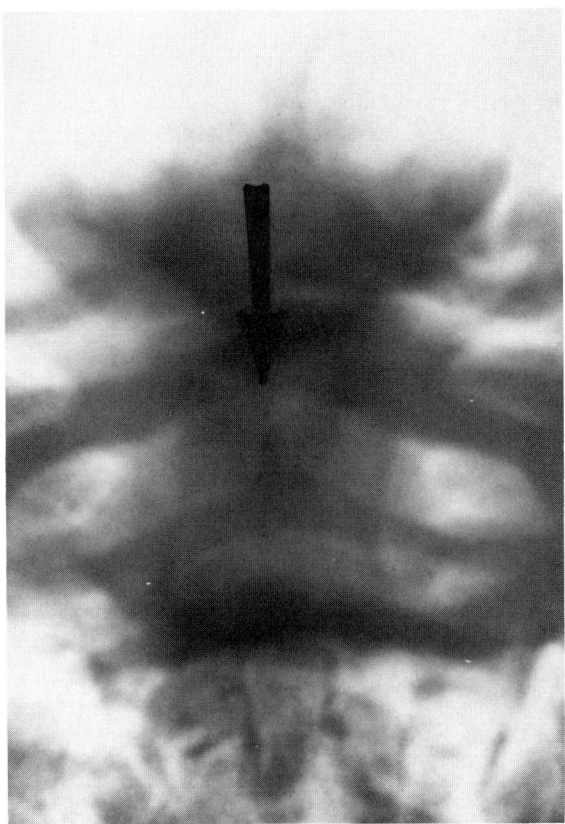

Figure 16.2 Normal appearances in the child's spine. (a) Open-mouth odontoid view in a six-month-old. The arrow indicates the synchondrosis between the two neural arches.

Other Normal Findings Or Variations

There are some other findings that might be interpreted as injury but are actually normal in children. One of these is that the cervical vertebral bodies are normally wedged anteriorly until about age eight (Figure 16.2e). There are also indentations in the vertebrae, both anteriorly and posteriorly that are normal in children. There is normally no lordotic curve in the cervical spine in 15 percent of children. (This would suggest muscle spasm and significant injury in an adult.)

Other Nontraumatic Findings

There are some other findings that are not normal but that are not traumatic in origin and need be of no concern in an emergency setting. Atlantoaxial instability often develops in Down's syndrome and in certain types of dwarfism (Figure 16.3a). There are also abnormalities associated with the formation of the odontoid process. Aplasia is the total absence of the odontoid, and hypoplasia is the incomplete

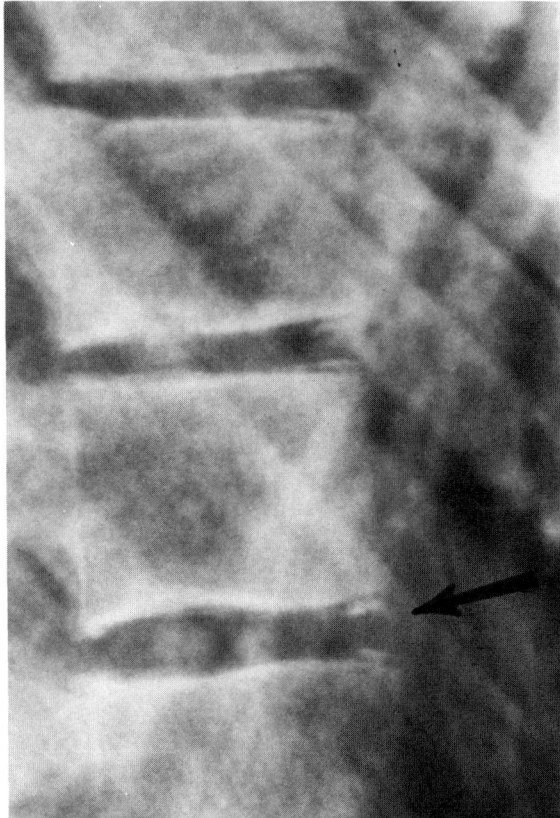

Figure 16.2 (continued)
(b) Ring apophysis. The arrow indicates the normal appearance. This is the site of the endplate fracture seen in adolescents although the injury involves the posterior portion of the ring.

formation of the odontoid. Either of these may be associated with atlantoaxial instability. Os odontoideum has the appearance of the tip of the odontoid being separated from its base. This is thought to be due to a nonunited fracture sustained earlier in childhood and is often associated with atlantoaxial instability (Figure 16.3b). The tip of the odontoid moves with the anterior arch of C1. Vertebra plana can be seen in eosinophilic granuloma and can be mistaken for a traumatic compression fracture (Figure 16.3c).

SPINE TRAUMA

Injury to the spine is usually apparent from the clinical picture, the presence of soft tissue swelling on radiographs, and the radiographic appearance of a fracture or dislocation. Neurologic findings may also be present. The following are some patterns of spine trauma that are commonly encountered.

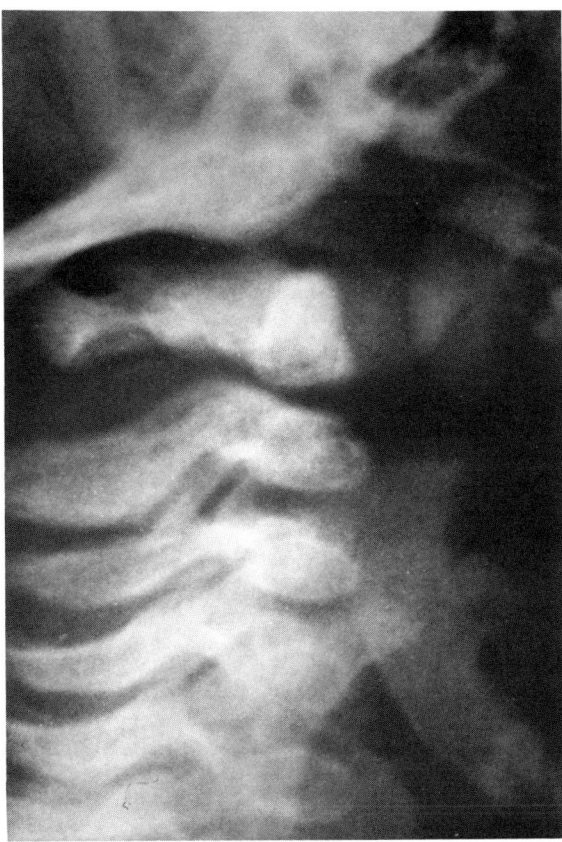

Figure 16.2 (continued)
(c) Odontoid growth plate can be mistaken for a fracture. In fact, most odontoid fractures in children occur through this area of weakness.

Spinal Cord Injury

Injury to the spinal cord or nerve roots is commonly associated with a fracture or dislocation. A neurologic injury may be present, however, without any apparent injury to the spine. There are varying degrees of neurologic injury. Most authors group SCIs into those that are complete and those that are incomplete. The incomplete injuries are then often subclassified by degree of neurologic involvement or by anatomic pattern of involvement. The prognosis for recovery is fairly good in an incomplete injury and dismal in a complete one, but this is not as certain in children as it is in adults.

Osseoligamentous Injuries/Fractures/Cervical Spine

Most injuries to the cervical spine in children are seen in the upper three segments, probably owing to the disproportionately large head and the poorly developed neck musculature in this age group. A fracture through the ring of C1

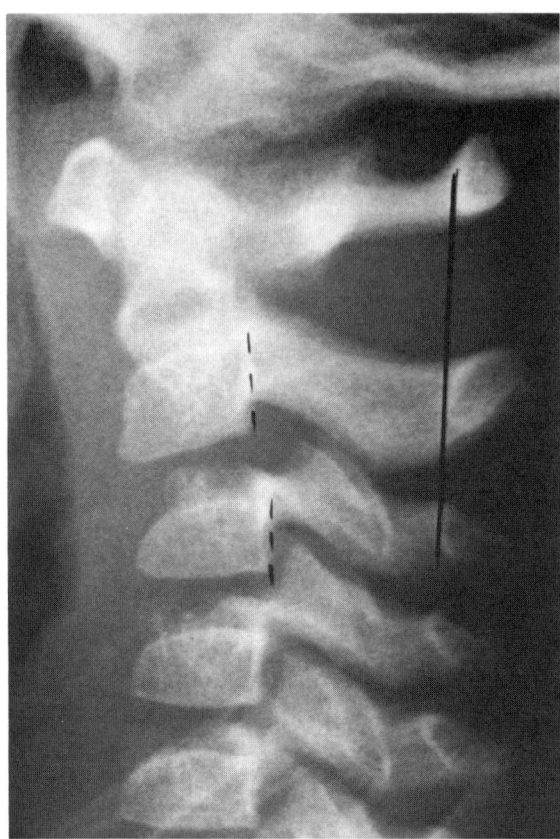

Figure 16.2 (continued)
(d) Pseudosubluxation in a 2½-year-old. Note the absence of soft tissue swelling anteriorly and that the posterior elements maintain their normal alignment.

posterior to the articular processes (Jefferson fracture) is an example (Figure 16.4a). Another is the *Hangman's fracture*, a failure of the posterior elements of the C2 vertebra sometimes associated with anterior subluxation of C2 on C3 (Figure 16.4b). Odontoid fractures are seen in children, but they usually fail through the growth plate, and their healing potential is better than it is in adults. There are some fractures that are peculiar to children. One example is an avulsion fracture that occurs through the ring apophysis as one might see in the cervical spine from a hyperextension injury. In children past the age of ten, the patterns more closely resemble those seen in adults; for example, more lower cervical spine injuries are seen. Anterior compression fractures are rarely seen in the cervical spine, and when they do occur, they are usually in the lower segments (Figure 16.4c). They are usually stable injuries. More often the appearance of wedging in a child's cervical spine is the normal pattern of ossification. Fracture-dislocations in the older age groups are seen in the lower segments and are virtually the same as adult injuries. Burst fractures are the result of axial compression and are often associated with encroachment on the spinal canal by retropulsed

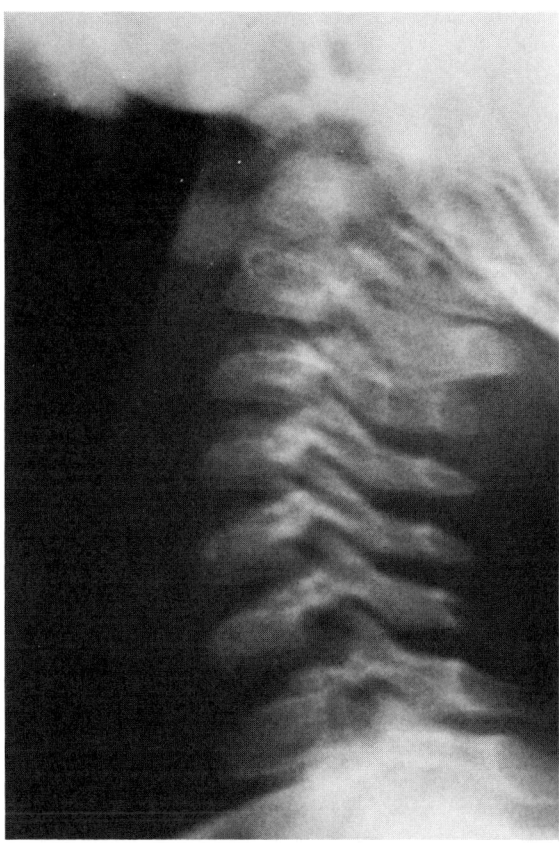

Figure 16.2 (continued)
(e) Normal wedged appearance of cervical vertebrae in a toddler.

fragments of the vertebral body. They are prone to late collapse and deformity and require prolonged traction or spinal fusion. They are usually seen only in patients who are past puberty.

Thoracolumbar Spine

Compression fractures and burst fractures are also seen in the thoracolumbar spine, although rarely in small children (Figure 16.4d). A flexion-distraction injury (Chance fracture) results when a passenger is thrown forward while restrained only by a lap seatbelt. The torso is flexed forcibly around the lapbelt with the axis of rotation anterior to the spine. The spine then fails in a tension mode. The fracture classically occurs through the interspinous ligaments posteriorly and through the disc space anteriorly, but the failure can occur through the spine at any level of the motion segment. Another injury peculiar to childhood is a fracture of the endplate, seen particularly in the lumbar spine in adolescents. These often mimic disc protrusions, and a CT scan, MRI scan, or myelogram is necessary to make the diagnosis.

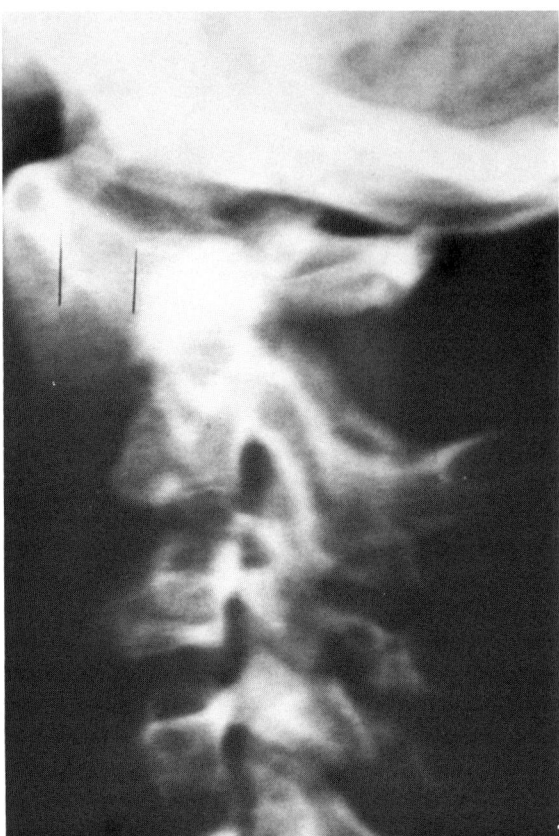

Figure 16.3 Nontraumatic abnormalities. (a) Atlantoaxial instability in a five year-old with Down's syndrome. Note the interval between the anterior cortex of the dens and the posterior cortex of the anterior ring of the atlas, which in this case measured 7 mm.

Dislocations

Dislocations commonly occur in conjunction with fractures and, when they do, are termed *fracture-dislocations*. It is very rare for them to occur by themselves in children. One instability pattern that *is* seen in childhood, however, is atlantoaxial instability. The transverse ligament is the first line of defense, and its rupture is denoted by an atlantodens interval (the distance between the anterior cortex of the dens and the posterior cortex of the anterior ring of the atlas on a flexion lateral radiograph) of greater than five mm. Only three mm is acceptable in an adult, but more of the dens and the atlas are cartilaginous in the child. Greater than 10 to 12 mm indicates that the alar, apical, and cruciate ligaments have also failed. Overriding of the atlas on the dens of as much as two-thirds on the extension radiograph is normal and is seen about 20 percent of the time. The *rule of thirds* states that the odontoid process occupies about one-third of the spinal canal as does the spinal cord, leaving one-third

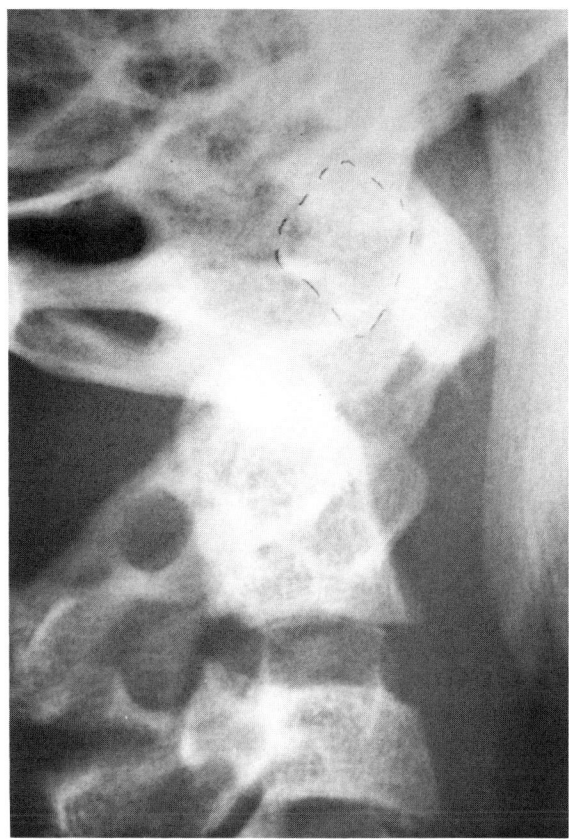

Figure 16.3 (continued)
(b) Os odontoideum (outlined) with C1–C2 instability. Note that the dens moves with the atlas.

empty. Knowing this and the amount of displacement, one can estimate the space available for the cord (SAC), thus determining if the position or the existing instability is acceptable.

Others
Atlantoaxial Rotatory Fixation

AARF is a condition in which one of the facets of C1 subluxes forward on C2, resulting in some amount of fixed rotation between C1 and C2. It often follows an upper-respiratory infection. It is usually apparent on plain radiographs, showing asymmetry of the lateral masses of C1, both in their size and in the distance between them and the odontoid process (Figure 16.5a). The lateral view shows a true lateral of the head and C1, but an oblique of the remainder of the cervical spine, or vice versa. The anterior ring of C1 on the lateral view appears larger than normal, because one is really viewing the lateral mass (Figures 16.5b and 16.5c). It is often impossible to obtain routine radiographic views because of the torticollis posture, but the diagnosis

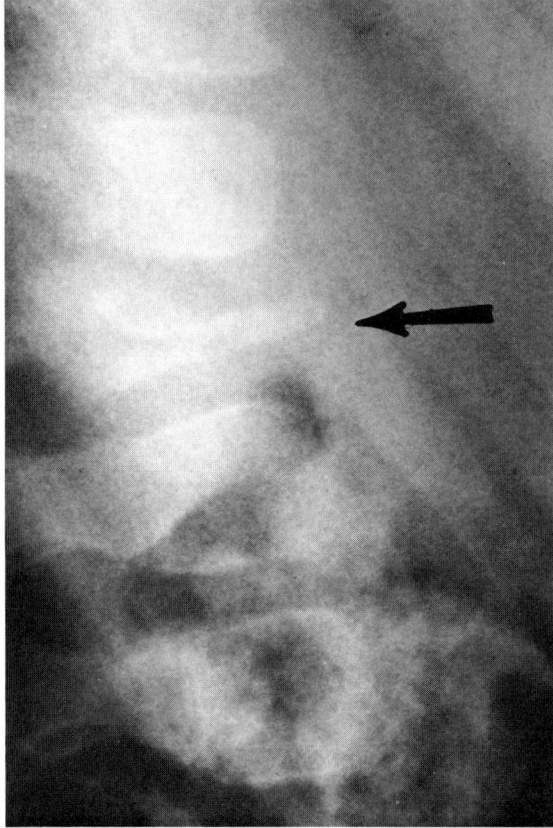

Figure 16.3 (continued)
(c) Vertebra plana of T12 (arrow) due to eosinophilic granuloma. This usually requires no treatment.

can be confirmed by CT or by cineradiography, either of which demonstrates that C1 is locked on C2 with respect to rotation in one direction or the other. Dynamic CT scanning is the most reliable modality.

Soft Tissue Injury

Soft tissue injury without instability, commonly known as *whiplash injury*, can occur in children as well as in adults. The etiology is unknown but probably results from tearing of soft tissue structures such as muscles and ligaments insufficient to cause demonstrable instability. Others may be due to occult fractures not seen with the modalities commonly employed. Just as in adults, the symptoms can become longstanding in children but usually respond to simple conservative measures and reassurance. Children generally do better than adults.

History and Physical Examination
History

It is invaluable to obtain an accurate history of what caused the injury from the patient or others present at the scene for determining the mechanism of an injury.

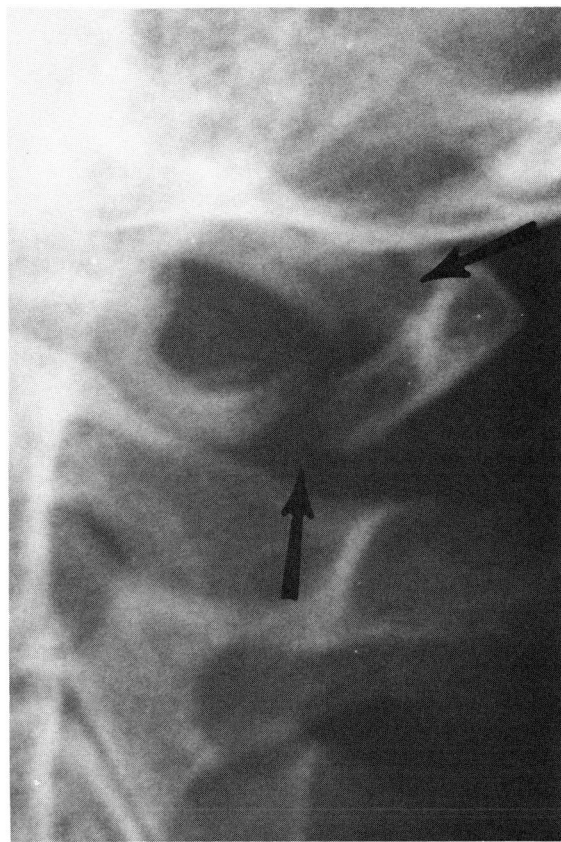

Figure 16.4 Traumatic appearances. (a) Jefferson fracture, two fractures with jagged edges are seen in the arch of C1.

Direct injury can occur from a direct blow or from a penetrating wound. Indirect injury can result from flexion, extension, axial loading, distraction, or flexion-distraction or from a combination of some or all these.

If there is no recognized trauma, one would want to know whether the patient has had any recent infections, particularly of the upper-respiratory tract. Next physicians should inquire about symptoms, particularly pain in the neck or back, and numbness or weakness, even if transient. Has the patient been able to void since the time of the injury? Those with upper cervical spine injuries sometimes complain of pain or numbness in the distribution of the occipital nerves.

Physical Examination

A thorough examination for other injuries must be done, especially in a patient with sensory loss or decreased level of consciousness. This helps to assess the general condition of the patient and may provide important clues regarding the likelihood and/or nature of spinal injury.

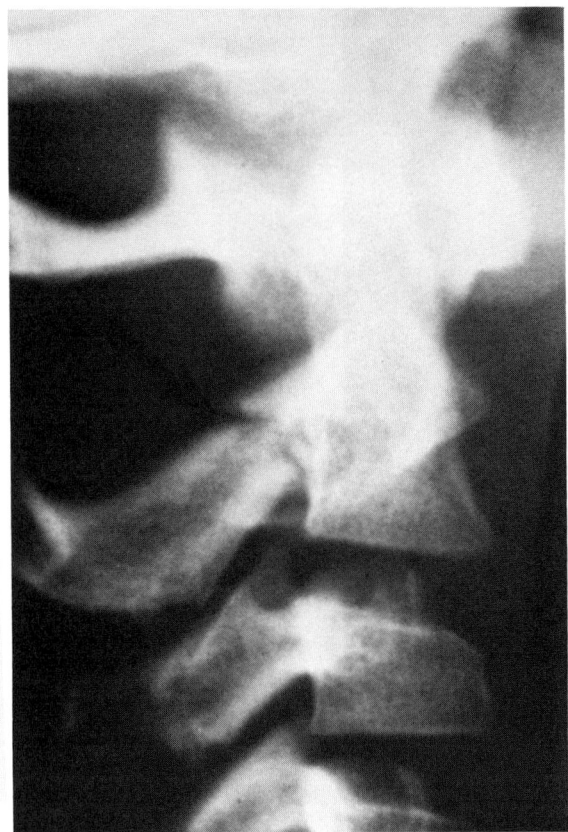

Figure 16.4 (continued)
(b) Hangman's fracture.

Signs of injury to other areas may give some information regarding the mechanism of injury. For example, a laceration, an abrasion, or a contusion on the forehead may indicate that the patient sustained a blow to the head that resulted in an extension stress to the neck. Similarly lap-belt marks should lead to suspect a flexion-distraction force.

There may be some local indicators in the area of the injury. Tenderness or ecchymosis should raise a high index of suspicion. Palpable ligamentous defects or step-offs can provide useful information regarding stability at the fracture site.

A thorough neurologic evaluation is mandatory. Motor and sensory levels should be determined and carefully recorded to serve as a baseline. Perianal sensation in patients with apparently complete injuries should be specifically tested because even a small amount of sparing indicates that the lesion is partial, vastly changing the prognosis. Also if an injury is apparently complete at first presentation, the clinician should look for reflexes, including abdominal, cremasteric, anal wink, and bulbocavernosus. As long as they are absent, the patient is in spinal shock, and the prognosis is indeterminate.

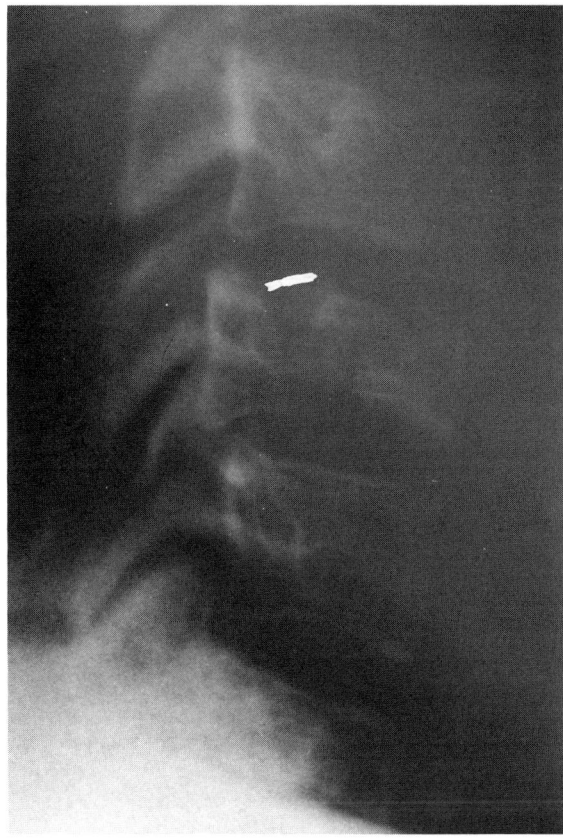

Figure 16.4 (continued)
(c) Compression fracture of C6 in a 20-year-old. This is basically an adult injury.

ADJUNCT STUDIES

Refer once again to Figure 16.1. Plain radiographs are usually sufficient to determine the presence or absence of significant spinal injury. The standard views generally obtained for the cervical spine are the AP, lateral, odontoid, and oblique views. It may not be necessary to obtain all of these views on every patient, depending on the level of suspicion. Every victim of blunt trauma from a motor vehicle accident should probably have a lateral view of the cervical spine, unless the victim is conscious and gives a reliable history of no neck injury. The lateral should include the C7 vertebra, which may be difficult to see in obese or heavily muscled patients. A swimmer's view, lateral linear tomography, or sagittal reconstruction from CT can be helpful in this instance. Lateral views in flexion and extension can demonstrate instability, but should only be performed in an awake patient, ideally with a physician in attendance, and should be curtailed if any neurologic symptoms occur.

If the plain radiographs are positive and clearly demonstrate the injury, proceed directly to treatment. If there is a question regarding stability, flexion-extension laterals or CT will be useful. If canal compromise is suspected, it can be evaluated by

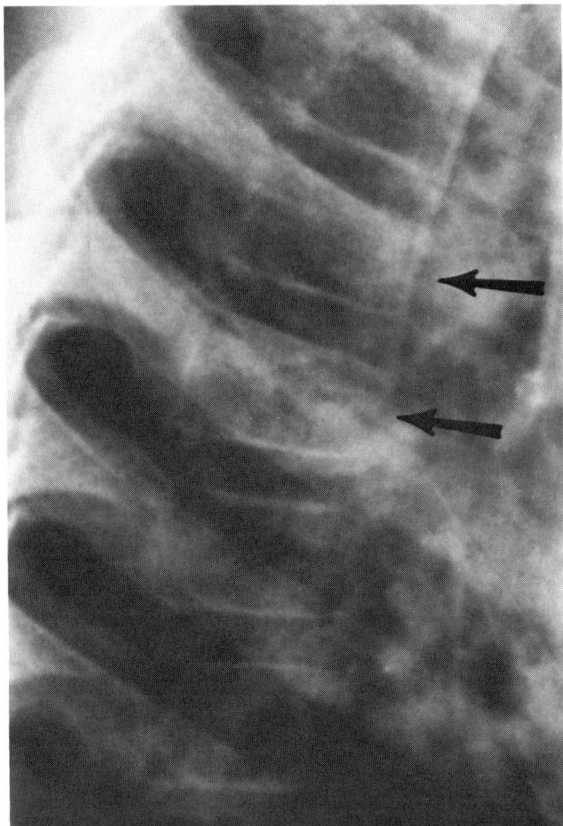

Figure 16.4 (continued)
(d) Compression fractures of T5 and T6 (arrows). Note the loss of anterior height compared to adjacent vertebrae.

CT, myelography, CT-myelography, or MRI scanning or in certain select cases by SSEP monitoring. To know whether the appearance is possibly that of a normal variant, computed or linear tomography may show a growth plate or the ragged edges of a fracture more clearly. If there is still uncertainty about whether the fracture is old or new, a bone scan may help but may not be positive for two or three days.

If the plain radiographs are normal and there is a low index of suspicion of significant injury, symptomatic treatment as with a soft collar and analgesics and follow-up are appropriate. If there is high suspicion of significant injury, CT is very useful in the cervical spine. Static images are good for delineating fractures; dynamic images may be necessary to show an AARF or to demonstrate an instability resulting in cord impingement. Linear tomography is better at showing fractures in the horizontal plane (for example, odontoid fractures). If these studies are negative and there is no spinal cord injury, proceed to treatment and follow-up. If a spinal cord injury is present, however, obtain an MRI scan and/or myelography. This may demonstrate a source of continuing cord impingement (such as a disc herniation or an endplate fracture) that would be amenable to surgery with a positive effect on the

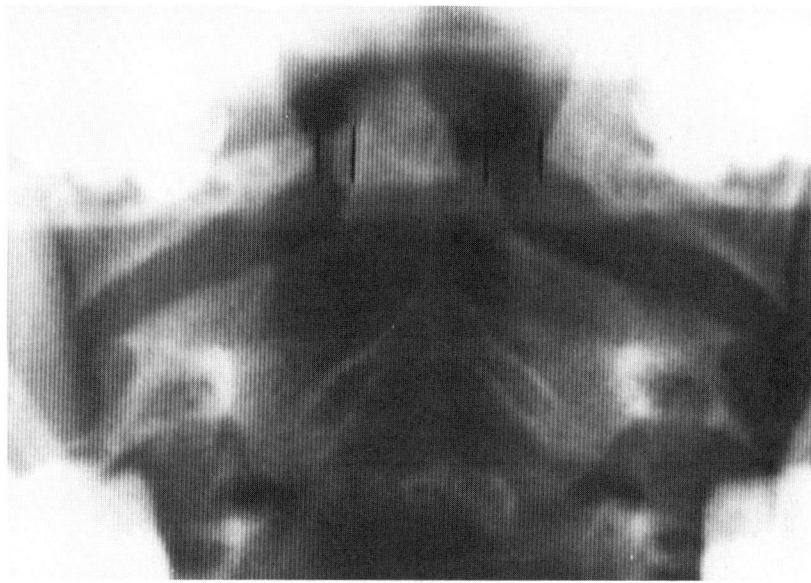

Figure 16.5 AARF. (a) Open-mouth odontoid view. Note the difference in the interval between the dens and the lateral masses.

long-term prognosis. These studies also will help to delineate the level of injury by the demonstration of bleeding or edema in the cord or by a block to flow or extravasation of contrast medium. Extravasation of contrast at the level of a SCIWORA injury carries an extremely poor prognosis. If a partial cord injury is recognized, a second episode of injury with catastrophic consequences can be prevented.

MANAGEMENT

The goals of management should be to prevent further injury, to relieve cord compression, to ensure stability, and to avoid deformity and pain in the future. Some differences in treating children are worth mentioning. First, they heal better and more quickly. Second, their potential for recovering useful function following a neurologic injury is greater. Even in an apparently complete injury, the prognosis is not necessarily nil at the time of initial presentation. Third, some deformities from fractures are able to remodel with growth. Finally, children tolerate prolonged immobilization and bedrest better than adults do. Therefore surgical treatment is less often necessary in children. On the other hand, children have a much greater tendency to develop spinal deformity following SCI. Therefore they are more likely to require long-term bracing or spine fusion for late deformity.

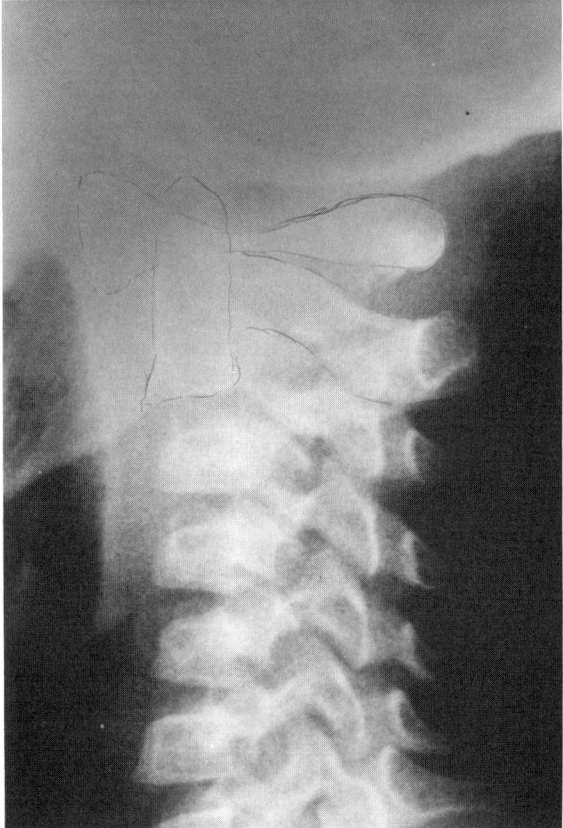

Figure 16.5 (continued) (b) Lateral view. Note how large the anterior ring of C1 appears (because one is really viewing the lateral mass).

Initial Management

The initial management should include optimal positioning to prevent further injury. The neck should be immobilized with a soft or hard collar and/or sandbags. The patient should be moved by log rolling and transported on a board. Extension of the neck for intubation should be avoided. In small children, the head is proportionately larger than it is in adults. Placing a child on a flat surface will tend to place the cervical spine in a flexed position or result in anterior translation at the site of injury. Therefore small children should be positioned with the head somewhat posterior to the trunk by placing bolsters under the trunk or the head in a depression.

For SCI patients, there is some evidence for the use of *methylprednisolone* in the acute management. All patients with SCIs should receive antacids to protect them from stress ulceration. A Foley catheter should be placed immediately, followed by an intermittent catheterization program if recovery of bladder function does not occur. Decubitus precautions should begin immediately.

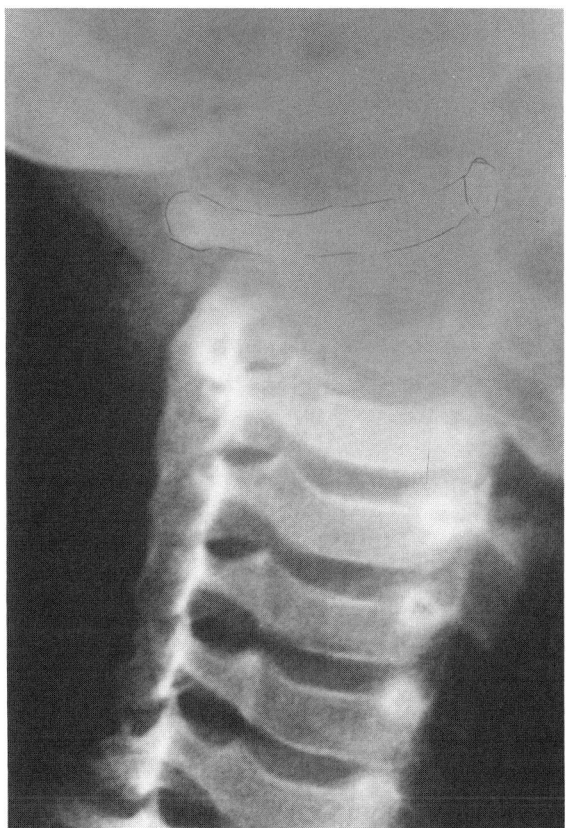

Figure 16.5 (continued)
(c) Oblique view. Note that a true lateral of the C1 vertebra is obtained with an oblique projection of the remainder of the cervical spine.

Surgical Management

Figure 16.6 presents an algorithm describing a reasonable approach to the management of spinal injuries. Usually the first consideration is whether the injury is displaced; if so, a reduction should be achieved. This can often be done by merely positioning the patient in such a way that the spine becomes better aligned. Sometimes traction is necessary to achieve a reduction, and rarely it may be necessary to perform an open reduction.

After the injury is reduced, one must maintain the reduction and provide stability if it is lacking. Some injuries are intrinsically stable and require only symptomatic treatment or a collar. Those that are less stable may require external support in the form of either a cast or orthosis or either prolonged bedrest or traction to maintain alignment while healing occurs. The halo brace can be considered a form of ambulatory traction. Surgical fusion is sometimes the best way to provide stability, particularly when an open reduction or decompression is necessary, when deformity

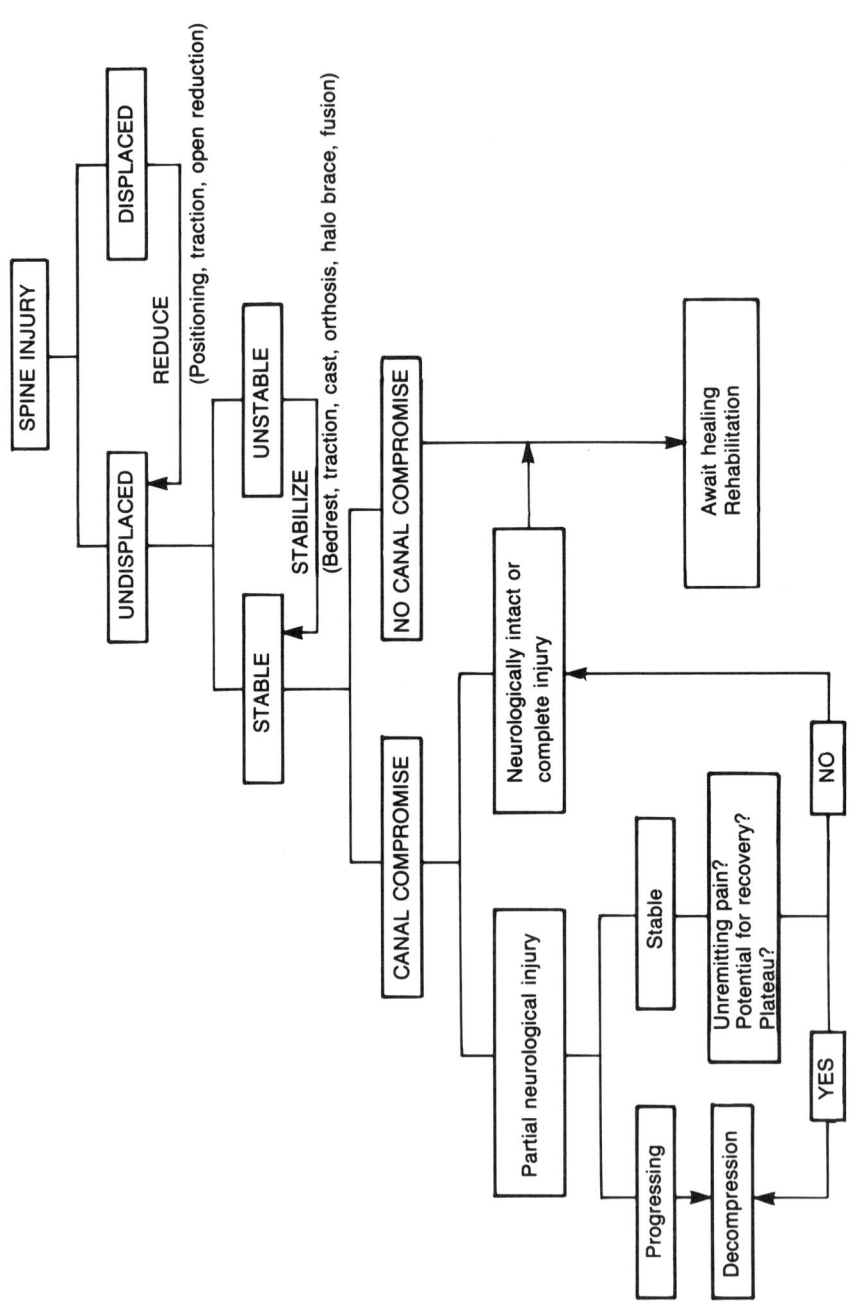

is present, or when rapid mobilization of the patient is desirable (as in a polytrauma patient or an SCI patient in need of rehabilitation).

The third consideration is compromise of the spinal canal and neural elements. The indications for decompression are a progressive neurologic deficit, possibly persisting compression of the cauda equina or conus medullaris (because of their increased potential for recovery), and possibly incomplete cord lesions with persistent compression, particularly if a plateau in neurologic recovery can be demonstrated. A final consideration might be canal compromise with intractable pain. Usually all that is necessary to decompress the spinal canal is realignment of the spine, especially when the injury is new. If decompression is necessary, a vertebrectomy through an anterior approach is more often appropriate. If an SCI is complete, the prognosis for recovery is very poor and probably is not improved by canal decompression. In this case, decompression is probably unwarranted, and consideration can be given to restoring alignment and providing stability.

The treatment of SCIWORA is no different from the treatment of SCI with fracture or dislocation, but it is very important to recognize partial injuries after the first episode, so that measures necessary to prevent further injury are taken.

Management of Specific Injuries
Atlantoaxial Rotatory Fixation

Most of these injuries are seen early and respond to bedrest, a soft cervical collar, and a mild relaxant such as diazepam or a nonsteroidal anti-inflammatory medication. If this is unsuccessful, a few days in head halter traction is usually successful. Some of these injuries are associated with temporary C1-C2 instability as is demonstrated on flexion-extension radiographs. They should be protected with a soft cervical collar for six weeks. When the condition has been present for longer than a month, it may not reduce, or it may recur after a reduction in traction. In this case or when instability persists for longer than six weeks, a C1-C2 posterior *in situ* fusion is occasionally indicated.

Atlas Fracture

Fracture of the atlas (Jefferson fracture) usually results from axial compression and is a stable injury. Most of these fractures will heal in a Minerva cast or a halo brace. Three months is usually sufficient for healing although six months may be necessary.

Axis Fractures

A fracture of the posterior elements of the C2 vertebra (hangman's fracture) will usually heal with a cast or brace but, if it is significantly displaced, may require a fusion.

Odontoid fractures can usually be treated with a halo brace or a Minerva cast for six to eight weeks, and surgery is seldom necessary. The results in older children are similar to those seen in adults. Fractures through the odontoid near the tip (type

I) and those through the body of C2 (type III) generally heal well. Those at the base of the odontoid (type II), however, frequently proceed to a nonunion and may require a fusion to restore stability.

Lower Cervical Spine

Fracture-dislocations in the lower cervical spine (C3-C7) are seen mainly in older children and are treated in a similar manner to treatment of the same injuries in adults. One should consider the mechanism of the injury since they can occur from flexion or extension. Most are adequately managed in a cast, an orthosis, or a halo. Surgery is usually done for flexion injuries, which can lead to late kyphosis, and generally consists of posterior wiring and fusion. Anterior fusion is not indicated because disruption of the anterior longitudinal ligament renders them more unstable. Primary anterior vertebrectomy and fusion is sometimes indicated for burst fractures from axial compression, because they commonly involve canal compromise, and because they have a tendency toward late collapse. Laminectomy is not indicated for any of these injuries because it produces further instability and may lead to a swan-neck deformity.

Ligamentous Disruption

Ligamentous disruption is less common in children than it is in adults. A loss of the normal lordosis and a stiff neck are constant features, but children commonly have no lordosis as a normal finding. Lateral radiographs in flexion may show a widened interspace posteriorly, a loss of parallelism of the facet joints, kyphosis of the disc space, posterior opening, or calcification of the disc space as a delayed feature. A delay in diagnosis is common, and it may be worthwhile to repeat the flexion film three to six weeks after the injury because increased mobility may be masked initially by splinting. Surgery is done for persistent or worsening deformity.

Thoracolumbar Injuries

Compression fractures occur at multiple levels more commonly in children than they do in adults. Pathologic fractures are seen in children and should be considered. They can result from an aneurysmal bone cyst, leukemia, or other myeloproliferative disorder. They are usually stable and can be treated with a cast or orthosis. Sometimes only symptomatic treatment is necessary. Most should be admitted to the hospital for observation because they are prone to developing ileus or urinary retention. They also often require pain management and should be observed for the development of a progressive neurologic deficit.

Flexion-distraction injuries (Chance fractures) are usually stable and can be managed by bracing although fusion may occasionally be required. One should also suspect injuries to visci from the lap belt.

Fracture of the vertebral limbus in adolescents occurs between the ring apophysis and the vertebral endplate. It most commonly involves the superior endplate in the midlumbar spine and often produces compression of the neural elements. Treatment is excision of the loose body through a laminotomy.

CONCLUSIONS

1. The recognition and understanding of spinal injuries in children is important if catastrophes are to be avoided.
2. Spinal injuries in children share some similarities with adult injuries but also have some important differences.
3. Significant neurologic sequelae are possible without radiographic abnormalities.
4. Treatment must be appropriate from the beginning to prevent complications.
5. Laminectomy should be avoided except in very special circumstances.

SUGGESTED READING

1. Cattell HS, Filtzer DL. Pseudosubluxation and other normal variations in the cervical spine in children. J Bone Joint Surg 1965;47A:1295.
2. Fielding JW, Hensinger RN. Fractures of the spine. In Rockwood CA, Wilkins KE, King RE, eds. Fractures in children. Philadelphia: Lippincott, 1984.
3. Ogden JA. Skeletal injury in the child, 2d ed. Philadelphia: Saunders, 1990;571–625.
4. Rang MC. Children's fractures, 2d ed. Philadelphia: Lippincott, 1983;331–345.
5. Sullivan JA. Fractures of the spine. In Green NE, Swiontkowski MF, eds. Skeletal trauma in children. Orlando, Fla.: WB Suanders, in press.

17

Coma and Altered Mental Status

James H. McCrory

Consciousness is a complex neurophysiologic process, involving the integrity of the reticular activating system in modulating interactions between the cerebral cortex and the brainstem. Suppression of the reticular activating system produces alterations in mental status leading to coma. The ultimate neurologic outcome and quality of survival depends on whether cellular integrity of the central nervous system (CNS) and supporting mylenation have been damaged during coma. In general, transient metabolic derangements of the CNS are well tolerated in children, provided that the flow of oxygen and glucose is uninterrupted.

PATHOPHYSIOLOGY

Loss of consciousness occurs after only six seconds of complete global ischemia and signifies the neurons' intolerance of anaerobic metabolism. The point at which irreversible damage from hypoxic-ischemic injury occurs is still controversial. Traditional clinical observations have noted irreversible damage occurring after approximately six minutes of complete global ischemia. Some children, after prolonged cardiac arrest, however, have a transient period of eye opening, recognition of parents, and response to verbal command followed by deterioration to brain death. Such clinical observations lend support to experimental evidence that irreversible neuronal injury occurs primarily during the period of reperfusion after complete global ischemia, due to the damage done to cellular membranes by superoxide radicals and by the influx of calcium ions.

Although the exact mechanism continues to be debated, there is universal agreement about the importance of preventing hypoxic-ischemic injury when possible by continuously delivering oxygen and glucose to the CNS. In addition to correcting hypoxemia, anemia, and hypotension, management of increased intracranial pressure is important in maintaining neuronal perfusion and integrity. Intracranial pressure (ICP) reflects a balance between the four intracranial fluids: blood, cerebrospinal fluid (CSF), interstitial fluid, and intracellular fluid.

After the sutures and fontanels close, the Kelly-Monroe hypothesis states that one of these fluids can increase only at the expense of the other three. During the early phases of cerebral edema, ICP remains normal or mildly elevated because of displacement of blood and CSF out of the intracranial compartment. The lateral ventricles collapse, and CSF is reabsorbed or displaced downward into the spinal canal where the dura has a limited capability of expansion. Cerebral blood volume, on the other hand, can be lowered by arterial constriction from hyperventilation or by increasing venous drainage with head elevation.

After compensatory mechanisms are exhausted, ICP elevates abruptly since liquids are not compressible substances. If the difference between the mean arterial pressure and the ICP falls to 30 torr, the electroencephalogram (EEG) becomes isoelectric, signifying global ischemia due to the collapse of small arterioles. Although it is invasive, monitoring of this type is used in children to determine the cerebral perfusion pressure as an indirect assessment of cerebral blood flow. Blood pressure and ICP are modulated to maintain the cerebral perfusion pressure in a safe range, usually above 50 torr.

Coma can also lead to either cardiopulmonary arrest or brain death. Respiratory failure progressing to arrest occurs secondary to suppression of the respiratory center in the medulla. Alterations in respiratory drive results in hypoventilation or central apnea, both of which present insidiously as a decreased work of breathing. Less commonly, coma can also be associated with a distributive form of shock. Thalamic dysfunction can produce decreased sympathetic tone and increased venous capacitance. The hemodynamic consequences are a relative hypovolemia, decreased venous return and decreased cardiac output.

CLINICAL PRESENTATION

The onset of altered mental status leading to coma is often insidious, producing vague symptoms from the parents, such as, "My child is acting funny or different," "She is not herself," "Something is wrong," or "He is not acting right." The first clinical task is to determine the child's level of responsiveness or consciousness. In the earliest phases of an abnormal physical examination, the child is awake and ambulatory, appears normal on first inspection, and answers questions appropriately. But on a closer look, the patient has an expressionless facies and appears dazed, perhaps glassy eyed. The ability to answer questions, though appropriate, is a bit sluggish. The term *cloudy sensorium* describes this condition. When it is associated with high fever, the neurotoxin produced by Shigella is one of the classic causes of this altered status, which can precede the diarrhea phase of the disease.

During the next lower phase, the patient is inappropriately sleepy, but can be aroused and is oriented. Failure to recognize parents is a cardinal symptom and sign which always points to a serious underlying disease process, whether it is due to coma, seizure, respiratory failure, or shock. At the beginning of this phase, the symptomatology is likely to be vague and perhaps even misleading, but if they are asked the specific question, "Does your child recognize you?" parents will respond "no" after a thoughtful pause. Failure to recognize parents is also a sign as judged by the nature of the child's eye contact and ability to follow their parents to whom they look for security. Ability to recognize and interact with parents can be judged and assessed as early as one month of age. Failure to recognize parents is often accompanied by being confused and combative, as well as by failure to respond to verbal commands. New onset of enuresis in a child who has been previously toilet trained can occur during this phase as well.

As the level of consciousness further deteriorates, the response to noxious stimuli becomes the critical factor. The degree of noxious stimuli can vary from light touch to moderate or severe pain. Failure of an infant to respond to a lumbar puncture or venipuncture rapidly alerts the clinician to a low level of consciousness.

Appropriate responses to pain vary in level of defensiveness. When *combative*, the patient is able to find and to fend off the noxious stimuli. *Localization* refers to the ability to reach and to touch the noxious stimuli, but the patient is too comatose to struggle against it. *Withdrawal* refers to a single extremity response to move away from the pain. If pain is applied to an extensor surface, the patient will flex away from it, and vice versa.

Withdrawal becomes an *inappropriate response to pain* when the patient flexes into pain applied on the flexor surface of the extremity. Inappropriate responses, however, are most obvious when the patient has a spastic, four-extremity reaction, which is nonpurposeful in nature. *Decorticate posturing* consists of extension of the lower extremities with simultaneous flexion of the upper extremities at the elbows. *Decerebrate posturing* involves extension of all four extremities. True posturing needs to be distinguished from appropriate withdrawal or combativeness with increased muscle tone. The distinction is usually obvious by the purposeful nature of the latter.

Decorticate and decerebrate posturing can be produced in laboratory animals by creating a surgical lesion at the level of cerebral hemispheres and brain stem respectively. In children, posturing rarely signifies a structural lesion such as a brainstem hemorrhage but is more commonly associated with a physiologic disturbance caused by a metabolic problem, inflammation, or increased ICP. In the deepest stages of coma, the child has no response to painful stimuli. The child's extremities are usually flaccid and areflexic at this point.

Children in shock, on the other hand, have a fluctuating level of consciousness. Their mental status can vary from being unresponsive during painful procedures to being alert and recognizing their parents. These fluctuations are indicative of the varying levels of cerebral blood flow and cortical perfusion. Obvious signs of posturing are usually absent during this process, so the severity of the child's condition can be underestimated if the clinician becomes falsely reassured by the child's best neurologic response instead of determining the reason for the child's worst neurologic response.

The clinical presentation of increased ICP varies. Subacute or chronic elevation of ICP presents as headaches, vomiting, and papilledema. Since papilledema takes 48 to 72 hours to develop fully, it is often absent in coma with acute increased pressure. In this situation, increased ICP is suspected when there is a rapid onset of coma with a working diagnosis compatible with this problem. It is especially suspected when the level of consciousness has deteriorated to the point of posturing or there are pupillary changes compatible with cerebral herniation.

Central herniation begins when bilateral pressure on the midbrain causes loss of sympathetic tone, and the pupils constrict in a pinpoint fashion. Uncal herniation occurs when pressure in one cerebral hemisphere causes a unilateral impingement on the third cranial nerve by the uncal gyrus at the level of the tentorium. Loss of parasympathetic tone causes dilation of the ipsilateral pupil. If the increase in ICP continues and is irreversible, both central and uncal herniation end in the pupils being irregular, fixed, and dilated in a midposition after both uncal gyri herniate downward through the tentorium.

The focus from which the pressure originates is also important in determining the clinical presentation. Increased ICP from hydrocephalus produces the *sunset sign*. Dilation of the lateral ventricles compresses nearby nerve tracts, causing a downward deviation of the eyes. This upper motor neuron sign presents as a gaze deficit, the earliest form of which consists of loss of upward gaze. Acute shunt obstruction in hydrocephalus can present as loss of upward gaze and altered mental status before progressing to coma.

Other forms of supratentorium increased ICP, such as that produced by the intracellular edema of Reye's syndrome, presents as *rostrocaudal deterioration*. In this situation, the level of consciousness deteriorates sequentially as has already been described, followed by progressive cranial nerve dysfunction, culminating in cerebral herniation. Compression of the respiratory center in the medulla finally leads to a permanent cessation of respiration. This process is exactly opposite of the return of function that can occur after a resuscitation from cardiac arrest. Return of respiration, followed by pupillary function and possibly by cortical function reflects the pattern of reperfusion.

Increased pressure, originating in the posterior fossa, is relatively uncommon but has a distinct clinical presentation. Etiologies include cerebellar infarction and tumors that cause secondary hemorrhage or edema. In the early phases, cortical perfusion remains intact. The patient is usually semialert but is confused or has an altered sensorium. The child is no longer ambulatory and can manifest unusual motor movements of the extremities that are neither posturing nor seizure activity. Occasionally pressure in the posterior fossa can slowly build to a critical point at which all circulation suddenly becomes compromised and global ischemia occurs. The patient has a sudden loss of consciousness with apnea. If it is witnessed, the respiratory arrest is rapidly reversible with assisted ventilation, but the neurologic examination reveals findings consistent with brain death.

Table 17.1 summarizes the rapid examination of the cranial nerves. Presence of the pupillary, oculocephalic, corneal, and gag reflexes confirms the basic function of all but the cranial nerves I and XI. Rapid lateral turning of the head stimulates a vestibular reaction and subsequent eye movement. This doll's eye maneuver is normal when eye movement occurs and is referred to as the *oculocephalic reflex*. The oculovestibular reflex has a similar motor component but is elicited by ice water irrigation of the tympanic membranes. For clarity of charting, these reflexes are best described as "present" when eye movement occurs or as "absent" when it does not. "Normal doll's eyes," on the other hand, means different things to different observers.

The presence of focal neurologic signs can be helpful in localizing discrete lesions when they are present or in signifying asymmetrical intracranial events. Examples of the latter include generalized seizures with prominent clonus on one side

Table 17.1 Rapid neurologic assessment

Level of consciousness		
Appropriate to verbal command	*Inappropriate response to pain*	
Alert, oriented	Decorticate	
Confused	Decerebrate	
Inappropriate to verbal command	No response	
Fails to recognize parents	*Focal neurologic signs*	
No response to verbal command	Anisocoria	
Appropriate response to pain	Hemiplegia	
Combative	Facial	
Localizes	Extremity	
Withdraws	Paraplegia	
	Quadriplegia	
Cranial nerve reflexes	*Sensory*	*Motor*
Pupillary reflex	II	III
Oculocephalic reflex	VIII	III, IV, VI
Corneal reflex	V	VI
Gag reflex	IX, X	IX, X, XII

The rapid neurologic assessment can be performed in less than two minutes and is helpful in determining the neurologic stability of the patient as well as in creating a differential diagnosis.

only and generalized cerebral edema with early uncal herniation. Focal cranial nerve signs include anisocoria, ophthalmoplegias, and facial asymmetry. Monoparesis, hemiplegia, paraplegia or quadriplegia can be detected by examination of the extremities for movement, tone, and reflexes.

DIFFERENTIAL DIAGNOSIS

The first diagnostic task is to separate the altered mental status leading to coma from those produced by seizures and postictal phenomenon. In the case of witnessed grand mal epilepsy, the distinction is clear. The physician only needs to check for return of purposeful responses to painful stimuli during postictal drowsiness to confirm that the seizure has stopped. If the patient fails to respond to painful stimuli appropriately, an EEG can be helpful in the diagnosis of ongoing electrical status without corresponding abnormal motor movements. Other forms of seizure activity, such as frequent petit mal and partial complex seizures, can present with altered mental status without the obvious abnormal motor movements and the loss of consciousness characteristic of grand mal. Once the possibility of seizures has been excluded, the differential diagnosis of coma can be divided into four categories, based on focal neurologic signs and increased ICP.

No Focal Signs and Normal Intracranial Pressure

This category contains the most common cause of childhood coma and is the least likely to be associated with any mortality or permanent sequella. It includes concussions from mild head trauma, toxins, metabolic abnormalities, mild CNS infections, and postictal states. Metabolic conditions include uremia, hyponatremia, hypernatremia, hypercapnia, hypocalcemia and global ischemia. The latter is usually associated with cardiac or respiratory arrest and can vary from transient to permanent. The severest forms, leading to brain death or survival in a persistent vegetative state, can be accompanied by a delayed onset of increased ICP after 12 hours or more. Managing this form of pressure with intracranial monitoring, however, has not been shown to improve outcome.

Children with small pupils and coma usually have a toxic ingestion that belongs in this category. Opiates produce these findings, but exposure to ethanol, phenothiazines, and organophosphates also presents in this fashion. The prognosis is usually favorable for all of these conditions. The possibility of pontine hemorrhage and early central herniation from cerebral edema also needs to be considered in these patients.

No Focal Signs and Increased Intracranial Pressure

This category has the highest mortality. It includes severe head trauma, Reye's syndrome, fulminant bacterial meningitis, and diabetic ketoacidosis. All of these conditions are reasonable candidates for monitoring intracranial pressure in order to prevent or minimize ischemic damage. Hydrocephalus with shunt obstruction also belongs in this category.

Focal Signs and Normal Intracranial Pressure

The most common cause in this category is benign. A Todd's paresis is a transient, postictal hemiparesis that resolves completely within 24 to 72 hours after the seizure. Cerebral vascular accidents, on the other hand, are relatively uncommon in the pediatric age group. The more frequent etiologies are sickle cell anemia and bacterial meningitis. Rare conditions include homocysteinuria and embolic phenomena from acute bacterial endocarditis or left atrial myxoma.

Focal Signs and Increased Intracranial Pressure

This category includes the mass lesions: intracranial hemorrhage, tumors, brain abscess, and arteriovenous malformations. Prognosis depends on location and surgical accessibility. Herpes encephalitis, which can produce cystic degenerations in the temporal region and generalized cerebral edema, also needs to be considered in this category.

PHYSICAL EXAMINATION

A rapid cardiopulmonary assessment is first performed in order to determine the adequacy of airway, breathing, and circulation (ABCs). If trauma is suspected, cervical immobilization should be performed simultaneously with this initial inspection. Next a rapid neurologic assessment should be performed to determine the child's level of consciousness, cranial nerve status, and the presence of any focal neurologic signs (Table 17.1). Determination of the exact heart rate, respiration, blood pressure, temperature, transcutaneous saturation, and glucose by bedside testing follows next.

With this information, the physician is able to build a working differential diagnosis based on one of the four categories already outlined. If the patient is neurologically and hemodynamically stable, the diagnosis can usually be made by taking a quick problem-oriented history from the parents. According to the index of suspicion that evolves from the working differential, questions can be directed toward recent onset of infectious symptoms, ingestion-related behaviors and risk factors, abnormal motor movement suggestive of seizures, complaints of headache and vomiting, changes in behavior, underlying medical illnesses, and occult forms of trauma. If the history is totally benign and does not help define the etiology of the coma, unwitnessed seizure, drug ingestion, and child abuse need to be given thorough consideration.

LABORATORY EVALUATION

Laboratory evaluation of altered mental status and coma can be thought of in terms of both general screening tests to be performed on all patients and specific tests directed at further defining the categories in the differential diagnosis already outlined. Basic screening tests include electrolytes, glucose, blood urea nitrogen, arterial blood gases, and at least one liver enzyme. In regards to the latter, the gamma Guatemala transferase (GGT) and serum glutamate pyruvate transaminase (SGPT) are more liver-specific than serum glutamic-oxaloacetic transaminase (SGOT), which can be found in skeletal and cardiac muscle as well. If hepatic coma is likely, determination of serum ammonia and prothrombin time (PT) is also important. Hyponatremia and hypernatremia can present as coma or seizures. Disturbances of potassium, calcium, and magnesium, however, are more likely to present as alterations in muscle tone and possibly as dysrhythmias.

For toxicology screenings, samples from the urine, blood, and gastric contents are important for analysis. Occasionally, a plain film of the abdomen can be helpful in quantifying the severity of the ingestion if a radiopaque substance such as iron tablets or substances containing lead are in question.

Lumbar puncture for diagnosis of meningitis and encephalitis is important but is deferred in situations in which the patient has focal neurologic signs or is suspected of having significant increased intracranial pressure. In severe meningitis with increased intracranial pressure, cerebral herniation and brain death can occur in the field or in the emergency department even before a lumbar puncture has been performed. If a child presents with a high fever, coma, and posturing, antibiotics can be started and the lumbar puncture postponed until it is clearly safe to perform it.

When increased intracranial pressure is suspected, an emergency computerized tomography (CT) or magnetic resonance imaging (MRI) scan is the procedure of choice, both to rule out mass effect and to document signs of cerebral edema. Obliteration of the quadrigeminal plate cistern correlates highly with pupillary changes of uncal herniation. Small lateral ventricles and obliterations of fissures can also indicate increased pressure.

MANAGEMENT

Supportive care of the comatose child is ultimately directed at continuous delivery of oxygen and glucose to the neurons while maintaining oxygenation, ventilation, and perfusion to the other organ systems (Table 17.2). Management decisions and interventions are made concurrently with performance of the physical examination. Once the initial assessment and stabilization have been performed, confirmation of the working diagnosis is performed by taking the history and performing selective laboratory procedures (Table 17.3).

Table 17.2 General management of children in coma

Rapid cardiopulmonary assessment	Rapid neurological asessment
Airway	Level of consciousness
Normal	Focal neurologic signs
Spinal immobilization if trauma suspected	Cranial nerve reflexes
Clear secretions	Increased intracranial pressure
Maintainable by simple maneuvers	*Quick history*
Chin lift or jaw thrust	*Initial blood work*
Nasopharyngeal airway	Dextrostix at bedside
Unmaintainable	Complete blood count (CBC)
Rapid oral intubation	Electrolytes and blood urea nitrogen (BUN)
Breathing	Glucose
Normal Spontaneous	Liver enzymes
Increase F_iO_2	
Maintainable by bag-valve-mask device	
Intubation necessary to	
Protect airway	
Maintain (hyper-)ventilation	
Circulation	
Normal	
Obtain vascular access	
Monitor heart rate	
Transcutaneous O_2 saturation	
Neurogenic Hypotension	
Trendelberg position	
Volume expansion	
Alpha agonists	

Table 17.3 Management based on four working diagnostic categories

1. *No focal signs and normal ICP*
   - Toxins — Blood and urine screen
   - CNS infections — CT scan for ICP signs
     - Lumbar puncture
   - Concussion — CT scan to rule out hemorrhage
   - Metabolic — Correct specific defect
   - Anoxic — Anticipatory counseling of family about outcome
   - Small pupils — Narcan for opiates
     - Also consider:
       - Ethanol
       - Phenothizines
       - Organophosphates
       - Pontine hemorrhage
       - Early central herniation

2. *No focal signs and increased ICP*
   - CT scan — Rule out mass effect
     - Rule out acute hydrocephalus
     - Evaluate basal cisterns
   - Medical therapy — Head elevation
     - Hyperventilation
     - Mannitol
     - Thiopental
     - Muscle relaxation

3. *Focal signs and normal ICP*
   - Todd's paresis — Reassure parents
   - Cerebrovascular accident — MRI scan
     - Possible angiogram

4. *No focal signs and increased ICP (CT scan)*
   - Hemorrhage — Emergent surgery
   - Tumor — Urgent surgery
     - Possible emergent ventriculostomy
   - Abscess — Antibiotics
     - Possible emergent surgery
   - AVM/subarachnoid hemorrhage — Observation
     - Delayed surgery
   - Herpes encephalitis — EEG
     - Lumbar puncture
     - Acyclovir
     - Monitor ICP

After stabilization of the patient, a working differential diagnosis of coma is based on categorization determined by ICP and focal neurologic signs. Specific diagnostic and therapeutic procedures follow and are summarized in this table.
AVM = arterial venous malformation

Table 17.4 Mnemonics for coma

Actions			Etiologies
D	Dextrostix (or give glucose)	A	Alcohol
O	Oxygen	E	Epilepsy/encephalopathy, electrolytes
N	Narcan	I	Insulin, intussusception, infection
T	Thiamine	O	Overdose
		U	Uremia

The above mnemonics, while created primarily for adults in coma, are helpful in summarizing the initial approach and etiologic considerations when managing a child in coma.

The degree of supportive care necessary in each case needs to be individualized according to the child's level of consciousness and the pathophysiology involved. The decision to perform endotracheal intubation to protect the airway, for instance, is based on the state of the child's protective reflexes more than on the level of consciousness and is modified by factors such as the presence of respiratory compromise or increased ICP.

CONCLUSION

The etiology of childhood coma can be either obvious (such as from witnessed trauma) or obscure and difficult to determine. In either event, initial stabilization in the emergency department (Table 17.4) is critical to prevent secondary cerebral ischemia whether it is from respiratory failure, shock, or increased ICP. (These mnemonics are helpful both for quick initial assessment and for management.) Once the patient is stabilized, the diagnostic work-up proceeds on lines determined by the presence or absence of increased ICP and focal neurologic signs. Except for anoxic encephalopathy incurred during an episode of asystole and for severe head trauma, the prognosis is usually favorable.

SUGGESTED READING

1. Ashwal S. Brain death in the newborn. Clin Perinatol 1989;169(2):501–518.
2. Coulter DL. Neurologic uncertainty in newborn intensive care. N Engl J Med 1987;316(14):840–844.
3. Drake B, Ashwal S, Schneider S, et al. Determination of cerebral death in the pediatric intensive care unit. Pediatrics 1986;78(1):107–112.
4. Frank LM, Furgiuele TL, Etheridge JE Jr. Prediction of chronic vegetative state in children using evoked potentials. Neurology 1985;35(6):931–934.
5. Goodwin SR, Friedman WA, Bellefleur M, et al. Is it time to use evoked potentials to predict outcome in comatose children and adults? Critical Care Medicine 1991;19(4):518–524.
6. Goitein KJ, Amit Y, Fainmesser P, et al. Diagnostic and prognostic value of auditory nerve brainstem evoked responses in comatose children. Critical Care Med 1983;11(2):91–94.

7. Groswasser Z, Sazbon L. Outcome in 134 patients with prolonged posttraumatic unawareness. Part 2: Functional outcome of 72 patients recovering consciousness. Neurosurg 1990;72(1):81–84.
8. Kanter RK. Evaluation and stabilization of the critically ill child. Clinics in Chest Medicine 1987;8(4):573–581.
9. Lutschg J, Pfenninger J, Ludin HP, et al. Brain-stem auditory evoked potentials and early somatosensory evoked potentials in neurointensively treated comatose children. American Journal of Diseases and Children 1983;137(5):421–426.
10. Nikas DL. Prognostic indicators in patients with severe head injury. Critical Care Nursing Quarterly 1987;10(3):25–34.
11. Plum F, Posner JB. The diagnosis of stupor and coma, 3d ed. Contemporary Neurology Series, Philadelphia: FA Davis, 1980.
12. Rowland TW, Donnelly JH, Jackson AH, et al. Brain death in the pediatric intensive care unit. A clinical definition. American Journal of Diseases of Children 1983;137(6):547–550.
13. Sazbon L, Groswasser Z. Outcome in 134 patients with prolonged posttraumatic unawareness. Part 1: Parameters determining late recovery of consciousness. Journal of Neurosurgery 1990;72(1):75–80.
14. Steinhart CM, Weiss IP. Use of brainstem auditory evoked potentials in pediatric brain death. 1985;13(7):560–562.
15. Strickbine-Van Reet P, Glaze DG, Hrachovy RA, et al. A preliminary prospective neurophysiological study of coma in children. American Journal of Diseases of Children. 1984;138(5):492–495.
16. Tasker RC, Boyd S, Harden A, et al. Monitoring in non-traumatic coma. Part II: Electroencephalography. Archives of Disease in Childhood 1988;63(8):895–899.
17. Tasker RC, Matthew DJ, Helms P, et al. Monitoring in non-traumatic coma. Part I: Invasive intracranial measurements. Archives of Disease in Childhood 1988;63(8):888–894.

18

Convulsive Status Epilepticus

Jeff Biehler

With a reported mortality rate of 8 percent to 15 percent, convulsive status epilepticus is a serious and potentially life threatening medical emergency (1,2). *Status epilepticus* is defined as continuous seizure activity lasting more than 20 or 30 minutes or as a series of recurrent seizures without a return of consciousness between episodes. Status epilepticus can be divided into two broad categories, convulsive and nonconvulsive. Convulsive status epilepticus is associated with the loss of consciousness and may be focal, focal motor, or generalized in nature. Convulsive status epilepticus necessitates immediate and definitive medical management. Nonconvulsive types of status epilepticus include complex partial or absence seizures (3). This chapter will be limited to the discussion of convulsive status epilepticus in the pediatric patient beyond the neonatal period.

Although a wide variety of serious complications may be associated with this disorder, a systematic approach to the initial evaluation and management of these children positively impacts patient outcome. Rapid evaluation, stabilization, and treatment of underlying disorders as well as the expeditious use of antiepileptic medications will reduce the morbidity and mortality associated with status epilepticus. It is therefore important that physicians involved in the emergency care of pediatric patients become skilled in the management of this disorder.

EPIDEMIOLOGY

There are many conditions that may play a causative role in the development of status epilepticus (Table 18.1). Patient age and a history of a previous epileptic disorder are the two most important factors when considering potential etiologies. A demonstrable etiology for seizure activity is more frequently found in children less than six months of age than in the older children or adults. In children with a known epileptic disorder, the lifetime occurrence rate of status epilepticus is approximately 16 to 24 percent.

Among all patients with status epilepticus, approximately one-half of the status episodes will have no identifiable specific etiology and are therefore labeled as idiopathic (3). Of the remaining one-half, 50 percent of patients will have an identifiable acute insult such as infection, traumatic injury, metabolic derangement,

Table 18.1 Etiologies of status epilepticus in children

	Percent
Idiopathic	53
Chronic encephalopathy	21
Known or suspected etiology	26
Withdrawal of antiepileptic drugs	
Infection	
Toxic exposure	
Metabolic derangement	
Head trauma	
Tumor	
Vascular malformation	
Congenital CNS* malformation	
Degenerative CNS* disease	
Neurocutaneous syndromes	

*CNS = central nervous system

hypoxia/anoxia, or acute substance ingestion. The etiology of status epilepticus in the remaining 25 percent of patients consists of static or chronic disorders such as encephalopathies of multiple etiologies, mass lesions, or vascular malformations (4,5).

When considering those children who present with status epilepticus for whom there is no identifiable cause for the seizures, approximately one-half will have a significant temperature elevation. This associated fever is most often found in children less than three years old. A portion of the febrile patients with status epilepticus may represent a prolonged febrile seizure; a careful search for a specific cause of the elevated temperature and other potential etiologies for the seizure activity, however, is warranted.

PATHOPHYSIOLOGY

Convulsive status epilepticus causes significant pathophysiolgic changes that may manifest in multiple adverse systemic derangements. These physiologic alterations may result in life threatening deviations of homeostasis and in variable degrees of neurologic damage. These systemic complications may effect virtually any organ system (Table 18.2).

Status epilepticus results in a dramatic activation of the autonomic nervous system. An initial increase in serum catecholamines is evidenced by systemic hypertension and tachycardia (6). Accompanying these changes are increases in pulmonary and systemic vascular resistance as well as an increase in cerebral venous pressure (7). Subsequently these physiologic alterations produce an increase in cerebral blood flow

Table 18.2 Systemic complications of status epilepticus

Autonomic nervous system	*Metabolic*
Hyperpyrexia	Lactic acidosis
Hypersecretion	Hypoglycemia
Nausea and vomiting	Hypernatremia
Hyperhidrosis	Hyperkalemia
Cardiovascular	Hyponatremia
Hypertension	*Renal*
Hypotension	Acute tubular necrosis
Bradycardia	Rhabdomyolysis
Cardiac arrest	Oligura
Respiratory	Acute renal failure
Hypoxemia	
Hypercarbia	
Apnea	
Neuogenic pulmonary edema	
Aspiration	

and variable degrees of increased intracranial pressure (ICP) (8). Secondary cardiovascular changes may include the sudden development of severe hypotension, bradycardia, and cardiac failure. Diminished cardiac output may compromise cerebral blood flow potentiating possible neurologic damage.

Respiratory compromise is one of the most common and serious complications of status epilepticus. Respiratory embarrassment may result from a combination of discoordinated contractions of respiratory muscles, the loss of central control of respiratory drive, and airway obstruction secondary to improper airway positioning or increased respiratory secretions. These conditions result in decreased ventilation and subsequent respiratory acidosis and hypoxia. Respiratory acidosis further compromises cerebral blood flow autoregulation and may result in worsening of intracranial hypertension and cerebral edema. Hypoxia contributes to neurologic damage encountered by seizure patients.

Sustained motor activity observed during convulsive status epilepticus results in a variety of systemic manifestations. Hyperthermia develops as a consequence of the increased heat production of repetitive muscle contractions. Increased serum lactate levels and subsequent lactic acidosis are also produced by excessive muscle activity. Protracted muscle activity may result in rhabdomyolysis and myoglobinuria with the subsequent development of nephrotoxicity and acute renal failure (9).

Metabolic derangements encountered during status epilepticus may include hypoglycemia, hyperkalemia, and abnormalities of serum sodium. Increased autonomic activity results in an hyperglycemia early in the course of status epilepticus. Hypoglycemia, however, may develop with prolonged seizure activity. Elevations in serum potassium are thought to be secondary to a combination of increased muscle activity and increased catecholamine secretion.

In spite of measures to minimize respiratory, hemodynamic, and metabolic derangements, injury to selected brain regions may occur during the course of status epilepticus. Brain injury on a cellular level may develop as a result of a combination of systemic complications (hypoglycemia, hypoxia, acidosis, and the like) and the excessive metabolic demands of repetitive neuronal discharge during a prolonged convulsive seizure (10,11,12).

CLINICAL PRESENTATION

The most common presentation of convulsive status epilepticus is a prolonged tonic, myoclonic, or tonic-clonic seizure. The persistence of a seizure or the rapid recurrence of repeated seizures differentiates status epilepticus from uncomplicated partial or generalized convulsive seizures (1). An abnormal level of consciousness, rhythmic or sustained involuntary muscle contractions, and physical findings provoked by abnormal sympathetic discharge make these forms of status epilepticus easily recognizable.

DIFFERENTIAL DIAGNOSIS

Because of the dramatic clinical presentation of childhood status epilepticus, the diagnosis is usually not difficult. Status epilepticus must be differentiated from nonepileptic disorders such as dystonic drug reaction, opisthotonic posturing, pseudoseizure, conversion reaction, or breath-holding spells (1,2).

Diagnostic efforts should be directed toward determining the etiology of seizure and other abnormalities that may affect patient outcome. Careful attention to the patient's medical history and physical examination should help the physician determine the contributing factors associated with the onset and continuation of seizure activity.

HISTORY AND PHYSICAL EXAMINATION

A thorough history and a physical examination are essential to the management of children presenting to the emergency department with status epilepticus. Careful documentation of antecedent events, of the condition of the patient at presentation to the emergency department, of responses to therapy, and of postictal condition is necessary.

At the time of presentation, a brief history should be obtained from the patient's caretaker or from transfer personnel. Questions should be asked regarding the patient's condition prior to the onset of the seizures, a history of previous seizures, current medications, recent head injury, and allergies to medications. After the patient has been stabilized, a complete medical and developmental history should be obtained. Special attention should be directed toward obtaining a thorough history of previous seizures and, if it is indicated, methods of seizure control. Information regarding a history of recent head trauma, headache, fever, visual change, and nausea or vomiting should be collected. Parents should be asked about potentially toxic substances the child may have ingested. Specific questions regarding aspirin, household cleaning solutions, prescription medications, illicit drugs, lead, and hydrocarbons should be addressed.

The initial physical examination should consist of a primary survey directed toward assuring that an unobstructed airway is being maintained and that adequate breathing and circulation is present. A rapid assessment of vital signs and overall neurologic status should be followed by complete exposure and a brief physical examination. After stabilization, a complete secondary survey with special attention to the neurologic examination should be accomplished.

LABORATORY AND RADIOLOGIC EVALUATION

Although the history and physical examination remain the most important tools in the evaluation of status epilepticus, supporting laboratory and radiologic information can also be invaluable. Initial laboratory tests should include a complete blood count (CBC), serum glucose (dextrostix), electrolytes, calcium, magnesium, urea nitrogen, and hepatic enzymes. A urine or serum metabolic screen should be considered in infants. If it is indicated, serum anticonvulsant levels should be determined and urine sent for toxicologic studies. Lumbar puncture for the evaluation of cerebrospinal fluid (CSF) should be considered in children with a history suggestive of CNS infection. To avoid potential complications, careful evaluation for increased ICP or mass lesions should be performed prior to lumbar puncture (13).

The indications for intracranial radiologic evaluation differ among experts. There is general agreement that patients with a history of recent head trauma, focal seizure activity, or persistent focal neurologic findings or with a history and physical examination suggestive of increased ICP, intracranial bleeding, or mass lesion should undergo computerized axial tomography. Radiologic studies should be delayed until after stabilization and adequate management of seizures has been accomplished. Pediatric neurology consultation regarding the evaluation and management of pediatric patients presenting with status epilepticus is suggested.

MANAGEMENT

As with any emergency, initial attention in the management of status epilepticus should be directed toward the establishment and maintenance of an adequate airway. The standard techniques of airway maintenance using proper head positioning (that is, sniffing position, head-tilt, or chin-lift) should provide adequate patency. Special attention should be directed toward stabilization of the C-spine in patients with associated head trauma. Many patients will benefit from the placement of an oral airway or nasopharyngeal airway. Following establishment of the airway, careful suctioning of oral secretions should be performed. When the above measures fail to provide an adequate airway, immediate consideration of endotracheal intubation is warranted.

Attention should next be directed toward the adequacy of ventilation and oxygenation. The physician should ensure that adequate ventilation is established. If ventilation is decreased or absent, assistance using a positive pressure ventilation (bag/mask or bag/endotrachial tube) device should be started. All patients should receive a high concentration of supplemental oxygen.

A rapid survey of the patient's vital signs should be the next step in patient management. An estimate of peripheral perfusion, as measured by capillary refill time, as well as respiratory rate, heart rate, blood pressure, and temperature should be measured. The placement of an electrocardiogram (EKG) monitoring device and a pulse oxymeter is also recommended.

Establishment of an intravenous (IV) line for the delivery of fluids and anticonvulsant medications should now be attempted. An indwelling peripheral IV line may be established at any available location. In patients with difficult IV access problems or with severe bradycardia or hypotension, the rapid placement of an intraosseous line should be considered. Once such a line is established, a continuous infusion of a 5 percent to 10 percent dextrose containing electrolyte solution should be started at a rate to meet 80 percent of maintenance requirements. If it is possible, blood samples for a determination of serum blood glucose and other laboratory tests should be obtained while placing the IV line.

Patients with metabolic derangements such as hypoglycemia, hypercalcemia, hypocalcemia, or severe hyponatremia require specific treatment directed toward correction of these abnormalities (Figure 18.1). Until these precipitating factors are corrected, poor response to anticonvulsive medications can be expected (1,14,15).

If seizure activity continues after the above measures, the patient should receive anticonvulsent medications. The selection of anticonvulsent medication depends on patient age, seizure type, ongoing chronic anticonvulsant therapy, and patient condition. Careful calculation of all antiseizure medication dosages is advised.

There is an increasing consensus that the drug of choice for the inital treatment of pediatric convulsive status epilepticus is IV lorazepam (for example, Ativan) (16). This rapidly acting benzodiazepine has a success rate of 80 percent to 100 percent when used in the treatment of status epilepticus (17). Termination of seizure activity is usually achieved within two to three minutes following administration of lorezepam (18). The recommended dosage is 0.05 to 0.1 mg/kg with a maximum dose of 4 mg (1). This dosage may be repeated as needed to a total of three doses. The anticonvulsant effect of lorazepam lasts approximately 3 hours in a majority of patients, but the effect may last as long as 72 hours (19). As with all benzodiazepines, close monitoring for respiratory depression and hypotension is a necessity. These side effects are less frequently seen with lorazepam than they are with diazepam.

If lorazepam is unavailable, diazepam (Valium) is an alternative medication useful for rapid treatment of seizures (20). The recommended dosage is 0.1 to 0.3 mg/kg with a maximum of 10 mg per dose. This dosage may be repeated at 15-minute intervals to a total of three doses. In patients without IV or intraosseous access, diazepam may be administered rectally at a dose of 0.5 to 0.75 mg/kg (21,22). Because the duration of antiepileptic effect is relatively short (20 to 30 min), a second long-acting anticonvulsant should be administered following initial seizure control. Potential adverse effects of diazepam are similar to those of lorazepam. Previously

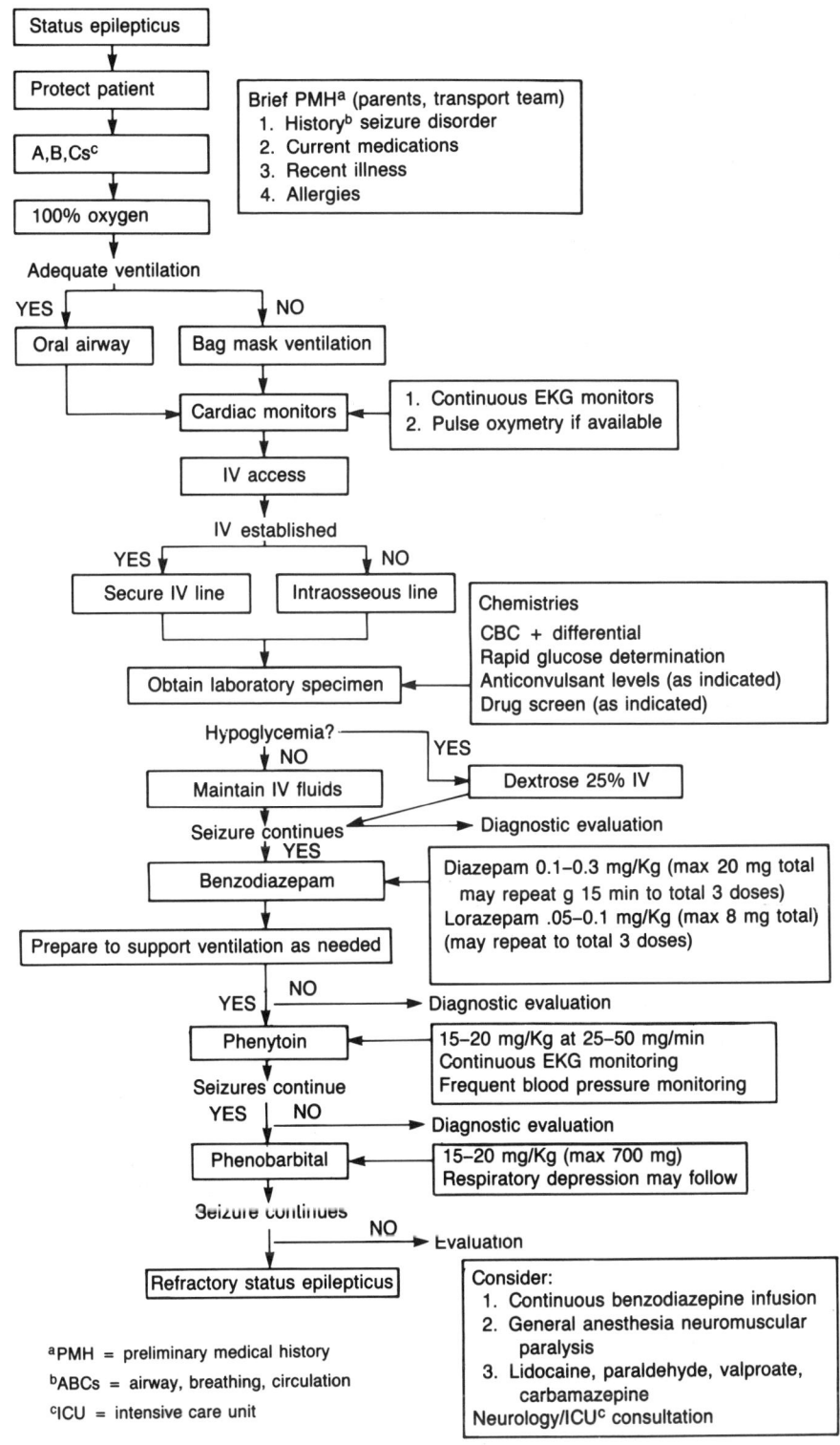

Figure 18.1　Status epilepticus management algorithm

administered barbiturates may potentiate the respiratory depression occasionally encountered with diazepam.

Phenytoin (for example, Dilantin) is also a useful medication for the treatment of status epilepticus. Considered by some to be the drug of choice in the treatment of seizures associated with head trauma, phenytoin may be used alone or in combination with a benzodiazepine. The long duration of action and lack of respiratory depression make phenytoin an excellent choice as a second medication in children previously treated with a benzodiazepine. The recommended initial loading dosage is 15 to 20 mg/kg, administered (in a nonglucose-containing solution) at a rate of 0.5 to 1 mg/kg/min (23). Phenytoin may be given by IV or by intraosseous infusion. Intramuscular injection of phenytoin is not an acceptable route of delivery for treatment of status epilepticus. Careful attention should be given to the monitoring of vital signs and cardiac rhythm during infusion of phenytoin. Rapid administration may precipitate cardiac dysrhythmia, hypotension, and respiratory depression (1). Peak CNS concentrations of phenytoin may not be achieved for 15 to 30 minutes after IV infusion, making the benzodiazipines a more desirable first choice for rapid treatment of seizures (24).

Phenobarbital is a medication familiar to most physicians experienced in the management of childhood seizures. It remains a useful alternative agent in the treatment of status epilepticus. When it is given as a bolus of 15 to 20 mg/kg intravenously, phenobarbital reaches peak CNS concentrations in 30 to 60 minutes. An additional dose of 5 to 10 mg/kg may be administered if the initial dose of phenobarbital fails to stop ongoing seizures. Because of this potentially prolonged time to achieve CNS levels necessary to control seizures, phenobarbital is considered a second choice adjunct to a benzodiazepine or as a third agent if a benzodiazepine and phenytoin fail to control seizures. Potential adverse effects of phenobarbital include sedation, hypotension, and respiratory depression. The incidence of respiratory depression is increased when phenobarbital is used in combination with a benzodiazepine.

Paraldehyde may successfully control seizures even after other antiseizure medications have failed. Because IV paraldehyde is no longer widely available, most physicians now use the rectal route of delivery when administering this medication. The recommended rectal dosage is 0.3 ml/kg of a solution diluted 3:1 with mineral, vegetable, or peanut oil. Absorption by rectal administration is rapid and estimated to be approximately 83 percent. Potential adverse effects include pulmonary edema, cardiorespiratory depression, and rectal inflammation (25,26,27). Because paraldehyde is metabolized in the liver and excreted by the lungs, its use should be avoided in patients with hepatic or pulmonary disease.

Valproate (28,29,30), carbamazepine, and lidocaine (31) have each been successfully used in the treatment of status epilepticus. The recommended dosage and and potential routes of delivery for these medications are provided in Table 18.3.

For patients with convulsive status epilepticus refractory to standard therapy and persistent for greater than one hour, general anesthesia is indicated (9). High-dose phenobarbital, short-acting anesthetic barbiturates (pentobarbital, thiopental, and methohexital), continuous IV diazepam infusion (32), and general inhalation anesthetics (halothane, isoflurane) (33) have each been used in the treatment of refractory

Table 18.3 Anticonvulsants for status epilepticus

Drug	Route	Dosage	Onset	Duration	Side Effects	Comments
Lorazepam	IV	0.05–0.1 mg/Kg max dose 4 mg/dose	2–10 min	>3 hours	Respiratory depression Sedation Hypotension	May repeat to total of 4 doses
Diazepam	IV Rectal	0.1–0.3 mg/Kg max dose 10 mg/dose	1–2 min	20–30 min	Respiratory depression Sedation Hypotension	May repeat to total of 4 doses
Phenytoin	IV	10–15 mg/Kg	15–30 min	T ½ > 20 hr	Bradycardia Hypotension	Must be given slowly (0.5 mg/Kg/min)
Phenobarbital	IV	15–25 mg/Kg	20–30 min	28–30 hr	Sedation Respiratory depression Hypotension	Increased respiratory depression when given in conjunction with benzodiazepines
Paraldehyde	Rectal	0.3 ml/Kg	?	?	Avoid with liver or respiratory failure	Diluted with mineral oil
Valproic Acid	Rectal	20 mg/Kg	?	?	Increase liver Increase phenobarbital levels	Dilute syrup 1:1 with water
Glucose	IV	0.25–1.0 g/Kg	Rapid			

status epilepticus. Use of these agents requires admission to an intensive care unit (ICU) so that ventilatory support as well as continuous monitoring of vital signs and electroencephalographic activity is available. Nondepolarizing neuromuscular blocking agents may be used as an adjuvant to general anesthesia in the management of status epilepticus. It is important to remember that these paralytic agents have no effect on the cerebral electrical activity of status epilepticus.

REFERENCES

1. Leppi IE. Status epilepticus. Neurologic Clinics 1986;4:633.
2. Lacey DJ. Status epilepticus in children and adults. J Clin Psychiatry 1988;49(Suppl):33.
3. McBride MC, Dooling EC, Oppenheimer EY. Complex partial status epilepticus in young children. Annals of Neurology 1981;4:526.
4. Aicardi J, Chevrie JJ. Convulsive status epilepticus in infants and children. Epilepsia 1970;11:187.
5. Chevrie JJ, Aicardi J. Convulsive disorders in the first year of life: Etiologic factors. Epilepsia 1977;18:489.
6. Meldrum BS, Horton RW. Physiology of status epilepticus in primates. Arch Neurology 1973;28:1.
7. Vining EP, Freeman JM. Status epilepticus. Pediatric Annals 1985;14:764.
8. Simon RP. Physiologic consequences of status epilepticus. Epilepsia 1985;26(Suppl 1):S58.
9. Delgado-Escueta AV, Wasterlein C, Treiman DM, Porter RJ. Management of status epilepticus. N Engl J Med 1982;305:1337.
10. Meldrum B. Psychological changes during prolonged seizures and epileptic brain damage. Neuropadiatrie 1978;9:203.
11. Delgado-Escuete AV, Bajorek JG. Status epilepticus: Mechanisms of brain damage and rational management. Epilepsia 1982;23(Suppl 1):S29.
12. Bleck TP. Therapy for status epilepticus. Clinical Neuropharmacology 1983;6:255.
13. Morriss FC, Cook JD. Status epilepticus. In DL Levin, FC Morriss, GC Moore, eds. A practical guide to pediatric intensive care. St. Louis: Mosby, 1984;41–46.
14. Sallman A, Goldberg M, Womholt D. Secondary hyperthyroidism manifesting as acute pancreatitis and status epilepticus. Arch Intern Med 1981;141:1549.
15. Henke JA, Thompson NW, Dauger H. Immobilization hypercalcemic crisis. Arch Surg 1975;110:321.
16. Walker JE, Homan RW, Vasko MR, et al. Lorazepam in status epilepticus. Annals of Neurology 1979;6:207.
17. Crawford TO, Mitchell WG, Snodgrass SR. Lorazepam in childhood status epilepticus and serial seizures: Effectiveness and tachyphylaxis. Neurology 1987;37:190.
18. Lacey DJ, Singer WD, Horwitz SJ, et al. Lorazepam therapy of status epilepticus in children and adolescents. Pediatrics 1986;108:771.
19. Homan RW, Walker JE. Clinical studies of lorazepam in status epilepticus. Adv Neurol 1983;34:493.
20. Tassineii Ca, Daniele O. Benzodiazepines: Efficacy in status epilepticus. Adv Neurol 1983;34:493.
21. Dulac O, Aicardi J, Rey E, et al. Blood levels of diazepam after single rectal administration in infants and children. J Pediatrics 1978;93:1039.
22. Albano A, Reisdorff EJ, Weigenstein JG. Rectal diazepam in pediatric status epilepticus. Am J Emerg Med 1989;7:168.
23. Cranford R, Leppik I, Patrick B, et al. Intravenous phenytoin: Clinical and phamacokinetic aspects. Neurology 1978;28:874.
24. Delgado-Escueta AV, Enrilo-Becsal F. Combination therapy for status epilepticus: Intravenous diazepam and phenytoin. Adv Neurol 1983;34:477.

25. Curless RG, Holzman BH, Ramsay RE. Paraldehyde therapy in childhood status epilepticus. Arch Neurol 1983;40:477.
26. Sinal, Crowe J. Cyanosis, cough, and hypotension following intravenous administration of paraldehyde. Pediatrics 1976;57:158.
27. Bostrom B. Paraldehyde toxicity during treatment of status epilepticus. Am J Dis Child 1982;136:414.
28. Snead III OC, Miles MV. Treatment of status epilepticus in children with rectal sodium valproate. J Ped 1985;106:323.
29. Manhire AR, Espir M. Treatment of status epilepticus with sodium valproate. Br Med J 1974;3:808.
30. Manhire AR, Espir M. Treatment of status epilepticus with sodium valproate. Br Med J 1974;3:808.
31. Hellstrom-Westas L, Westgren U, Rosen I, et al. Lidocaine for treatment of severe seizures in newborn infants. Acta Paediatr Scand 1988;77:79.
32. Bell HE, Bertino JS. Constant diazepam infusion in the treatment of continuous seizure activity. Drug Intell Clin Pharm 1984;18:965.
33. Kofke WA, Young RKS, Davis P, et al. Isoflurane for refractory status epilepticus: A clinical series. Anesthology 1989;71:653.

19

Acute Meningitis

Richard Stuntz
Terrence Morton, Jr.
Robert Schafermeyer

Meningitis strikes children of all ages. A variety of etiologic agents are responsible, but the majority of cases and almost all of the morbidity and mortality are due to acute bacterial meningitis. Despite significant advances in the understanding and treatment of this disease process, the case fatality rate is still over 5 percent and the morbidity rate is still 20 to 30 percent.

PATHOPHYSIOLOGY

Acute bacterial meningitis most commonly results from hematogenous seeding of the meninges. The usual source of bacteremia is nasopharyngeal colonization or infection, though any other site of infection may also serve as the source. Spread from a contiguous site of colonization or infection is also well known. Such sites include the paranasal sinuses, the nasopharynx via basilar skull fracture, and meningomyeloceles.

Several host factors are known to predispose an individual to meningitis. Males are affected more frequently than are females. Those less than four years old are affected more often and more severely than are older children. Newborns, because of the immaturity of their immune defenses, are particularly vulnerable. Other conditions that predispose to sepsis and meningitis include the use of irradiation or other antineoplastic agents, functional or anatomic asplenia or splenectomy, malnutrition, sickle cell disease, cystic fibrosis, and renal and adrenal insufficiency.

Bacterial virulence also plays a role in the ability of certain organisms to initiate infection. The most common offending organisms are: group B *streptococcus* and *E. coli* in the newborn and *H. influenzae*, *S. pneumoniae*, and *N. meningitidis* in infants and older children. The presence of specific capsular polysaccharide antigens appears to confer added virulence to some of these organisms.

The pathologic changes of meningitis have been described since the preantibiotic era. In necropsy specimens, these consist of a widely distributed purulent meningeal exudate, thrombosis of small cortical veins, and patchy or diffuse necrosis of cerebral cortex.

Recently a great deal has been learned about meningeal inflammation at the cellular and molecular levels (1). Elements of the bacterial cell wall (peptidoglycan and teichoic acid in gram-positive organisms, lipopolysaccharide in gram-negative ones) appear to be strong initiators of inflammation in the cerebrospinal fluid (CSF). In response to these and other stimuli, humoral factors are elicited by macrophages, monocytes, and other cells. Among the many factors being investigated, high CSF levels of tumor necrosis factor alpha (cachectin) and interleukin-1 beta have been shown to correlate with the degree of inflammation and with poor outcome. As the role of these inflammatory mediators becomes clearer, so will the implications of therapies aimed at blocking them.

CLINICAL PRESENTATION

Evidence of meningitis may be vague and nonspecific especially in neonates and infants. Poor feeding, lethargy or irritability, and paradoxical irritability when they are being held may be observed. As the child becomes older, vomiting, headache, photophobia, and positive Kernig's and Brudzinski's signs are seen. Fever is usual, but may be absent, or there may even be hypothermia, especially in infants. Response to acetaminophen does not reliably distinguish sepsis or meningitis from other illnesses. Increased intracranial pressure (ICP) is common and is manifested by headache in the older child or bulging fontanelle in the infant, but papilledema is not usually seen. Seizures and focal neurological signs are not uncommon. As the symptoms and signs are nonspecific, diagnosis of meningitis should be seriously considered in any ill-appearing infant or child with high fever.

DIFFERENTIAL DIAGNOSIS

A variety of infectious and noninfectious conditions must be differentiated from acute bacterial meningitis. These include: tuberculous, fungal, and viral meningitis; brain and epidural abscess, bacterial endocarditis with embolism, pneumonia, otitis media, pharyngitis, toxic ingestions, adrenal hypoplasia, and heart disease. Finally children with simple febrile seizures often present a diagnostic dilemma for the clinician. Most clinicians agree that fever and a seizure in a child less than six months of age requires that meningitis be ruled out by lumbar puncture (LP). In older children, this is debatable because of the frequency of uncomplicated febrile seizures.

LABORATORY EVALUATION

The LP is the essential diagnostic test if meningitis is suspected. If there is evidence of increased ICP, a computerized tomography (CT) scan of the head may be done before the LP, but treatment should not be withheld during this time. Table 19.1 outlines the usual diagnostic tests performed on CSF and their interpretation.

Countercurrent immunoelectrophoresis (CIE) is a useful technique for the rapid detection of most of the common bacterial pathogens. Latex particle agglutination (LPA) is more sensitive than CIE for the detection of *H. influenzae* in CSF, but

Table 19.1 CSF values

Test	Normal Value	Abnormality/Interpretation	
Opening pressure	70–180 mm H_2O	High:	Meningitis, cerebral edema, combative patient, many others
		Low:	Obstruction of needle by meninges
Color	Clear	Xanthochromic:	Meningitis, subarachnoid hemorrhage, jaundice, hemolysis
Cell count	0–5 WBC[a]/cmm All lymphocytes	10–1000 WBC/cmm: <20% PMNs:	Viral, fungal or TBM[b] Partially treated bacterial meningitis
	All monocytes	>1000 WBCs/ccm:	Bacterial meningitis
Glucose	50–80 mg/dl	<40 mg/dl or <60% of serum value:	Bacterial, fungal, TB, viral meningitis, hypoglycemia, other CNS disorders
Protein	15–45 mg/dl	Normal to moderately elevated (<500 mg/dl):	Viral, fungal, or TBM[b]
		>500 mg/dl:	Bacterial meningitis
Lactate	<3 mmol/liter	<3 mmol/liter:	Normal or viral meningitis
		3–6 mmol/liter:	Nondiagnostic, or partially treated bacterial meningitis
		>6 mmol/liter:	Bacterial meningitis
Gram stain	No organisms	Gram-negative diplococci:	N. Meningitidis
		Small Gram negative bacilli:	H. influenzae
		Gram positive cocci:	S. pneumoniae, other streptococcus, staphyllococcus

Note: CSF should always be cultured even if all values are normal.
[a]WBC = white blood cell count
[b]TBM = tuberculous meningitis
[c]PMN = polymorphonuclear neutrophil leukocytes
[d]TB = tuberculosis

nonspecific agglutination limits its specificity. CIE and LPA are most effective when CSF, serum, and concentrated urine are examined concomitantly. Both techniques may be useful in patients who have been pretreated with antibiotics.

MANAGEMENT

As with any life-threatening condition, initial priorities should include management of the airway, administration of oxygen, and treatment of shock. Seizures must be treated promptly, and fever should be controlled. Once these priorities have been addressed, LP should be performed without delay. If the LP must be delayed for any reason, appropriate antibiotics should be given before the LP. Initial antibiotics are given empirically based on the most likely pathogens in a particular clinical situation. These may be altered as culture results and sensitivity become available. Traditional antibiotic management for many years has included Ampicillin and Gentamycin for neonates and Ampicillin and Chloramphenicol for infants and children. Convincing data is now available that some of the newer cephalosporins are equally effective (2,3). Table 19.2 summarizes current recommendations (4,5).

Although corticosteroids have long been used by some in the treatment of meningitis, only recently has convincing evidence been provided of their usefulness. It now appears that dexamethasone (0.15 mg/kg q 6 hr for 4 days) given prior to or

Table 19.2 Potential pathogens by age group

Age	Likely Pathogens	Recommended Antibiotic Choice
0–1 mo	Group B Streptococci Gram neg. bacilli Listeria, Enterococcus	Ampicillin + Gentamicin Ampicillin + Cefotaxime
1–2 mos	As above, plus H. influenzae, S. Pneumoniae, N. meningitidis	Ampicillin + Chloramphenicol Ampicillin + Cefotaxime Ampicillin + Ceftriaxone
2 mos–15 yrs	H. influenzae, S. pneumoniae, N. meningitidis	Ampicillin + Chloramphenicol Cefotaxime Ceftriaxone
Above 15 yrs	S. pneumoniae, N. meningitidis	Penicillin G Cefotaxime Ceftriaxone

Doses: Ampicillin 100 mg/kg q8h (0–1 month)
Ampicillin 50 mg/kg q8h (over 1 month)
Gentamicin 2.5 mg/kg q8–12h
Cefotaxime 50 mg/kg q6h
Ceftriaxone 50 mg/kg q12h
Chloramphenicol 25 mg/kg q6h
Dexamethasone 0.15 mg/kg q6h × 4 days

with the initial dose of antibiotics serves to attenuate the inflammatory response to the release of endotoxin in the CNS. Benefits include decreased mortality and reduced rates of major neurological morbidity, including deafness (1,6).

PREVENTION

H. influenzae, type B vaccine protects against the most common cause of childhood meningitis. Unfortunately it is ineffective in children under 18 months of age in whom it is most needed. Use is individualized. In close household contacts or in those providing mouth-to-mouth contact with victims of meningococcal meningitis, rifampin may be given for prophylaxis.

ACUTE ENCEPHALITIS

Encephalitis is an inflammation of brain parenchyma that may involve other areas of the central nervous system (CNS). The spectrum of encephalitis is quite varied in presentation, etiology, and area of the CNS involved. The disease is usually worse in children under one year of age, however, and viral etiologies predominate. Herpes simplex encephalitis (HSE) will be given special attention because it may be treated effectively if it is diagnosed early.

PATHOPHYSIOLOGY

Encephalitis is classically subdivided into two categories based on the type of CNS damage that occurs (7). The first group is composed of agents that cause direct invasive cytotoxic damage. These include herpes viruses, rabies, and the arboviruses. The second category of injury results from immune-mediated damage and may be referred to as postinfectious, secondary, or allergic encephalitis (7,8). Injury of this type is seen following immunization for tetanus, diphtheria, pertussis, scarlet fever, meningococcus, and others. Immune-mediated damage also follows active infection with measles, rubella, varicella zoster, and mycoplasma (7,8). Clusters of encephalitis often occur concurrent with arbovirus and enterovirus epidemics in late summer or early fall. Thus the diagnosis is usually presumptive and based on the clinical picture and current epidemiology.

The mode of entry into humans differs among the viral etiologies (Table 19.3). Arbovirus infections are transmitted by an arthropod vector, usually a mosquito. The rabies virus in contrast is transmitted in the saliva of infected mammals and travels up sensory nerves into the CNS.

Herpes simplex virus (HSV) may reach the CNS from hematogenous routes, retrograde from ganglia, or across the cribriform plate from the nasopharynx (9). Man is the only source for the herpes viruses.

Table 19.3 Etiology of acute encephalitis

Viral	Arboviruses, enteroviruses, herpes viruses, rabies, mumps, measles, rubella, influenza A, HIV
Bacterial	*Haemophilis influenza, Streptococcus pneumoniae, Neisseria meningitis,* rickettesia, mycoplasma
Other infections	Spirochetal, fungal, protozoal, mycoplasma
Vaccines (post infectious encephalitis)	Rabies, influenza, measles, pertussis, yellow fever, typhoid fever
Toxins	Heavy metals, pesticides, alcohol, drugs

CLINICAL PICTURE

There is considerable variation in the clinical presentation depending on age, specific pathogen or toxin, immunocompetence and other host factors, and the area of involved brain. HSE presents differently in the newborn than it does in older infants and is a more severe disease. The neonate is born normal but transmission occurs at, or just preceding, birth. In the first two weeks, many infants will develop a vesicular rash that is localized. The illness begins with poor feeding, jaundice, irritability, and subtle CNS changes. Later fever evolves with seizures and focal neurologic changes (9). The most common HSV infection in children and infants older than two months is gingivostomatitis. HSE is, however, the most common cause of fatal encephalitis in the western world (9,10).

DIFFERENTIAL DIAGNOSIS

The differential diagnosis of encephalitis should include five major categories of illness (Table 19.4). These include disease or injury causing increased intracranial pressure, infectious diseases, metabolic derangement, demyelinating disease, and toxins (9).

Table 19.4 Differential diagnosis of encephalitis

Increased ICP	Tumor, trauma, CNS bleed (AVM), Abuses, Hydrocephalus
Infectious diseases	Viral, bacterial, fungal, mycoplasmal, chlamydial, parasitic
Metabolic disorders	Hepatic encephalopathy, uremia, hypoglycemia, SIAD
Demyelinating disease	Multiple sclerosis
Toxic encephalopathy	Lead, hexachlorophine, drugs, Reye's syndrome

AVM = Arteriovenous malformation
SIAD = Secretion of inappropriate antidiuretic hormone

HISTORY

A detailed history is invaluable and will often yield the diagnosis. The patient or family must be questioned about any exposure in the preceding three to four weeks to viral illnesses, animals (especially horses), ticks, and travel outside the United States. The child's immunization history should be reviewed, and the possibility of toxic exposure must be addressed. The child's immune status and any risk for human immunodeficiency virus (HIV) infection must be considered (9,10,11).

PHYSICAL EXAMINATION

The physical examination should be thorough and all inclusive with particular attention to the neurologic status. Document the presence of papilledema and the presence or absence of venous pulsations, nuchal rigidity, and any change in mental status.

LABORATORY EXAMINATION

Hematologic testing provides evidence for a nonspecific infection, and a metabolic profile will delineate electrolyte abnormalities. An LP is always part of the work-up of encephalitis though some patients may need a head CT prior to the LP. Antibiotic therapy should begin early and continue until bacterial etiologies are eliminated.

HSE presents with a CSF pleocytosis ranging from 0 to 2000 WBC with PMNs predominating early and monocytes predominating late in the course. Because HSE causes a hemorrhagic encephalitis, red blood cell counts (RBCs) are expected on an LP even with a non-traumatic tap. The CSF glucose is normal, and protein is normal to modestly elevated (7,9,11). Cultures of CSF, blood, nasopharynx, urine, and stool should be sent.

The head CT may demonstrate a mass, demyelination, edema, or vasculitis and will help delineate those patients who need a biopsy (9). Brain biopsy will yield a diagnosis early and should be done when HSE is suspected. The relative safety of brain biopsy, however, is not universally accepted. An electroencephalogram (EEG) will be abnormal initially in 80 to 90 percent of patients with encephalitis, especially those with HSE. The finding of paroxysmal lateral eleptiform discharges though not pathognomonic are typical of HSE (8,9).

MANAGEMENT

Most patients with encephalitis have an undiagnosed viral etiology and require only supportive care. The clinician must be prepared to treat seizures, cerebral edema, increased ICP, electrolyte abnormalities, and disseminated intravascular coagulation (DIC) (7,8). Antiviral therapy with acylovir is started early until HSE can be eliminated. Acyclovir is a safe and effective medication that has reduced mortality from 70 to 20 percent. Vidarabine is an acceptable alternative (11,12,13).

The use of steroids has long been advocated for the reduction of ICP. Their use in encephalitis remains controversial and may be contraindicated in active viral disease.

CONCLUSION

Encephalitis is an inflammatory brain disease with a myriad of potential etiologies. Diagnosis is made by combining a thorough history, clinical findings, and local epidemiology. Although treatment is primarily supportive, antiviral therapy with acyclovir is effective for HSE.

REFERENCES

1. Saez-Llorens X, Ramilo O, Mustafa MM, et al. Molecular pathophysiology of bacterial meningitis: Current concepts and therapeutic implications. J Peds 1990;116:671-684.
2. Peltola H, Anttila M, Renkonen OV, et al. Randomised comparison of chloramphenicol, ampicillin, cefotaxime, and ceftriaxone for childhood bacterial meningitis. Lancet 1989;1:1281-1287.
3. Jacobs RF. Cefotaxime treatment of gram-negative enteric meningitis in infants and children. Drugs 1988;35(Suppl 2):185-189.
4. Committee on Infectious Diseases. Treatment of bacterial meningitis. Pediatrics 1988;81:904-907.
5. McCracken GH. Current management of bacterial meningitis. Pediatr Infect Dis J 1989;8:919-921.
6. Committee on Infectious Diseases. Dexamethasone therapy for bacterial meningitis in infants and children. Pediatrics 1990;86:130-133.
7. Krugman S, Katz SL, Gershon AA, et al. Encephalitis in infectious diseases in children, 8th ed. St. Louis: Mosby, Princeton, 1985;32-41.
8. Cherry JD. Encephalitis and meningoencephalitis. In Feigin RD, Cherry JD, eds. Textbook of pediatric infectious disease, 2d ed. Philadelphia: Saunders, 1987;484-496.
9. Rudolph A, Hoffman J. Acute viral encephalitis in pediatrics, 18th ed. Norwalk, Conn.: Appleton & Lange, 1987.
10. Kohl S. Herpes simplex virus encephalitis in children. Pediatric Clinics of North America, 1988;35:465-483.
11. Georges P. Herpes simplex. In Committee on Infectious Diseases, AM Accady Peds, 22d ed. Elk Grove, Ill.: AM Accady Peds, 1991;259-268.
12. Jenista J, Tam J. Practical decision making regarding antiviral therapy: The future is now. Emergency Medicine Reports 1991;12:42-48.
13. Whitner RJ. Herpes simplex infections of the central nervous system, a review. Am J Med 1988;85:61-67.

PART VII

Gastrointestinal

20

Gastrointestinal Bleeding

David Fisher

Gastrointestinal bleeding presents as a highly emotionally charged and difficult-to-control situation. There is usually a great deal of parental anxiety that must be eliminated to facilitate control of the clinical situation. Many significant upper gastrointestinal bleeding events can be expected as a result of portal system hypertension and resultant varices. Lower gastrointestinal (GI) bleeding, however, usually results from a previously unsuspected disease process such as Meckel's diverticulum or polyp. There are also reports of GI bleeding as a result of blunt abdominal trauma or foreign body injury from child abuse. A recent article described a child with suspected GI bleeding that was later found to be factitious. The child's mother was discovered lacerating herself and applying her own blood to the patients' mouth and in the baby's diaper to mimic gastrointestinal bleeding. GI bleeding should be evaluated in a logical sequence, first to differentiate internal from external sources and then to identify upper- or lower-tract locations.

PATHOPHYSIOLOGY

Assuming a normal coagulation system that may well be compromised in the patient with hepatic abnormalities, the causes for GI bleeding usually include ingested blood, infection, abnormal venous pressures, mucosal disruption, ischemia, and arterial injury. The effects of major blood loss differs depending on general health and age group. An infant can sustain a 50 percent blood loss and still recover without major injury. Other pediatric groups parallel the adult population wherein a 20 percent loss is significant.

The resulting loss of heme volume and the subsequent loss of oxygen carrying capacity account for most of the injury from GI bleeding. Volume depletion with accompanying shock triggers additional neural and hormonal mechanisms that shunt blood flow to vital organ areas. Although the changed distribution of blood flow is initially helpful, the end result is a decreased perfusion of the mucosal barrier in the gut leading to further injury potentiating sepsis. The continuing diminishment of perfusion impairs renal and hepatic function, creating terminal events of multiple systems failure and death. Presently our efforts are directed toward control of hemorrhage and restoration of volume. Additional therapeutic modalities may be developed to control the distribution of blood flow.

Blood acts as a cathartic in the GI system and may impede absorption and impair nutrition. Poor GI function will also affect coagulation status. The bacterial degradation of blood in the gut elevates the serum blood urea nitrogen (BUN) and may be useful in predicting upper or lower GI bleeding sources. Ventilatory compromise may occur as a result of aspiration with significant sequela.

CLINICAL PRESENTATIONS

GI bleeding in children is classified according to source and age group. The cause for blood loss is easier to isolate in this fashion. Bright red blood indicates a current high flow rate bleed. Coffee-ground emesis usually indicates that the bleeding has stopped; it may also result from nasogastric tube placement not sampling the area of duodenal bleed but only recovering the contents that reflux into the stomach. Testing for bile in the aspirate will help document duodenal contents. Melena and hematochezia may be seen with both upper and lower GI tract sources. Melena indicates that the bleeding is several hours old, but ongoing blood loss may still occur. Melena usually indicates a blood loss of at least 50 to 100 cc in 24 hours.

After protection of the airway and control of ventilatory status with oxygen supplementation, the circulatory status is evaluated. Clinical evaluation of shock is difficult, particularly in children. The classic findings: poor capillary refill, tachycardia, narrowed pulse pressure, and changed mental status are late findings and require immediate intervention to salvage the patient. The increased cardiac reserves make it more difficult to detect the early phases of hemorrhagic shock. Intravenous (IV) access should be obtained early; delayed attempts, after the patient demonstrates collapse, may be impossible. Intraosseous routes should be used if prompt peripheral IV lines cannot be instituted.

Following initial airway and circulatory stabilization, bleeding cause should be delineated. To eliminate factitious bleeding sources and for confirmation of true GI bleeding, bedside observation may be required. The patient is examined for extra GI causes such as epistaxis, hemoptysis, coagulopathy, foreign body or toxin irritation, and ingestion of maternal blood. Then the age group is identified. Commonly the pediatric population is divided into four groups; the neonate (0 to 30 days), the infant (30 days to 1 year), the child (1 to 12 years), and the adolescent. This separation of age groups combined with differentiation of upper and lower bleeding sources allows better prediction of clinical course and care requirements (Table 20.1).

The general bleeding area is identified by placement of a nasogastric tube. Positive aspiration of blood, confirmed by a positive guaiac testing appropriate for low pH testing (Gastroccult by Smith Kline Corporation), localizes the source to above the ligament of Treitz. An upper GI bleeding source can also be monitored for ongoing blood loss by this technique. Saline lavage may also decrease the mucosal blood flow and decrease blood loss. Upper GI bleeding can also be better delineated, and therapeutic interventions performed, through endoscopy. Lower GI sources should also be evaluated with a primary examination of the anus and rectum with a test tube in the neonate and with an anoscope in the older age groups. Colonoscopy is

Table 20.1 Common causes of gastrointestinal bleeding by age group and site

	Upper GI	Lower GI
Neonate (0–30 days)	1. Idiopathic (uninvestigated) 2. Gastritis (investigated) 3. Esophagitis 4. Peptic ulcer disease 5. Ingested maternal blood	1. Benign anorectal lesions 2. Upper GI bleeding 3. Milk allergy 4. Necrotizing enterocolitis 5. Mid-gut volvulus
Infant (30 days–1 year)	1. Gastritis/idiopathic 2. Esophagitis 3. Peptic ulcer	1. Benign anorectal lesions 2. Idiopathic intussusception 3. Meckel's diverticulum 4. Infectious diarrhea 5. Upper GI bleeding 6. Milk allergy 7. Lymphonodular hyperplasia of the colon
Child (1–12 years)	1. Esophageal varices 2. Esophagitis 3. Peptic ulcer disease	1. Benign anorectal lesions 2. Juvenile polyp 3. Intussusception 4. Meckel's diverticulum 5. Infectious diarrhea 6. Upper GI bleeding
Older Child and Adolescent	1. Esophageal varices 2. Esophagitis 3. Peptic ulcer disease	1. Juvenile polyps 2. Benign anorectal lesions 3. Inflammatory bowel disease 4. Upper GI bleeding

Adapted with permission from Emergency Medical Concepts and Clinical Practice, 3d ed. 1992;2824.

extremely helpful in the population group with a history of colonic polyps but requires sedation and is not as useful in an acute bleeding episode. Ancillary evaluation is frequently useful to confirm source and plan therapy.

ANCILLARY EVALUATION

Primary laboratory emphasis is on work-up necessary for replacement of volume and stopping the hemorrhage. Clotting parameters must be studied. Blood is typed and cross-matched as soon as possible. The further evaluation then depends on the suspected source of bleeding. The recommendations for laboratory analysis are separated for upper and lower GI sources. Consider the BUN to creatinine ratio; if the clotting and renal functions are normal, a ratio of 30:1 suggests an upper rather than lower bleeding source.

In upper GI sources, the neonate should have gastric aspiration and the contents should be examined by the Apt test to rule out ingestion of maternal blood. The neonate rarely requires further evaluation unless the bleeding is severe or recurrent. In the infant, child, or adolescent, further evaluation is usually necessary. A significant bleed—one that is recurrent—is continuously bleeding or one that creates a 20 percent drop in blood volume and requires endoscopy for further delineation of the cause. If the source is not identified with endoscopy, arteriography or nuclear studies will frequently define the cause. A combination of these approaches will offer a diagnosis in 95 percent of cases. An abdominal flat plate may help eliminate foreign bodies, duplication abnormalities, or bowel perforation.

In lower GI sources, the neonate should also be examined first for the possibility of ingested maternal blood. If minimal bleeding is noted in an infant, suspect more serious causes such as duplication abnormalities or necrotizing enterocolitis. These infants usually have accompanying signs of significant disease. Infectious causes should be sought with examination and cultures of the stool. Painless bleeding may suggest Meckel's diverticulum as the cause; occasionally the patient will present with severe pain and bleeding if the diverticulum forms a lead point for an intussusception and resultant obstruction. These cases will be best identified with a technetium scan unless the diverticulum does not contain gastric mucosa, the bowel is hypermotile, or the hemorrhage is marked or if other areas of uptake overlay the area. Barium studies should be done last as they will interfere with evaluation by other modalities. Barium may be helpful for identification of juvenile polyps or the reduction of an intussusception. Colonoscopy will help in the identification of juvenile polyps and in the patient with unexplained and persistent lower tract bleeding. Colonoscopy requires anesthesia or sedation and is not very helpful in the acute bleeding event.

TREATMENT

As was previously discussed, primary attention is directed to provision and protection of the airway. Supplemental oxygen is provided to improve tissue oxygenation. Two large bore peripheral IV lines should be secured to restore volume. If peripheral constriction has already occurred, consider cut-downs or intraosseous lines, the latter in a child under four years of age. A patient in profound shock will require the immediate transfusion of O negative blood. Continuous monitoring both clinically and by EKG is indicated. A pulse oximeter will help with early warning of decompensation.

After stabilizing maneuvers, a nasogastric tube is placed. Irrigate with saline to detect source and monitor rate of blood loss. Consider saline washout if an active upper-tract source is identified. If cooled solutions are used, the patient's temperature should be monitored closely. A stressed patient may become hypothermic rapidly with resultant multiple system changes including clotting parameters.

In the upper GI source, institute local measures to protect the mucosa. Antacids are started in an attempt to increase the gastric pH to over five. Cimetidine at a dosage of 20–30 mg/kg/24 hrs may also help to control pH of the gastric contents. If massive bleeding continues, rapid surgical intervention may be required. Procedures may include truncal vagotomy, antrectomy, and oversewing of the bleeding site. Vasopressin may be needed to quell a severe variceal bleed. Start with an initial bolus of .3 units/kg, with a maximum bolus of 20 units infused over 20 minutes. Then institute a drip at .01 units/kg/min. Increase the drip rate every 2 hours to a maximum of .1 units/kg/min. If these maneuvers are ineffective, balloon tamponade or surgical intervention with sclerosis or shunting may be necessary to control the hemorrhage.

The lower-tract source requires the same stabilization measures. Prompt surgical and radiographic consultation should be obtained. A slow blood loss may be identified with the use of contrast studies, nuclear scan techniques, or arteriography. Stool cultures should be obtained as infectious causes are frequently identified with a lower GI bleeding source. Antibiotic therapy can then be guided by the culture results for a more specific therapeutic intervention.

SUGGESTED READING

1. Bailey MA, Rosenthal P. Insurability of pediatric gastrointestinal disorders. Clin Pediatr 1991;28(2):60–63.
2. Berezin S, Newman LJ. Lower gastrointestinal bleeding in infants owing to lymphonodular hyperplasia of the colon. Pediatr Emerg Care 1987;3(3):164–205.
3. Bernard O, Alvarez F, Brunelle F, et al. Portal hypertension in children. Clin Gastroenterol 1985;14(1):33–55.
4. Brophy C, Seashore J. Meckel's diverticulum in the pediatric surgical population. Conn Med 1989;53(4):203–205.
5. Cox K, Ament ME. Upper gastrointestinal bleeding in children and adolescents. Pediatrics 1979;63(3):408–413.
6. Cynamon HA, Milov DE, Andres JM. Diagnosis and management of colonic polyps in children. J Pediatr 1989;114(4):593–596.
7. Felber S, Rosenthal P, Henton D. The BUN/creatinine ratio in localizing gastrointestinal bleeding in pediatric patients. J Pediatr Gastroenterol 1988;7:685–687.
8. Fonkalsrud EW. Treatment of variceal hemorrhage in children. Surg Clin N Amer 1990;70(2):475–487.
9. Hyams JS, Leichtner AM, Schwartz AN. Recent advances in diagnosis and treatment of gastrointestinal hemorrhage in infants and children. J Pediatr 1991;106(1):1–9.
10. Nanjundiah P, Lifschitz CH, Gopalakrishna GS, et al. Intestinal strictures presenting with gastrointestinal blood loss. J Pediatr Surg 1989;24(2):174–176.
11. Oldham KT, Lobe TE. Gastrointestinal hemorrhage in children. Pediatr Clin North Am 1986;32(5):1247–1263.
12. Quintero E, Pique JM, Bombi JA, et al. Upper gastrointestinal bleeding caused by gastroduodenal vascular malformation. Dig Dis Sci 1986;31(9):897–905.
13. Richards RJ, Donica MB, Grayer D. Can the blood urea nitrogen/creatinine ratio distinguish upper from lower gastrointestinal bleeding? J Clin Gastroenterol 1990;12(5):500–504.
14. Tam PKH, Saing H. Pediatric upper gastrointestinal endoscopy: A 13-year experience. J Pediatr Surg 1989;24(5):443–447.
15. Tam PKH, Saing H, Lau JTK. Diagnosis of peptic ulcer in children: The past and present. J Pediatr Surg 1986;21(1):15–16.
16. Terblanche J, Burroughs AK, Hobbs KEF. Controversies in the management of bleeding esophageal varices. N Eng J Med 1989;320(21):1393–1398.
17. Towbin RB, Ball WS. Pediatric interventional radiology. Radiol Clin North Am 1988;26(2):419–440.

21

Intussusception

Phyllis T. Doerger
Jonathan Singer

Intussusception is the most frequent cause of intestinal obstruction between the ages of two months and five years, occurring in about two children per 1000 live births. Mortality has declined to almost nil over the 300 years since it was first recognized as a disease in the seventeenth century (1). The diagnosis, however, may not be considered for several reasons. These include young or old age, prolonged symptomatology, and normal physical examination. Intussusception in children remains a challenge to the emergency physician (2,3).

Intussusception involves the invagination of a proximal portion of the bowel, commonly the terminal ileum, into a more distal segment, usually the colon. The innermost layer is called the *intussusceptum*. The structures brought along with it in its distal passage are enveloped in the *intussuscipiens* (the distal portion of bowel). The mesentery and vasculature of the intussusceptum is compressed within the intussuscipiens especially at the points of fold. This results in a very rapid vascular engorgement and edema that leads to further venous compression and on to necrosis if it is not relieved.

The classic "currant jelly" or "prune juice" stool, a cardinal feature in some cases of intussusception, is a mixture of mucus extruded from engorged goblet cells and blood oozing from the distended submucosal venules (4).

Intermittent pain results from peristaltic waves pushing against the obstruction created by the infolded bowel. Bowel contents distal to the intussusception may be evacuated as normally formed stools or diarrhea.

The pathophysiologic origin of the lethargy often associated with intussusception is unknown. Several theories have been advanced including toxic metabolites released from the compromised bowel (5) or endogenous opiate poisoning reversible by the administration of naloxone (6) but the latter was not supported in cases reported by Hickey (7), Singer (8), or McCabe (9), and the former theory has never actually been studied.

Several types of intussusception have been described including ileojejunal and jejuno-, appendico-, and colocolic forms, but greater than 95 percent begin near the ileocecal valve making the ileocolic variant the most common. Colocolic intussusception is rare in children but occurs in up to 2.1 percent of all ages (10). Ileo-ileal forms are more difficult to reduce and are more often associated with specific anatomical defects.

The etiology of 85 to 90 percent cases of intussusception is unknown. Little advance has been made in the understanding of the cause of these idiopathic cases since Adams declared in 1910 that "all authorities agree the causative factor is irregular peristalsis" (11). Before Adam, Hess originated the idea that an area of intestinal spasm became a fixed lead point resulting in intussusception and noted that there is a different rate of growth of the ileum and colon occurring during the age when intussusception is most common (12).

One of the most popular theories remaining today emphasizes the influence of an antecedent upper-respiratory infection causing mesenteric lymphoid hyperplasia. Adenovirus (13,14) or other viruses (15,16,17) are proposed to increase the likelihood of creating a lead point for intussusception but various authors (1,18,19) have found no correlation with peak virus season, and Ravitch (20) cautions that enlarged lymph nodes produced in his study on dogs may be the result, rather than the cause, of intussusception. Others have proposed that *E. coli* infection predisposes intussusception (21).

True anatomic lead points are most likely in older children and adults or in cases of recurrent intussusception (1,22,23). Some feel that polyps are the most common (10,24), but others champion Meckel's diverticulum as the leading cause (19).

Other demonstrable causes for intussusception have been found in 2 to 15 percent of reviews. These include lymphoma, duplication, and Henoch-Schoenlein purpura (25,26,27). The postoperative period following many different abdominal surgeries appears to be a time of special risk (1,28,29,30) as does the medical diagnosis of cystic fibrosis (31).

CLINICAL PRESENTATION
Epidemiology

Several epidemiologic features are important in intussusception. The peak occurrence in virtually every large review is between three and nine months of age, while two-thirds to three-quarters of cases were found to occur in infants less than one year of age (1,19). Males are affected twice as often as females (3,19,22), and this difference becomes even more pronounced in children over four years of age, rising to an 8:1 ratio (22).

Geographic location, season, and race are of considerably less significance. While Thorbjarnarson (23) found incidence varying with geography in his study with both children and adults, most other research has not indicated this. Likewise seasonal incidence was inconsistently reported as having peaks in spring and summer (3,19) or none (18). Race was not found to influence occurrence in any study.

Symptoms

Intussusception classically creates a triad of clinical symptoms: colicky pain, vomiting, and bloody stools (3,18). The pain is usually described as intermittent and severe but can be totally absent (19). The intermittent nature of the pain with the child appearing quite well between bouts is often an important clue and should be given due weight in the history. Pain may be recognized more readily in the older child, but if irritability is included, the majority of the patients will have this symptom regardless of age (32). In about one-half of cases reported by Ravitch, pain was the initial complaint, while vomiting was the chief complaint in almost one-half at the time of the evaluation (2). Vomiting, occurring sometime during the course of the illness, was found in a majority of patients (3). Blood per rectum is among the chief complaints in 40 percent of affected patients. Hematochezia is the initial complaint in only 5 to 10 percent of patients (2,3).

Associated findings can occur in combination with the classic triad, or they may occur alone, contributing to diagnostic error (2). Anorexia is an almost universal but nonspecific symptom. Diarrhea was thought by the early medical practitioners to exclude intussusception. It has been found in 7 to 12 percent of cases, and its presence by no means excludes the diagnosis (2,19).

Altered mental status ranging from lethargy to frank coma can be an accompaniment of the gastrointestinal symptoms (6–8,32–34) or can precede gastrointestinal complaints (35,36) leading to the suggestion by McCabe and colleagues that intussusception be addended to the list of causes of coma with the mnemonic AEIOU-TIPS (9). The late appearance of lethargy was felt by some authors (19,37) to relate to developing shock, but recently authors stress that altered consciousness may be an early symptom. Increased awareness on the part of emergency practitioners is necessary to prevent diagnostic delay (8,33,34).

PHYSICAL EXAMINATION

The general appearance of the victim of an intussusception may vary from cheerful and interactive to lethargic and poorly perfused. The vital signs can also vary widely. Hypotension may be seen secondary to hypovolemia from vomiting and/or extravasation of fluids and blood. Even hypertension has been reported, probably related to pain (38). Low-grade fever is common only in younger patients but not invariably present.

With the exception of variable mental status changes, positive physical findings are limited to the abdominal exam. Hess's statement in 1905 remains true: "the tumor of invagination is the most important physical sign from the diagnostic standpoint" (12). The classic sausage-shaped mass has remained a prominent feature of intussusception, being found in 60 to 95 percent of cases (1,39). Unfortunately, a mass may be missed if it occurs in a subhepatic location. The mass may be palpated on rectal exam or on the rare occasion the intussusception may actually protrude from the anus (40). An interesting historical eponym, Dance's sign, describing an empty right lower quadrant of the abdomen because of invagination of the cecum up into the colon (37,40) may be the physical equivalent of the empty right lower quadrant seen on plain film (41). It was present in only 5 percent of patients reported by Bruce (42), and is not specifically commented on elsewhere.

The rectal examination attains additional importance in the early search for blood. Gross blood may not be noted by the parent, but becomes apparent on the examining finger. Occult blood is a more common finding (39).

Other findings such as abdominal distension, hypoactive bowel sounds, or abdominal tenderness are less frequent manifestations of intussusception.

DIFFERENTIAL DIAGNOSIS AND LABORATORY

With a classic presentation of intermittent pain, vomiting, abdominal mass, and heme-positive stools the differential diagnosis is narrow. As only 10 percent of cases will exhibit the complete constellation, the remaining cases have a more extensive differential including gastroenteritis, dysentery, appendicitis, toxic, metabolic and infectious disease, tumor, and ulcer. If lethargy is a prominent component, trauma, hypoxia, fluid imbalance, electrolyte abnormalities, and central nervous system (CNS) pathology must be considered.

No laboratory values are singularly representative of intussusception but laboratory assessments may be used to exclude other diagnoses and to assist in evaluation of the general condition of the child. For the patient likely to be hypovolemic, electrolytes and a type-and-cross would be important as well as a complete blood count (CBC), blood urea nitrogen (BUN), and a glucose test and a urinalysis. If the diagnosis is unclear and altered mental status is present, a toxicology screen, bedside blood glucose test strips, liver function tests, ammonia, arterial blood gas and cultures of blood, urine, and cerebrospinal fluid (CSF) are obtained.

Radiologic Evaluation

Plain abdominal radiographs are the first step in the radiologic assessment of the child with a history and physical examination causing suspicion of intussusception.

Plain radiographs are essential to look for complete obstruction or other contraindication to hydrostatic reduction. Some degree of intestinal obstruction may be apparent in 23 to 50 percent of cases (3,18). School-aged children almost always show some bowel obstruction with air fluid levels (43). Brondum's observations that long duration of pain made abnormal findings more likely is consistent with previous literature (44). The findings of bowel obstruction, mass lesion, little gas in the bowel combined with little or no solid large bowel content are consistent with intussusception (39). The most characteristic finding is the abnormally scant amount of intestinal gas with small bowel loops displaced to the right. The intussusception itself may be visible in up to one-half of patients (41). Abnormal findings that may point the physician to the correct diagnosis are present in up to 89 percent of cases (41,45) although a normal plain film cannot reliably rule out the disease (41,44).

A barium enema was initially considered to have only diagnostic importance (37,40). More recent reviews concur in both the diagnostic and therapeutic benefits of a barium enema when proper criteria and techniques are employed. Ravitch pioneered this method (2) and still strongly champions its use (1). Diagnostically the intussusception is seen on the barium enema as a cervix-like convexity outlined by the advancing rim of barium.

Ultrasonography of the abdomen, while not routinely employed to diagnose intussusception, has shown utility in atypical cases (34,38,46). This diagnostic tool

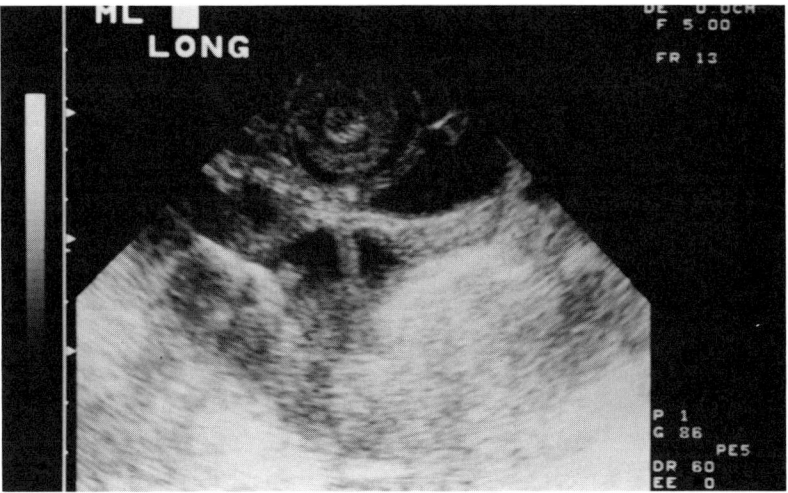

Figure 21.1 Real-time echogram "donut sign."

may provide prognostic implications for the success of reduction by hydrostatic means (47). Characteristically the ultrasound shows a sonolucent doughnut on cross section and a pseudokidney appearance on longitudinal section (Figure 21.1). The rim in either case represents the edematous head of the intussusception. If this rim is thickened, the chance of hydrostatic reduction is less likely as opposed to a greater likelihood of reduction when the intussusception is loose and the rim exhibits concentric rings (cross section) or layering (longitudinal section).

MANAGEMENT

The child with intussusception who presents in shock or with peritonitis or sepsis must be resuscitated as any other critically ill child with attention to the ABCs (airway, breathing, circulation). The patient must be kept NPO (*nil per os* = nothing by mouth) while fluid boluses and blood are given as needed for resuscitation. In septic children, a nasogastric tube is inserted and antibiotics are administered while surgical consultation is being obtained. Plain films are ordered, and both the radiologist and surgeon are involved in the determination of the feasibility and type of attempts at nonoperative reduction or the decision to perform immediate surgery (see Figure 21.2).

If the child is stable, the use of hydrostatic or barometric means of reduction is warranted regardless of age or duration of symptoms (1,18). Nonoperative reduction is the best therapeutic option to reduce morbidity if the anticipated rate of success is greater than 14 percent (48). It has the advantage of avoidance of anesthesia and laparotomy. Even if only partial reduction is obtained by barium enema, there is a

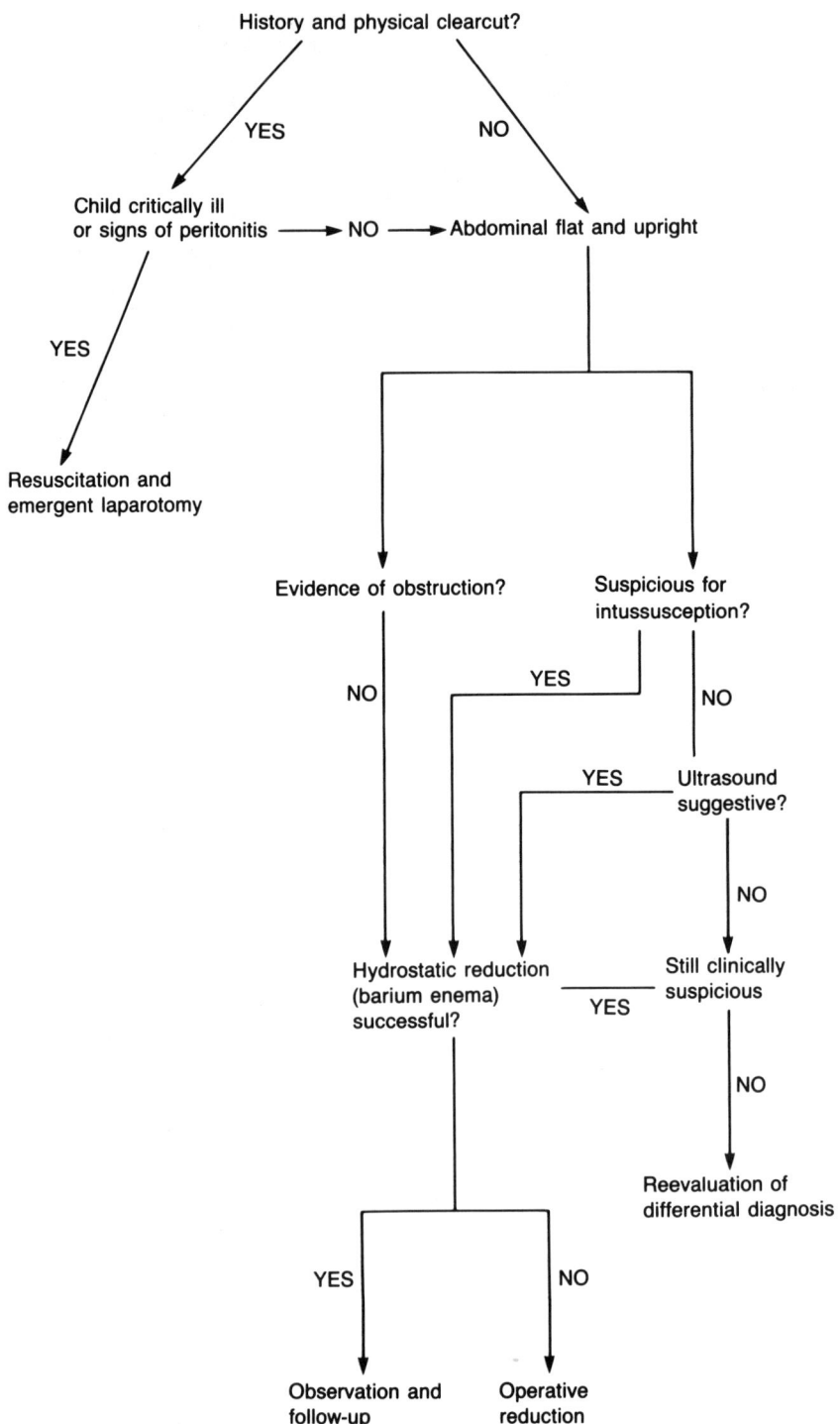

Figure 21.2 Management algorithm.

decreased frequency of postoperative complications, adhesions, and bowel resection, and shorter operating time (1). Success rates of hydrostatic reduction vary from around 45 percent to 75 percent (1) but often depend on which criteria are used to enroll the patient in the attempt at hydrostatic reduction instead of primary operation. Longer duration of symptoms and older children show decreased success rates (19,43). Sedation may be helpful in increasing success rates (22,46).

Air or barium may be used to nonoperatively reduce an intussusception. Air reduction has become popular at several institutions. It offers reduced exposure to radiation and decreased potential for peritoneal contamination in the event of perforation, with success rates equivalent to barium enema reduction (49–51).

A generally accepted contraindication to hydrostatic reduction is ileo-ileal intussusception with its propensity for late diagnosis and its frequent causative lesions. Bowel perforation with and without peritonitis and generalized sepsis is also a contraindication. Other criteria are not as universally followed: poor general condition of the child; duration of symptoms for longer than 48 hours when they are accompanied by rectal bleeding (52); and complete small bowel obstruction as evidenced by abdominal distension, hyperresonance, abnormal bowel sounds, air-fluid levels, and grossly distended bowel loops.

If hydrostatic reduction is successful, most surgeons will admit the child for a 24-hour observation period. Immediate recurrence is rare; recurrence within several months following discharge, however, has been reported. It is therefore important for the parent to recognize all variations of expression of intussusception. If hydrostatic reduction is unsuccessful, operative reduction is necessary.

SUMMARY

Early recognition of intussusception is an important goal for the emergency physician. The disease is less likely to be missed if it is kept in the differential for all children with abdominal pain or vomiting or for those who present with a change in mental status. Careful abdominal and rectal examination and liberal use of abdominal radiographs will aid in timely diagnosis. Along with early diagnosis, stabilization of the critically ill child with prompt mobilization of radiologic and surgical consultants are the primary roles of an emergency specialist.

REFERENCES

1. Ravitch MM. Intussusception. In Welch KJ, Randolph JG, Ravitch MM, et al, eds. Pediatric Surgery, Chicago: Yearbook Publishers, 1986;868–882.
2. Ravitch MM. Consideration of errors in the diagnosis of intussusception. AMA J of Dis of Children 1952;84:17.
3. Fanconi S, Berger D, Aldose PP. Intussusception: A classic clinical picture? Helv Paediat Acta 1982;37:345–352.
4. Reijnen JAM, Mravunac M, Festen C. Intussusception complicated by bowel perforation during hydrostatic reduction. Z Kinderchir 1989;45:219–221.
5. Miller LD, Mackie JA, Rhoads JE. The pathophysiology and management of intestinal obstruction. Surg Clin North Am 1962;42:1285.

6. Tenenbein M, Wiseman NE. Early coma in intussusception: Endogenous opioid induced? Pediatr Em Care 1987;3:22–23.
7. Hickey RW, Sodhi SK, Johnson WR. Two children with lethargy and intussusception. Ann Emer Med 1990;19:390–392.
8. Singer, J. Altered consciousness as an early manifestation of intussusception. Pediatrics 1979;64:93–95.
9. McCabe JB, Singer JI, Love T, Roth R. Intussusception: A supplement to the mnemonic for coma. Pediatr Em Care 1987;3:118–119.
10. Ippolito RJ, Touloukian RJ. Colocolic intussusception in an older child. Clin Pediatr 1978;17:720–726.
11. Adam JE. The clinical aspect of intussusception. The Practitioner 1910;85:679–695.
12. Hess JH. Intussusception in infancy and childhood, with collection of 1,028 cases, with statistics. Arch Pediatr 1905;22:655–683.
13. Dennison WM, Shaker M. Intussusception in infancy and childhood. Br J Surg 1970;57:679–684.
14. Ross JG, Potter CW, Zachary RB. Adenovirus infection in association with intussusception in infancy. Lancet 1962;2:221.
15. Nicholas JC. A one-year virological survey of acute intussusception in childhood. J Med Virology 1982;9:267–271.
16. Mulcahy DL. A two-part study of the etiological role of rotavirus in intussusception. J Med Virology 1982;9:51–55.
17. Gardner PS, Knox EG, Court SDM, et al. Virus infection and intussusception in childhood. Br Med J 1970;2:697.
18. Gierup J, Jorulf H, Livaditis A. Management of intussusception in infants and children: A survey based on 288 consecutive cases. Pediatrics 1972;50:535–545.
19. Ein SH, Stephens CA. Intussusception: 354 cases in 10 years. J Pediatr Surg 1971;6:16–27.
20. Ravitch MM, McCune RM. Reduction of intussusception by hydrostatic pressure: An experimental study. Ann Surg 1948;128:904.
21. Lopez EL, Devoto S, Woloj M, et al. Intussusception associated with *Escherichia Coli* 0157:H7. Ped Infect Dis J 1989;8:471.
22. Bergdahl S, Hugosson C, Lauren T, et al. Atypical intussusception. J Pediatr Surg 1972;7:700–705.
23. Thorbjarnarson B. Intussusception. Hosp Med 1975;58–71.
24. Castleman B, McNeely BU, eds. Case 47–1970. Case Records of the Mass Gen Hosp 1970;283:1101–1107.
25. Strang R. Intussusception in infancy and childhood. Br J Surg 1959;46:484.
26. Beck AR, Leichtling JJ. Intussusception in Henoch-Schoenlein's purpura. Mt. Sinai J Med 1972;39:397.
27. Emmanuel B, Lieberman AD, Rosen S. Intussusception due to Henoch-Schönlein purpura. Ill Med J 1962;122:162.
28. LaSalle AS, Andrassy RJ, Page CP, et al. Intussusception of the appendiceal stump. Clin Pediatr 1980;19:432–435.
29. Stevenson EOS, Hays DM, Snyder WH. Postoperative intussusception in infants and children. Am J Surg 1967;113:562.
30. McGovern JB, Gross RE. Intussusception as a post-operative complication. Surgery 1968;63:507.
31. Holsclaw DS, Rocmans C, Shwachman H. Intussusception in patients with cystic fibrosis. Pediatrics 1971;48:51.
32. Heldrich FJ: Lethargy as a presenting symptom in patients with intussusception. Clinical Pediatrics 1986;25:363–365.
33. Rachmel A, Rosenbaum Y, Amir J, et al. Apathy as an early manifestation of intussusception. Am J Dis Child 1983;137:701–702.
34. Swischuk LE. Lethargy and vomiting in an infant. Pediatr Emer Care 1991;7:97–98.

35. Braun P, Germann-Nicod I. Altered consciousness as a precocious manifestation of intussusception in infants. Z Kinderchir 1981;33:307–309.
36. Goetting MG, Tiznado-Garcia E, Bakdash TF. Intussusception encephalopathy: An underrecognized cause of coma in children. Pediatr Neuro 1990;6:419–421.
37. Gross RE, Ware PF. Intussusception in childhood. NEJM 1948;239:645–652.
38. Barton LL, Koteswararao C: Intussusception associated with transient hypertension. Pediatr Emer Care 1988;4:249–250.
39. Losek JD, Fiete RL: Intussusception and the diagnostic value of testing stool for occult blood. Am J Em Med 1991;9:1–3.
40. Ladd WE, Gross RE. Intussusception in infancy and childhood. Arch Surg 1934;29:365–384.
41. Eklöf O, Hartelius H. Reliability of the abdominal plain film diagnosis in pediatric patients with suspected intussusception. Pediatr Radiol 1980;9:199–206.
42. Bruce J, Huh YS, Cooney DR, et al. Intussusception: Evolution of current management. J Pediatr Gastroenterol Nutr 1987;6:663–674.
43. Matlack M quoted in. Unusual intussusception. Pediatr Emer Trends 1987;3.
44. Brondum V, Lopez H, Lindequist S, Teisen H. Intussusception in children: Plain abdominal radiograph and reduction by barium enema in relation to clinical features. Röntgen-Bl 1990;43:471–474.
45. Bisset GS, Kirks DR. Intussusception in infants and children: Diagnosis and therapy. Radiology 1988;186:141–145.
46. Swischuk LE: Acute vomiting and abdominal pain in an infant. Pediatr Emer Care 1986;2:201–202.
47. Swischuk LE, Hayden CK, Boulden T. Intussusception: Indications for ultrasonography and an explanation of the doughnut and pseudokidney signs. Pediatr Radiol 1985;15:388.
48. Leonidas JC. Treatment of intussusception with small bowel obstruction: Application of decision analysis. AJR 1985;145:665–669.
49. Palder SB, Ein SH, Stringes DA, Douglas A. Intussusception: Barium or air? J Pediatr Surg 1991;26:271–275.
50. Gu L, Altson GL, Daneman A, et al. Intussusception reduced by rectal inflation of air. Pediatr Radiol 1987;17:353.
51. Todan T, Sato Y, Watanabe Y, et al. Air reduction for intussusception in infancy and childhood: Ultrasonographic diagnosis and management without x-ray exposure. Z Kinderchir 1990;45:222–226.
52. Reijnen JAM, Festen C, van Roosmalen RP. Intussusception: Factors related to treatment. Arch Dis Child 1990;65:871–873.

22

Hypertrophic Pyloric Stenosis

David Fisher

Hypertrophic pyloric stenosis was first accurately described by Hirschprung in 1877. Since then, there have been many technical advances that are helpful in diagnosis and treatment of the persistent vomiting infant. The cornerstone in the evaluation process, however, remains the carefully obtained history and the physical examination. The reported incidence varies from 3 to 6.4/1000 live births. In America, the most recent literature suggests the lower incidence. This still amounts to over 11,000 cases per year. Male infants are affected approximately four times as often as are females. Recent studies suggest that there is no correlation with maternal age, blood factors, or season of birth. The diagnosis may be delayed for the black or female infant if the clinician relies too heavily on epidemiology in diagnostic considerations. Early diagnosis, before major electrolyte disturbances occur, allows surgical correction under more stable conditions. The clinician should consider this condition in every infant with persistent and projectile nonbilious vomiting. Hypertrophic pyloric stenosis is most commonly seen in the infant under three months of age, but cases of adult hypertrophic stenosis have also been reported.

PATHOPHYSIOLOGY

There has not been a clearly defined cause for the development of hypertrophic stenosis. Recently, prostaglandin dysfunction has been implicated in the development of pyloric abnormalities in adult peptic ulcer disease. Prenatal gastric dilation without polyhydramnios has been associated with the later finding of pyloric stenosis. Fourteen hundred newborns underwent ultrasound evaluation without detection of the nine infants that subsequently developed pyloric stenosis.

Pathologic examination of the infant with hypertrophic stenosis demonstrates a pyloric region with a marked elongation of the sphincter and a hypertrophy of the circular fibers. These findings correlate well with the measurement changes seen on ultrasound evaluation of the patient. The affected infant has a resulting gastric outlet obstruction with gastric dilation and incessant postprandial vomiting. This creates an increased abdominal tone and dehydration that compromises bile flow. Starvation also affects glucoronyl tranference activity creating a mild jaundice. The loss of electrolytes and the disruption of the body's acid-base balance results from the abnormal pyloric sphincter preventing concurrent loss of the alkaline contents of the small bowel. As the process of vomiting gastric contents continues, the loss of potassium, chloride, and hydrochloric acid creates the classic finding of hypochloremic hypokalemic alkalosis usually reported in hypertrophic pyloric stenosis. With improved diagnostic approaches, the incidence of alkalosis or hypochloremia is thought to be less than 50 percent. The increased risk of anesthesia in the alkalotic patient requires correction of metabolic abnormalities prior to surgery.

CLINICAL PRESENTATION

The most easily recognized presentation is that of the 2 to 6 week old male infant with persistent projectile vomiting and dehydration. There may also be an accompanying family history of pyloric stenosis. The classic case also will demonstrate a palpable epigastric mass or "olive." These historical and clinical findings need little further evaluation and the clinical scope should change to preparation of the patient for surgical intervention. The most pertinent areas of the clinical history involve the timing, characteristics, and effects of the vomiting spells.

Unfortunately there are many atypical historical presentations of the disease process. The patient frequently does not have the vomiting history, and clinical exam fails to reveal a palpable mass in 20 percent of cases. Moreover as was previously described, one cannot rely on epidemiologic criteria in entertaining this diagnosis. Many cases will require ancillary modalities to confirm the clinical suspicion of this diagnosis.

In the patient with an atypical presentation consider an antral web, pyloric duplication, or pylorospasm. An acute gastroenteritis may closely mimic hypertrophic stenosis necessitating a radiographic evaluation to exclude the diagnosis.

Physical diagnosis is most accurate if one combines the observation of a vomiting event with the careful examination of the abdomen. Clinical evaluation of the degree of vomiting is also essential to guide the replacement therapy in preparation for surgery. An experienced examiner, usually the pediatric surgeon, can diagnose the condition on abdominal exam alone 80 percent of the time. A palpable epigastric "olive" has a specificity of virtually 100 percent in the detection of hypertrophic stenosis. Many surgeons believe that a patient with such a palpable mass requires only electrolyte correction followed by surgery without the need of performing ultrasound or radiographic examinations.

After observation of a regurgitant event, the examiner should stand on the right side of the patient. Using the left hand to support the infant's head and torso and flexing the legs on the examination table, palpate with right hand. Then use the index and middle fingers to palpate in the epigastrum at the right rectus abdominis muscle carefully. There have been rare reports of palpable masses that were subsequently found to represent atypical hepatic borders or accompanying volvulus. If there is any question of the origin of the palpated mass, the clinician should proceed to use ultrasound or radiography to confirm the impression.

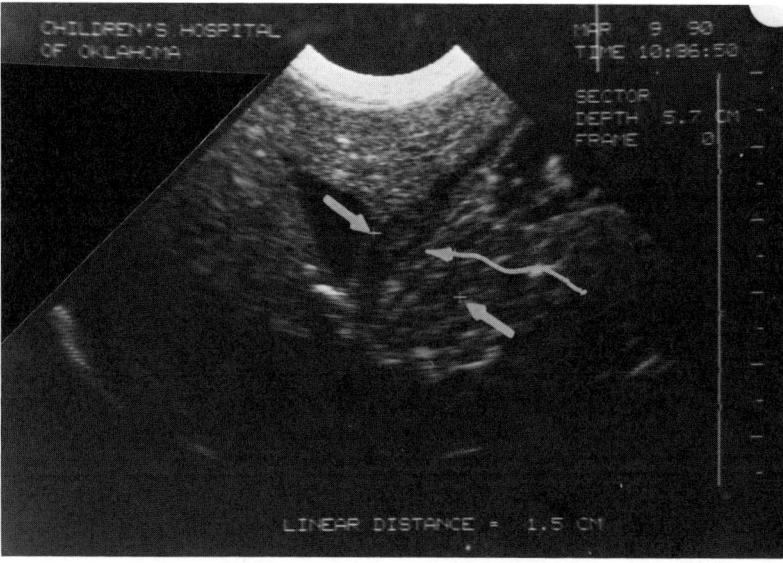

Figure 22.1 Ultrasound: The shorter arrows show the width of the pyloric channel—1.5 cm (normal 1.3 cm). The distance between the upper short arrow and the curved arrows represent wall thickness (>1 cm—normal < 3mm). (Adapted with permission from Amer Med Concepts & Clinical Practice; 3:2820.)

ADJUNCT EVALUATIONS

Ancillary studies may be required to confirm a diagnosis of pyloric stenosis. The infant with a palpable mass, confirmatory history, and stable electrolyte balance requires little further preparation for surgery. Twenty percent of patients with a strongly suggestive history and an ultimate diagnosis of pyloric stenosis do not have a palpable mass. These patients will usually be diagnosed by ultrasound (Figure 22.1). If ultrasound does not show an elongated and hypertrophied pyloric sphincter, an upper gastrointestinal (GI) series should be done (Figure 22.2). An upper GI barium study has virtually 100 percent specificity and sensitivity. There is a potential though rare complication of aspiration prior to ordering of the upper GI barium study.

Once pyloric stenosis is confirmed, the goal is to proceed to a prompt and safe surgical correction. The emergency physician will usually institute volume and electrolyte repletion to help prepare the infant for surgical intervention. The infant with hypochloremic hypokalemic alkalosis usually demonstrates a CO_2 of greater than 27 mEq/l. The usual surgical procedure to correct hypertrophic pyloric stenosis does not invade the bowel mucosa, and blood replacement is rarely needed. The clotting parameters should be evaluated prior to surgery. Alkalosis will increase the anesthetic risk, and correction with frequent monitoring of acid base balance will minimize potential complications. With improved preoperative care, the mortality of pyloromyotomy is less than 1 percent.

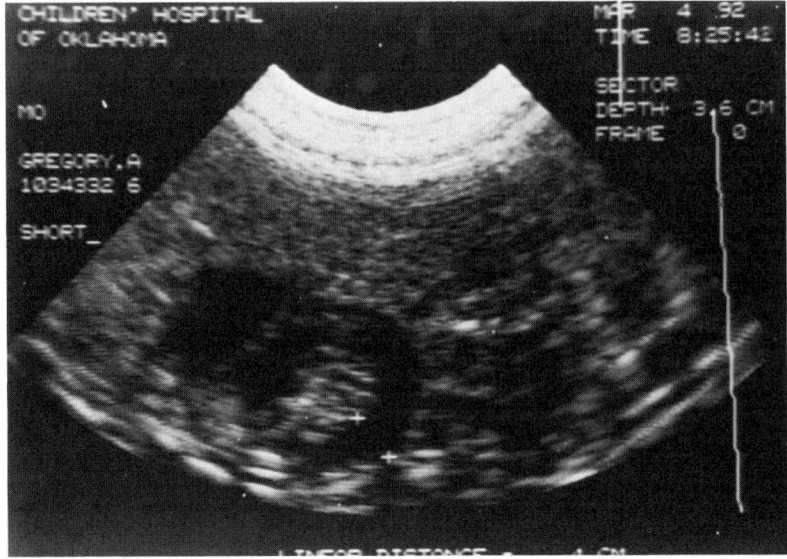

Figure 22.2 A two-month-old male with projectile vomiting and weight loss. Real-time echogram shows wall thickness of 0.4 cm normal < 0.3 cm.

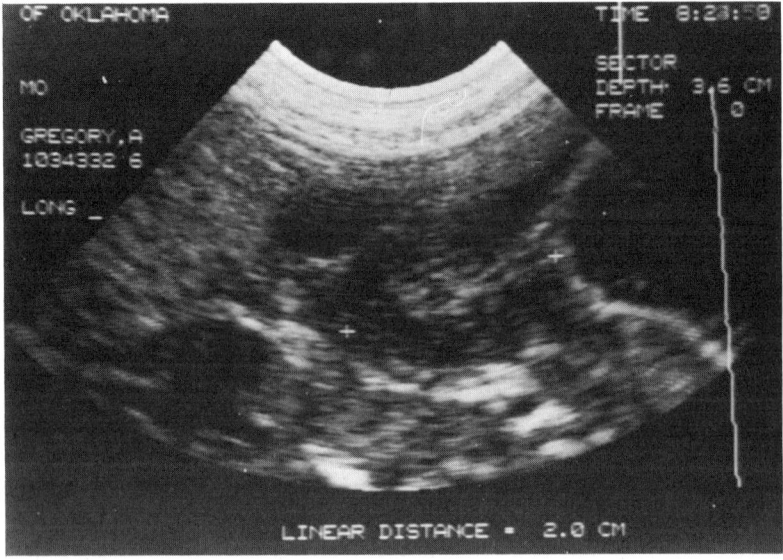

Figure 22.3 A two-month-old male with projectile vomiting and weight loss. In this real-time echogram, a pyloric channel measures 2 cm in longest length. There is retained gastric content.

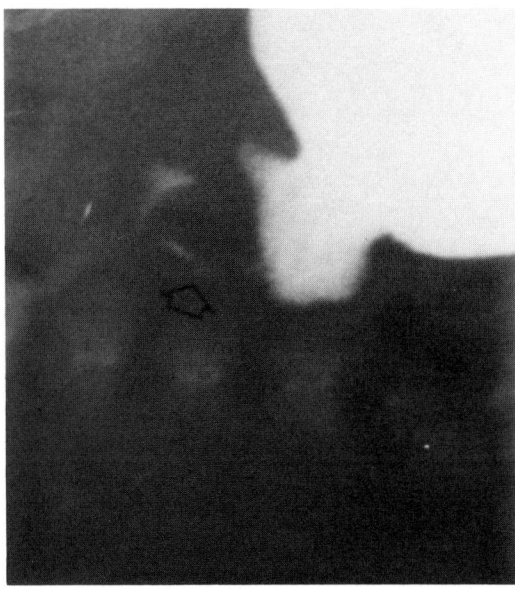

Figure 22.4 Barium study shows elongated pyloric channel "string sign."

Treatment

Further stimulation by attempting to feed the affected infant orally only increases the electrolyte and acid base disturbances. There is also a risk of aspiration with continued attempts to feed. Many other clinicians also feel that nasogastric intubation, sedation, and antiemetics increase the aspiration risk. Therefore all volume repletion should be given parentally.

Early surgical consultation should be obtained. A surgeon may palpate or confirm the epigastric mass that would preclude further diagnostic studies. One should begin fluid replacement as soon as the diagnosis is suspected and complicating congenital abnormalities have been detected and evaluated. Fluid and electrolyte management are easiest to determine after taking into consideration volume status, solute concentration disturbance, acid base balance, renal status, and potassium loss. Prophylactic antibiotics are indicated for the patient with a cardiac murmur history.

A moderately dehydrated infant may require 10 to 15 mEq/kg of sodium in addition to maintenance, to correct the total deficit. Potassium may be more difficult to calculate. In the presence of normal renal status a moderately dehydrated infant should receive 3 to 5 Meq/kg of potassium chloride to the calculated daily needs. A serum bicarbonate of less than 30 Meq/l will lessen the effects of rapid CO_2 changes during anesthesia. An infant with a long-term deficit will require frequent electrolyte determinations to guide replacement therapy.

All infants with a suspected diagnosis of pyloric obstruction should be hospitalized to prevent aspiration and provide fluid resuscitation. Early consultation from

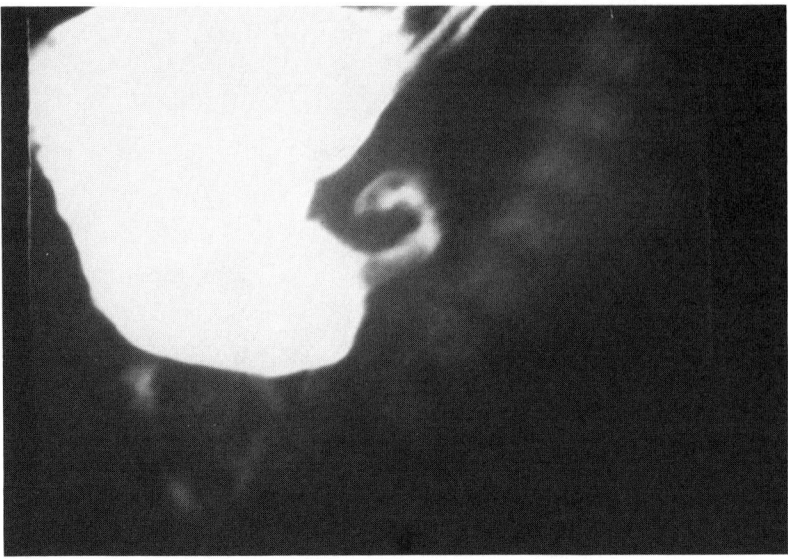

Figure 22.5 Barium showing elongated upturning pylorus.

surgery and radiology will provide optimal patient care rapidly and will also improve outcome. Early diagnosis will allow more informed family involvement and less resistance to prompt surgical correction. The procedure of choice remains a Ramstedt's Pyloromyotomy with a complication rate of less than 8 percent and a mortality rate of less than 1 percent. The advent of intraluminal instrumentation may soon be available in the therapy of hypertrophic pyloric stenosis.

SUGGESTED READING

1. Blumhagen JD, Maclin L, Krauter D, et al. Sonographic diagnosis of hypertrophic pyloric stenosis. AJA 1988;150:1367–1370.
2. Breaux CW, Georgeson KE, Royal SA, et al. Changing patterns in the diagnosis of hypertrophic pyloric stenosis. Pediatrics 1988;81(2):213–217.
3. Breaux CW, Hood JS, Georgeson KE. Embryologic and developmental anomalies. J Pediatr Surg 1989;24(12):1250–1252.
4. Forman HP, Leonidas JC, Kronfeld GD. A rational approach to the diagnosis of hypertrophic pyloric stenosis: Do the results match the claims? J Pediatr Surg 1990;25(2):262–266.
5. Goldman G, Tiomny E, Kahan PJ, et al. Prostaglandin E2 in pyloric stenosis. Arch Surg 1989;124:724–726.
6. Katz S, Basel D, Branski D. Prenatal gastric dilatation and infantile hypertrophic pyloric stenosis. J Pediatr Surg 1988;23(11):1021–1022.
7. Latchaw LA, Nabil NJ, Harris BH. The development of pyloric stenosis during transpyloric feedings. J Pediatr Surg 1989;24(8):823–824.
8. Okorie NM, Dickson JAS, Carver RA, et al. What happens to the pylorus after pyloromyotomy? Arch Dis Child 1988;63:1339–1340.

9. Rasmussen L, Green A, Hansen LP. The epidemiology of infantile hypertrophic pyloric stenosis in a Danish population, 1950–1984. Int J Epidemiol 1989;18(2):413–417.
10. Rasmussen L, Hansen LP, Ovist N, et al. Infantile hypertrophic pyloric stenosis and subsequent ulcer dyspepsia. Acta Chir Scand 1988;154:657–658.
11. Rasmussen L, Hansen LP, Pedersen SA. Infantile hypertrophic pyloric stenosis: The changing trend in treatment in a Danish county. J Pediatr Surg 1987;22(10):953–955.
12. Rollins MD, Shields MD, Quinn RJM, et al. Pyloric stenosis: Congenital or acquired? Arch Dis Child 1989;64:138–147.
13. Sleisenger MH, Fordtran JS. Gastrointestinal Disease. Philadelphia: Saunders, 1973;485–493.
14. Stringer MD, Brereton RJ. Current management of infantile hypertrophic pyloric stenosis. Brit J Hosp Med 1990;43:266–272.
15. Stunden RF, LeQuesne GW, Little KET. The improved ultrasound diagnosis of hypertrophic pyloric stenosis. Pediatr Radiol 1986;16:200–205.
16. Tam PKH, Saing H, Koo J, et al. Pyloric function five to eleven years after Ramstedt's pyloromyotomy. J Pediatr Surg 1985;20(3):236–239.
17. Vilmann P, Hjortrup A, Altmann P, et al. A long-term gastrointestinal follow-up in patients operated on for congenital hypertrophic pyloric stenosis. Acta Paediatr Scand 1986;75:156–158.
18. Westra SJ, deGroot JC, Smits NJ, et al. Hypertrophic pyloric stenosis: Use of the pyloric volume measurement in early US diagnosis. Radiology 1989;172:615–619.

23

Acute Appendicitis

David Tuggle

Appendectomy for acute appendicitis is one of the most common surgical procedures in the North American continent (1). Approximately 250,000 cases of appendicitis occur annually, accounting for 1,000,000 hospital days per year (1). The lifetime risk of appendicitis is 8.6 percent for males and 6.7 percent for females. In males, the incidence of nonperforating appendicitis rises from 44 per 100,000 population in the 0 to 9 years of age group, to a peak of 170 cases per 100,000 in the 10 to 19 years of age group (2). Yet the etiology and epidemiology of appendicitis remain poorly understood. The evaluation of abdominal pain where appendicitis is a consideration is without doubt one of the most common problems encountered in emergency departments today.

PATHOPHYSIOLOGY

In most instances, obstruction of the lumen of the appendix is the event that leads to appendicitis. It has been recognized that chronic and recurrent appendicitis does occur (3). In the usual case, however, the appendiceal lumen becomes acutely obstructed by a fecalith. Less common causes are lymphoid tissue hypertrophy, bacterial infections, inspissated barium, seeds, intestinal worms, edema, or foreign bodies. As obstruction progresses, the appendix becomes distended, leading to periumbilical pain. The appendiceal mucosa may suffer ischemic damage with increasing luminal pressure. When the integrity of the appendiceal wall has been compromised, bacteria invade the wall, and infection contributes to continued appendiceal damage. Ultimately gangrene or perforation may occur, allowing spill of grossly contaminated material.

When the appendiceal wall becomes inflamed, the nearby peritoneum is irritated, and pain is localized to the right lower quadrant (McBurney's point). If perforation occurs and is not well contained, diffuse peritonitis ensues.

CLINICAL PRESENTATION

Appendicitis in children presents with a widely varying clinical spectrum. In preschool children, the classic triad of pain, vomiting, and fever is not always readily apparent. Older children tend to have a more obvious presentation, but younger children may have a more confusing picture that necessitates more extensive evaluation (Figure 23.1).

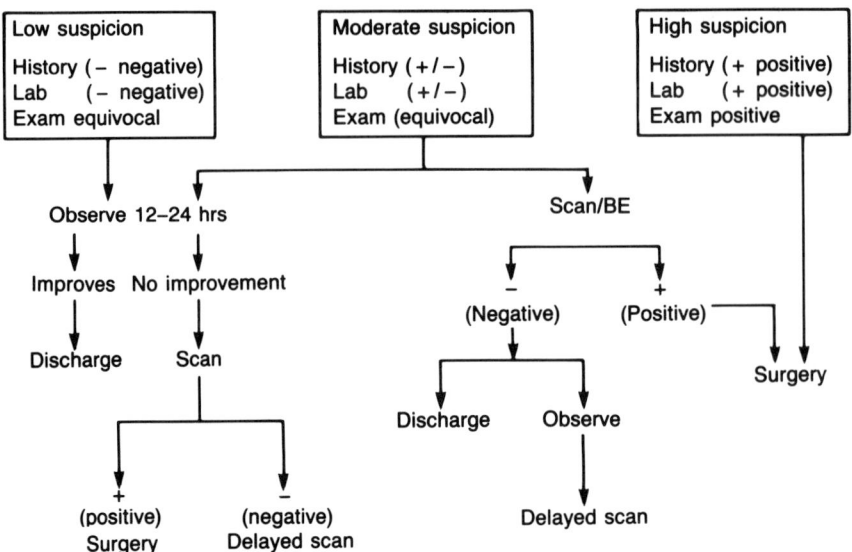

Figure 23.1   Abdominal pain.

History

Abdominal pain is the predominant symptom of appendicitis. In a classic case, pain begins as a vague discomfort in the periumbilical region, relocating to the right lower quadrant 1 to 12 hours later. This pain may persist for 24 to 48 hours. Occasionally the pain may subside then reappear with a more diffuse pattern consistent with perforation. Delays in diagnosis, however, are not uncommon due to variations in the location of the appendix (4) such as retrocecal or pelvic locations or coexistent malrotation. This may occur in up to one-third of cases.

Anorexia commonly accompanies appendicitis. It is more often variable in children than in adults, however. In otherwise healthy teenagers, appetite may not be negatively influenced so that close questioning is vital. Vomiting occurs in 75 percent of patients but rarely more than once or twice prior to surgery unless bowel obstruction is present. Obstipation or diarrhea may accompany other symptoms but are not reliable enough to offer help in the differential diagnosis. In older patients, the typical sequence of symptoms is anorexia, followed by pain and nausea or vomiting. In younger patients, this sequence of events is more variable.

Physical Examination

Observation of the child with appendicitis will more often be revealing than actual physical examination. The typical child with appendicitis is reluctant to move. A bumpy ride to the hospital is painful. Tapping the heels or rocking the bed elicits abdominal pain. The child may limp while ambulating or be unable to extend the right leg.

Bowel sounds may be normal with acute appendicitis. Bowel sounds with perforation may suggest bowel obstruction with high-pitched tinkles or be completely silent with an ileus. The chest should be carefully auscultated to rule out pneumonia mimicking appendicitis.

Gentle abdominal examination will be more rewarding than vigorous evaluation. It is best to start the exam in a quadrant away from the source of pain. A very light percussive tap on the abdomen is all that is required to identify peritonitis because of the child's abdominal wall being thinner than an adult's. Obese children will require more aggressive evaluation since their body habitus may mask many of the signs of appendicitis. If the appendix lies in proximity to the psoas muscle, the psoas sign will be positive. The sign is elicited by having the child lie on the left side and hyperextending the right thigh. This maneuver stretches the psoas muscle; a positive response suggests an inflamed appendix overlying the muscle. The *obturator sign* maneuver consists of internal rotation of the flexed right thigh while the child lies in the supine position. A positive result occurs when this maneuver produces hypogastric pain. Rectal examination may demonstrate right-sided tenderness.

Rectal examination is of value in about 50 percent of children with abdominal pain. It is more likely to be helpful in the adolescent female who presents with right lower quadrant pain. A positive psoas or obturator sign suggests a retrocecal inflammatory process.

Signs of trauma or abuse should be looked for. Occult or overt trauma can mimic appendicitis. Evidence for other causes of abdominal pain such as petechiae (Henoch Schoenlein purpura), abdominal masses, or insect bites should be sought.

Complications

Rupture of the appendix is the major complication of the disease and occurs more commonly when diagnosis and surgery is delayed. As compared with uncomplicated cases, rupture typically produces tenderness that is more diffuse, a higher fever, and a greater degree of leukocytosis. As peritonitis progresses, the child typically lies quietly supine because the slightest movement causes pain. The child will often complain of pain over the entire abdomen rather than just in the right lower quadrant. In older children, the perforation may wall off to form an appendiceal abscess. If this abscess ruptures or progresses to severe peritonitis, the child will show signs of extreme toxicity and sepsis.

Laboratory and X-ray

The white blood cell count (WBC) may or may not be elevated in early appendicitis. As many as 20 percent of patients may have a normal WBC upon presentation. Frequently a high band count or a left shift will be noted. Urinary examination may reveal a few white or red blood cells per high-powered field. Other laboratory determinations have not been routinely helpful.

Radiologic examination may be helpful in many cases, but with clear-cut appendicitis, it is not routinely necessary. Radiologic signs suggestive of appendicitis include a fecalith (Figure 23.2), right lower quadrant ileus, scoliosis, a psoas shadow, and small bowel obstruction. In selected cases, work-up with adjunctive studies is appropriate. Ultrasonography has been widely used to evaluate the child with abdominal pain (Figure 23.3) (5,6). The typical ultrasonic finding is a cystic ovoid hypoechoic area with internal debris surrounded by strong echoes. The more intense the inflammation, the more clearly it is demonstrated. Other important ultrasonic findings are an inflamed appendix, pelvic fluid collection, and paralytic ileus. With graded compression to the lower abdomen, the inflamed appendix is recognized as a sausage-shaped blind-ended structure on longitudinal imaging and as a target lesion on transverse section. The appendiceal wall in all abnormal cases is greater than two mm thick and the wall layers are less distinct than normal. The appendiceal lumen may or may not be dilated. Appendicoliths are recognized with greater frequency than they are with plain films. Sonography is also useful in suspected appendiceal perforation and abscess. It is useful but not infallible. It does not involve X-rays, but the results are operator-dependent, limiting its usefulness in certain locals. Barium enema has also been helpful in selected cases (7). Radiolabeled autologous white blood cell

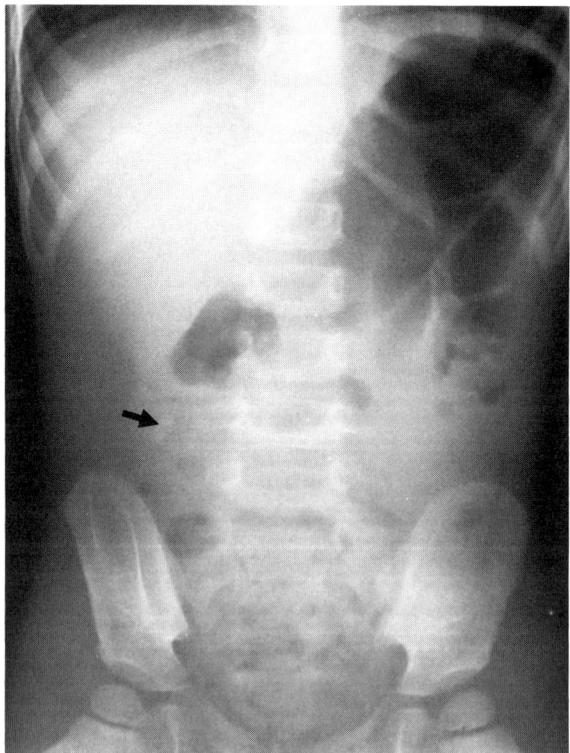

Figure 23.2 A child with fever and acute abdominal pain. Plain film abdomen showing (arrow) "appendicolith."

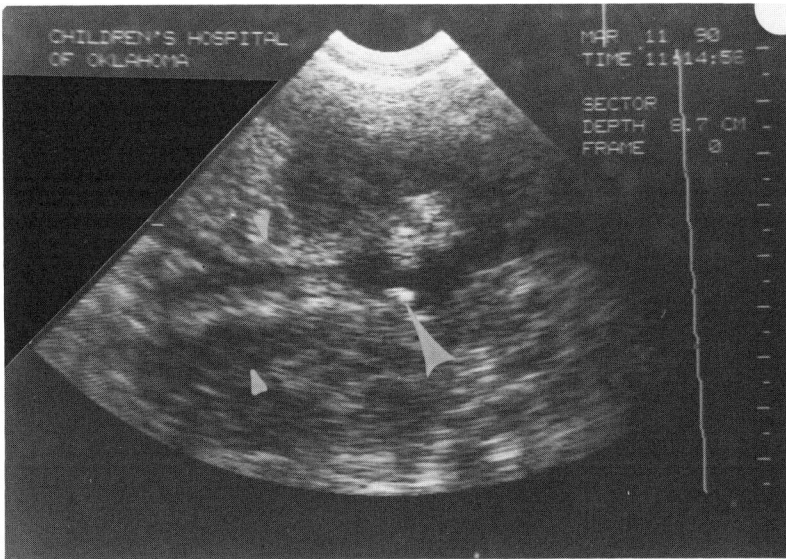

Figure 23.3 Ultrasound: large arrows showing appendicolith.

scans have recently become very useful and may be more specific and sensitive than ultrasound or a barium enema would be (8).

DIFFERENTIAL DIAGNOSIS

Many other illnesses can mimic appendicitis in children. Specific facets of the history or physical examination may lead the physician to a different diagnosis. Common illnesses that mimic appendicitis include pneumonia, bacterial or viral gastroenteritis, acute pharyngitis, urinary tract infections, and gynecologic disorders in adolescent females. Unusual causes of abdominal pain may also mimic appendicitis (Table 23.1).

Table 23.1 Unusual causes of right lower quadrant pain

Hirschsprung's enterocolitis	Volvulus of a wandering spleen
Foreign body bowel perforation	Acute ileitis
Internal hernia with volvulus	Tumor of the organ of Zucker-Kandl
Acalculus cholecystitis	Burkitt's lymphoma
Torsion of the ovary	Streptococcal pharyngitis

A partial list of other illness mimicking appendicitis at the Children's Hospital of Oklahoma 1987–1991.

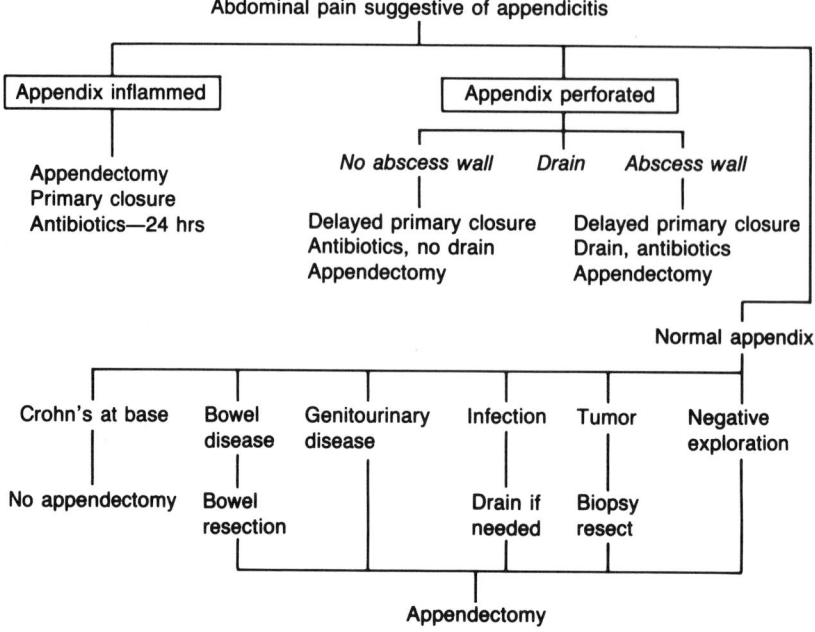

Figure 23.4 Algorithm.

MANAGEMENT

The management of appendicitis is usually straightforward. Removal of the appendix is indicated whether it is inflamed or not. If Crohn's disease is involving the base of the appendix or if the cecum is so friable that appendectomy would cause more harm than good, appendix removal should be reconsidered or avoided. If perforation has occurred, abscess drainage is indicated if the abscess wall is intact. Even with appropriate management of a perforated appendix, abscess recurrence is noted in 1 to 20 percent of patients. Most of the complications of perforated appendicitis are related to infection, and the use of antibiotic therapy to treat enteric bacteria and anaerobes is appropriate (Figure 23.4).

CONCLUSION

The identification of appendicitis in childhood requires a thorough knowledge of abdominal physiology and diagnostic probabilities. Even in this era of sophisticated radiologic evaluation of patients with abdominal pain, a negative exploration rate of 10 to 20 percent is still appropriate because of the high incidence of perforation in children. Selective use of imaging modalities may lower this rate slightly, but the morbidity of a missed appendicitis mandates the removal of an occasional normal appendix.

REFERENCES

1. Addiss DG, Shaffer N, Fowler BS, et al. The epidemiology of appendicitis and appendectomy in the United States. Am J Epidemiology 1990;132:910–925.
2. Luckmann R. Incidence and case fatality rates for acute appendicitis in California: A population-based study of the effects of age. Am J Epidemiology 1989;129:905–918.
3. Crabbe MM, Norwood SH, Robertson HD, et al. Recurrent and chronic appendicitis. Surg Gynecol Obstet 1986;163:11–13.
4. Poole GV. Anatomic basis for delayed diagnosis of appendicitis. South Med J 1990;83(7):771–773.
5. Puylaert JB, Rutgers PH, Lalisang RI, et al. A prospective study of ultrasonography in the diagnosis of appendicitis. NEJM 1987;317:666–669.
6. Rubin SZ, Martin DJ. Ultrasonography in the management of possible appendicitis in childhood. J Pediatr Surg 1990;25(7):737–740.
7. Garcia C, Rosenfiled NS, Markowitz RI, et al. Appendicitis in children: Accuracy of the barium enema. AJDC 1987;141:1309–1312.
8. Delaney AR, Raviola CA, Wever PN, et al. Improving diagnosis of appendicitis: Early autologous leukocyte scanning. Arch Surg 1989;124:1146–1152.

24

Acute Abdominal Pain

Edwin Ide Smith

Twenty percent of all children will seek medical help for abdominal pain by the age of 15 years. It is estimated that 5 percent of the group will require hospitalization or surgical intervention (1). A study of patients 2 to 16 years of age, seen in a pediatric emergency facility for acute abdominal pain, found that nine diagnoses accounted for 84 percent of the patients seen. Medical conditions accounted for 56.5 percent, surgical 8.5 percent, and nonspecific abdominal pain 35 percent. Appendicitis was the only surgical condition to appear in more than 1 percent of the patients (2). Patients with severe pain lasting more than six hours have a high probability of having a condition requiring surgical therapy.

Appropriate diagnosis depends on the basic tools—clinical history and physical examination aided or confirmed by appropriate laboratory and radiological studies. Early diagnosis is reflected in lessened morbidity and mortality. In the appropriate management of the pediatric patient with acute abdominal pain, it is necessary that an attempt be made to make a defensible tentative diagnosis and that operation is not considered on the basis that the abdomen represents a "surgical abdomen" with the disease and site unspecified. Early surgical consultation is of value in order that several examinations over time are possible. Progression of the disease can be appreciated at an earlier stage.

PATHOPHYSIOLOGY

Acute abdominal pain arises from three nervous pathways: parietal, referred, and visceral. Parietal pain is the "first pain" which is carried by somatic nerves. This somatic pain can be cutaneous, superficial, or deep pain from muscles or tendons. The retroperitoneal, retroileal area beneath the mesentery and the pelvic areas do not generate parietal pain, and are "silent areas." Referred pain occurs when pain fibers converge on a spinal tract or higher with resultant pain in the referred area. An example is the shoulder pain with diaphragmatic irritation. Visceral pain is carried by sympathetic and parasympathetic fibers and is poorly localized. Visceral pain may be caused by ischemia, some chemical mediators as in inflammation or trauma, stretching and distension, and extremes of thermal change.

While the pathophysiology of the various conditions causing acute abdominal pain varies, several generalizations are present. Organs inflamed either primarily or secondarily by contact tend first to hyperfunction and then to hypofunction. Trauma or inflammation within the free peritoneal cavity tends to produce gastrointestinal symptoms and signs. Obstruction of a tubular organ causes hypertrophy and enlargement proximally and usually results in emptying distally. Colicky pain is usually associated with obstruction, while constant pain is associated with ischemia and necrosis.

The anatomy of the peritoneal cavity and its organs is important in the interpretation of signs and symptoms. In general the pain representation of the stomach and small intestine tend to be supraumbilical with the appendix and the large bowel being infraumbilical.

CLINICAL PRESENTATION

The clinical presentations of the common conditions causing acute abdominal pain in infants and children are shown in Figure 24.1. The first three considerations for the clinician are (1) the age of the patient; (2) the duration and the severity of the pain; and (3) the presence of other gastrointestinal, urinary, respiratory, and genitourinary signs and symptoms.

DIFFERENTIAL DIAGNOSIS
Infants (Newborn to Two Years of Age)

The major differential diagnosis in the infant (not the neonate) includes medical conditions such as acute viral or bacterial (Shigella, Salmonella) gastroenteritis, pneumonia, colic, milk allergy, and constipation with a localized impaction. The primary surgical conditions to rule out are midgut volvulus associated with incomplete rotation and intussusception.

Acute volvulus usually presents in the first year of life with over half of the patients being under 30 days of life. The onset is usually sudden with bilious vomiting, apparent pain, and abdominal distension. With vascular compromise, a bloody stool may be passed. The patient can progress rapidly to hypovolemia and shock. Babies with midgut volvulus tend to appear ill. The abdomen is distended and firm. Anemia from intraluminal bleeding is common. Usually a contrast study from below delineates the volvulus and incomplete rotation.

Intussusception usually occurs in a previously well infant who is a good eater and often has the history of a recent viral infection. Fifty percent of patients with intussusception are 6 to 12 months of age, and 85 percent are seen before the age of 2 years (3). Characteristically the infant begins with intermittent colicky pain during which the legs are drawn up. The intermittent episodes of pain become more frequent and severe. A bloody or "currant jelly" stool may be passed. On examination, a sausage-shaped mass may be palpated in the right side or upper abdomen. Listlessness and lethargy are also frequent in babies with intussusception. The majority of intussusceptions are ileocolic and idiopathic. Lead points such as a Meckel's diverticulum or ileocecal lymphoma are more common in older children. A contrast study

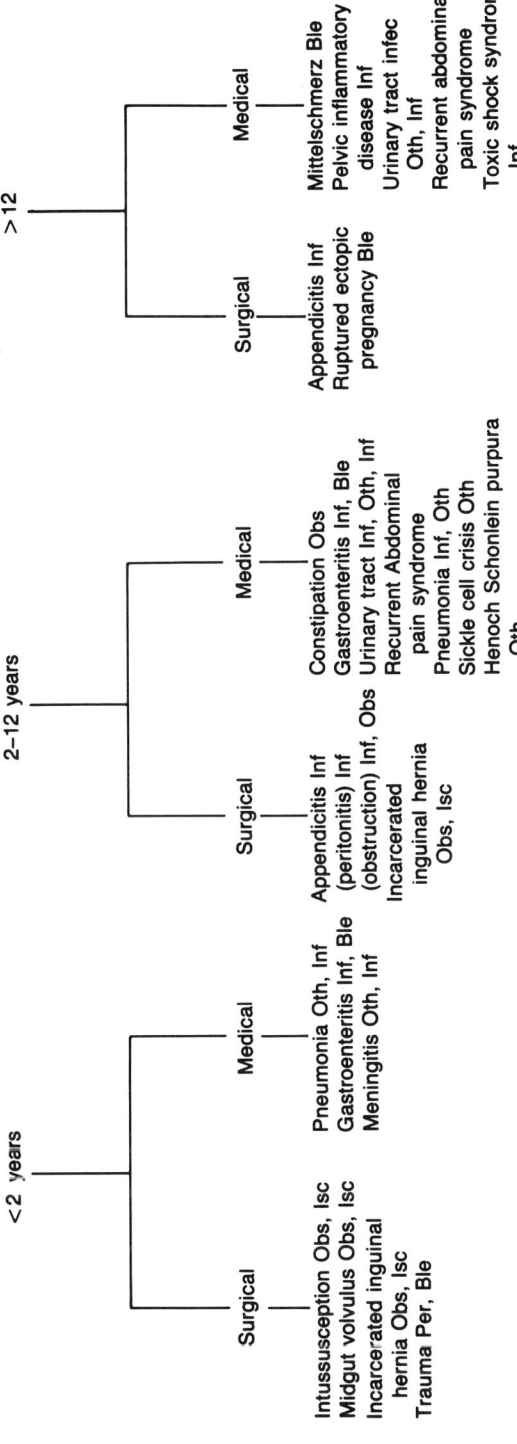

Figure 24.1 Acute abdominal pain, clinical presentation by age (Inf = Inflammation [pain, hyperfunction—hypofunction, fever], Obs = Obstruction [pain, vomiting, distension, absence stools], Oth = Other [respiratory, urinary], Isc = Ischemia [pain, blood GI tract], Ble = Bleeding [pain, anemia, ?hypovolemia], Per = Perforation [pain, fever]).

is necessary for the diagnosis and may achieve therapeutic reduction. Contraindications for a contrast study are pneumatosis, signs of peritoneal irritation, and possibly symptoms lasting longer than 48 hours.

Incarcerated inguinal hernia is also common, and often difficult to see immediately in well-nourished infants.

Children (2 to 12 Years of Age)

In this age group, acute appendicitis is the chief surgical condition to be ruled out. Trauma in childhood is very often occult and should be considered even in the absence of a positive history. Medical conditions include constipation, acute viral or bacterial enteritis, urinary tract infections, recurrent abdominal pain syndrome, pneumonia, sickle cell disease, and Henoch-Schonlein purpura. Apley has pointed out that 10 percent of all children have recurrent abdominal pain (4).

In *acute appendicitis* in childhood, the classic time sequence of abdominal pain followed by vomiting may be altered. Twenty percent of children with acute appendicitis have been found to have a history of recent respiratory or gastrointestinal infection in the two previous weeks, and 24 percent had symptoms on admission (5). The physical examination is the key to the diagnosis of acute appendicitis.

Adolescents (More Than 12 Years of Age)

Appendicitis remains a major consideration, but with the onset of puberty, gynecological considerations become important in the adolescent female and include mittelschmerz or bleeding from a follicle cyst, pelvic inflammatory disease with tubo-ovarian abscess, and ectopic pregnancy. Biliary tract disease and inflammatory bowel disease must also be included in the differential diagnosis.

HISTORY AND PHYSICAL EXAMINATION

Taking the history from the child depends considerably on age. Many times the secondhand history of the parent must be relied upon, a history that varies in accuracy. The onset of the present illness begins with the change from a well to a different child. The nature of the abdominal pain and its onset are important as is any means of relief. Sudden pain with a bump in the road is a good sign of peritoneal irritation. Disturbances of gastrointestinal (GI) function such as anorexia, vomiting, and alteration of bowel function are common in acute appendicitis.

Small children have no significant omentum, and they may have diarrhea or dysuria with an inflamed appendix that is adherent to the ileum (high-output diarrhea), the sigmoid (low-output diarrhea), or the bladder (dysuria, retention). Localization of pain in the small child is often not exact. Midline and even left-sided symptoms can be seen.

The physical examination should be complete. The critical examinations should be performed first and the troublesome examinations such as the pharyngeal and rectal last. It helps to sit down as one examines a small child, thus removing some of the scariness. Inspection of the child is valuable—sick or not, moving actively or lying quite still. Combative and hyperactive children rarely have peritonitis in which case they are more likely to remain still and to resist movement. Inspection of the conjunctivae, the skin, and the mucous membranes is very helpful with the viral infections, Henoch-Schonlein purpura, and streptococcal disease. The abdomen is examined for distension, for visible loops of bowel, and for an incarcerated inguinal hernia. Palpation should be very gentle, and the avoidance of pain is critical to a successful examination. It often helps to start with the child pointing to the area of greatest pain. Very light palpation is performed using the two sides of the abdomen as controls. Eight points, upper and lower rectus bilaterally, upper outer muscle groups, and lower outer muscle groups, are palpated. The degree of rigidity and/or spasm on one side is compared with the other side. Guarding and abdominal tenderness are the most important findings in acute appendicitis (2). Percussion is used in preference to rebound tenderness to elicit peritoneal irritation. While palpating or percussing the child, the eyes and face are carefully observed as indicative of a positive response. Bowel sounds are of limited value.

There are three rules for the diagnosis of appendicitis: (1) The abdominal examination in acute appendicitis should equal the vital signs of pulse, respiration, and blood pressure (rule of relativity). (2) Peritonitis in the child is acute appendicitis until it is proven otherwise. (3) Intestinal obstruction in the child without a history of an abdominal operation is acute appendicitis until it is proven otherwise.

The rectal examination is of greatest importance in demonstration of a mass or a fecal impaction and of less importance in determining tenderness. The male genitalia should be carefully examined. Both testis should be carefully palpated as torsion of an undescended testis may present with abdominal pain.

LABORATORY EVALUATION

Blood studies should include a routine complete blood count (CBC) with a differential and a sickle cell preparation when one is indicated. Although extremes in the leukocyte count may be helpful, this count is often not helpful in the difficult diagnostic situation. White blood cell counts (WBC) of 15,000 to 18,000/mm^3 are not uncommon with gastroenteritis. A routine urinalysis is necessary to look for acetonuria, glycosuria, bacturia, and pyuria. Routine electrolytes and a blood urea nitrogen (BUN) should be performed in patients who have had significant vomiting or who are dehydrated. A pregnancy test is advised for all female patients past puberty.

Radiological and Other Special Studies

The radiological examination is quite helpful, particularly in the smaller child; however, it is not necessary in every case. Specific abdominal findings in appendicitis are an appendiceal fecalith and intraluminal appendiceal air. Nonspecific signs are a generalized or localized ileus, scoliosis concave to the right, masses, and extraluminal air in an abscess. The abdominal roentgenogram also gives information concerning the location of the cecum. If a fecal impaction is suspected in the absence of acute peritoneal irritation, a low saline or hypertonic enema can be given (6). Pneumonia in a dehydrated child may show little X-ray evidence of consolidation until rehydration has occurred.

Ultrasonography is used increasingly in the diagnosis of acute abdominal pain in children and adolescents. A recent series had a sensitivity of 89 percent and a specificity of 92 percent. It proves most helpful in the patient with an unclear diagnosis, particularly in the adolescent female where there is high accuracy in delineating gynecological disease (7).

Barium enema examination of the child with abdominal pain may also be employed where the diagnosis is not clear. Complete filling of the appendix should exclude acute appendicitis, but it is often difficult to determine the entire extent of the appendix.

MANAGEMENT

The management of the patients with abdominal pain depends on the urgency of treatment, particularly that involving an operation (Figure 24.2). In some patients, the diagnosis can be made readily and a treatment plan formulated. An example of this would be a midgut volvulus where an emergency operation would be clearly indicated. A second group of patients will have a tentative diagnosis but will need stabilization and observation prior to surgical correction. The major areas that may need correction are fluid deficits, infection, and pain. A third group of patients remain with an unclear diagnosis and require observation within the emergency department or in the hospital. These patients require several points on their "illness curve" to clarify their probable diagnosis.

Resuscitation should proceed concomitant with diagnosis. When the patient is dehydrated and perhaps hypovolemic, initial resuscitation with intravenous fluids—either Ringer's lactate or normal saline dependent on site of loss—or with colloid is begun early, usually 20ml/kg as a bolus. Analgesia should be withheld until a tentative working diagnosis is established. Temperature elevation is controlled with rectal or oral acetaminophen.

Infant

Resuscitation of the infant is doubly important as fluid losses and hypovolemia can produce hypovolemic shock. These should be initiated prior to special studies. Observation of some infants may be necessary to rule out an intraperitoneal process. Sedation of the infant will often make demonstration of the abdominal mass possible. If hospitalization is planned, the earlier the patient can be transferred to the nursing unit the more desirable it is for the infant.

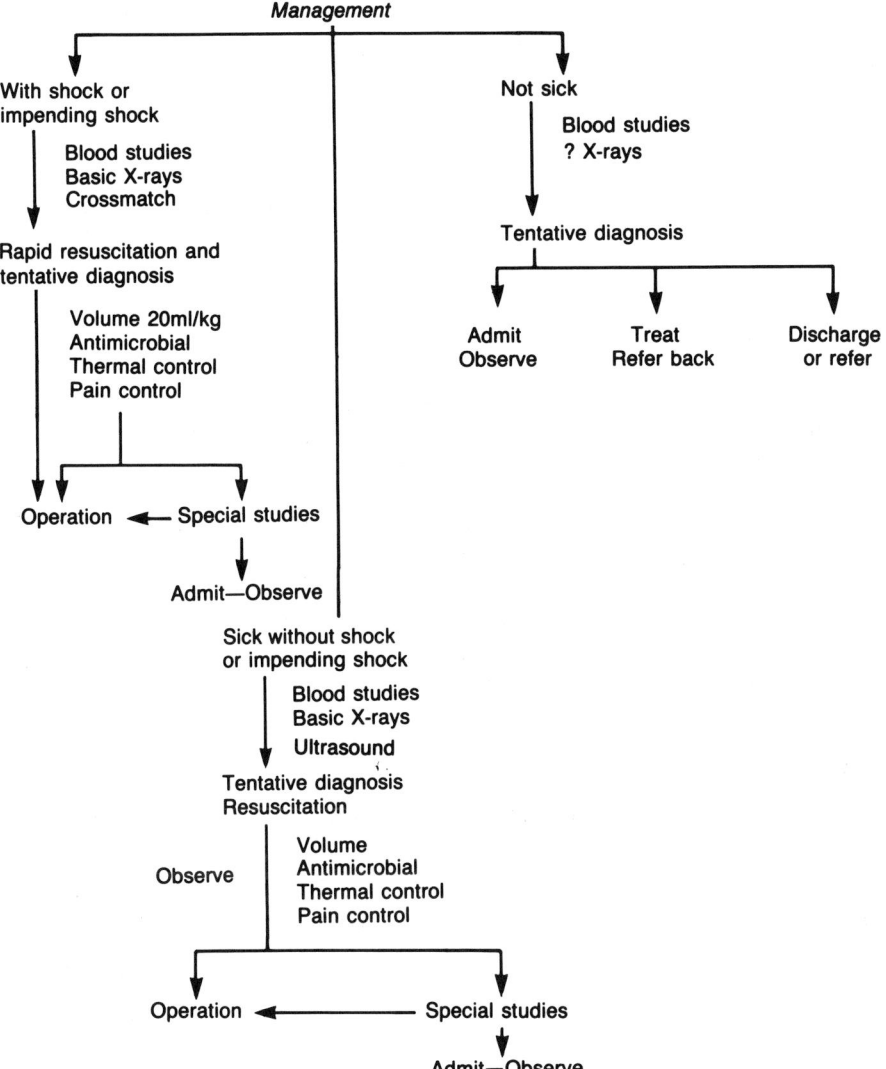

Figure 24.2 Acute abdominal pain

Child

Resuscitation again should be started promptly. Short periods of observation to assist in diagnosis are important. Where exploration for possible appendicitis has been decided on, antibiotics should be begun. Choice of drugs should provide both gram negative and positive coverage. Addition of a drug effective against anaerobic infection is necessary where an abscess or diffuse peritonitis exists.

The patient should be made NPO (*nil per os*), have a nasogastric tube inserted and have intravenous (IV) fluids begun. Temperatures should be taken axilliarily or orally if there is a pelvic abscess.

Adolescent

In management of the adolescent, appropriate attention should be given to the special needs. Often sedation and observation are very helpful. In the adolescent, female use of ultrasonography to examine the adnexae can be particularly helpful.

CONCLUSIONS

The diagnosis and management of acute abdominal pain in children and adolescents continues to pose a challenge to the emergency physician. While the majority of the patients seen will probably have nonsurgical disease, often self-limited, the identification of patients with surgical or probably surgical disease, particularly acute appendicitis, is critical. One hundred percent accuracy is not possible, and one should err on the side of inclusion into the surgical group. Ancillary laboratory and diagnostic technological examinations are adjunctive and should be used to support or to rule out tentative diagnoses that have been made on the basis of the history and physical findings. Age is a major determinant of the probable cause of the symptom-sign complex with which the patient presents.

REFERENCES

1. Buchert GS. Abdominal pain in children: An emergency practitioner's guide. Emer Med Clin NA 1989;7:497–517.
2. Reynolds S, Jaffe D, Lavigne J. Abdominal pain in a pediatric emergency department (abstract). Pediatr Emerg Care 1988;4:297.
3. Leape LL. Patient care in pediatric surgery. Boston: Little Brown, 1987;313–316.
4. Apley J. The child with abdominal pains. Springfield, Ill.: Charles C Thomas, 1959.
5. Jackson RH, Gardner PS, Kennedy J, et al. Viruses in the etiology of acute appendicitis. Lancet 1966;2:711–715.
6. Smith EI. Appendicitis and peritonitis. In Kelley VC, ed. Practice of pediatrics. Philadelphia: Harper and Row, 1982;1–13 (Chapter 32).
7. Rubin SZ, Martin DJ. Ultrasonography in the management of possible appendicitis in childhood. Jour Pediatr Surg 1990;25:737–740.

PART VIII

Renal/Genitourinary

25

Dehydration and Electrolyte Problems

A. Eugene Osburn

Dehydration is the result of a decrease in body water. The manner in which an individual is affected by dehydration is determined, however, not only by how much volume is lost but also by which fluid compartments of the body are most involved and by the effectiveness of the compensatory mechanisms the person is able to muster against the losses. The contribution of individual fluid compartments is determined primarily by the sodium concentration of the extracellular fluid.

Management of dehydration in children requires an understanding of how shifts in fluid compartments occur, how such shifts are compensated for physiologically, and how such events are reflected in physical examination and laboratory findings. It also requires a knowledge of safe ranges for correcting the derangements that have accrued in the patient.

PATHOPHYSIOLOGY

Disruption of fluid and electrolyte balance can occur from multiple causes (Figure 25.1). Dehydration occurs when water intake plus water produced by oxidation fails to equal fluid losses. The distribution of the fluids between intracellular and extracellular spaces is determined primarily by the osmolality of the fluids in these compartments. This distribution in turn influences the clinical interpretation of hydration status significantly, since the customary signs of dehydration are based on an assessment of the normalcy of the extracellular volume.

As dehydration evolves, compensatory mechanisms are invoked to lessen its disruption on homeostasis. These compensations are mediated primarily by the kidney. Antidiuretic hormones (ADHs) reduce the volume of urinary free water excreted, and the renin-angiotensin-aldosterone axis effects sodium retention. Blood urea nitrogen (BUN), serum creatinine (Cr) and urine sodium concentration are helpful parameters to facilitate assessment of these compensatory mechanisms. There are limits to these compensatory mechanisms, however, therefore the clinician must monitor for evidence of renal failure because its development requires subsequent adjustments to the fluid management.

Dehydration is a clinical diagnosis. Laboratory findings can help determine what kind of dehydration has occurred. Clinical criteria are used to estimate the severity of

286 | SYNOPSIS OF PEDIATRIC EMERGENCY CARE

TOTAL BODY WATER	DECREASED			NORMAL OR INCREASED	
Serum Sodium Concentration	Decreased	Normal	Increased	Decreased	Increased
Physiologic Derangement	Hypotonic Dehydration	Isotonic Dehydration	Hypertonic Dehydration	Water with Sodium Retention	Sodium with Water Retention
Urine Sodium	<10 mEq/L / >20 mEq/L	Variable	<10 mEq/L / >20 mEq/L	<10 mEq/L / >20 mEq/L	<10 mEq/L / >20 mEq/L
Causes	GI Losses / Vomiting / Diarrhea / Fistulae / Third Space Losses / Burns / Peritonitis / CSF Drainage || Adrenal Insufficiency / Sodium Losing Nephropathy / Bicarbonaturia / Metabolic Alkalosis / Renal Tubular Acidosis / Diuretic Excess / Post Obstructive Diuresis		Diabetes Insipidus / Sweating / Diarrhea / Vomiting / Fever / Thyrotoxicosis / Cystic Fibrosis	Osmotic Diuresis	Nephrotic Syndrome / Cardiac Failure / Hepatic Failure / Acute Water Loading	Excess ADH / SIADH / Renal Failure / Hypothyroidism / Glucocorticoid Deficiency	Cardiac Failure / Cirrhosis / Nephrosis	Primary Hyper-Aldosteronism / Cushing's Syndrome / Salt Ingestion / NaHCO₃ Excess / Chronic Renal Failure
Treatment	Isotonic Saline	1/2 NS	1/3 NS	Water Restriction	Sodium Restriction / Diuretics / Dialysis

Figure 25.1

the dehydration before laboratory results are available. That estimate can then be modified when the serum sodium is known.

In assessing the severity of dehydration, a designation of mild, moderate, or severe is commonly used and assumed to correspond to a 5 percent, 10 percent, or 15 percent fluid deficit respectively. These percents refer to findings of isotonic loss of water and sodium and of the effects an isotonic fluid loss will have on extracellular volume. Dehydration that results in hypotonic extracellular fluids will cause the same progression of clinical findings as does isotonic dehydration. They appear after less total body water loss, however, because of shifts of water into the cells at the expense of the extracellular and vascular spaces. Conversely hypertonic dehydration can mask the clinical findings used to characterize the degree of dehydration even though a dangerously large percent of total body water loss may have occurred because of shifts of fluid from the intracellular space into the extracellular, and hence vascular, space. By the time a patient with hypertonic dehydration demonstrates clinical signs of significant dehydration, there may be little in the way of fluid reserves left.

Recognition of the role of electrolyte derangements in evaluating the clinical significance of dehydration is important. It is also critical to understand that all electrolyte derangements are not dehydration. Dehydration is water loss. The hydration status of an individual at any given time is the net result of loss versus intake of both water and electrolytes. Water loss can occur at a lesser, equal, or greater rate than the electrolytes it contains with a resulting state of hypotonic, isotonic, or hypertonic dehydration. If hyponatremia is present in a patient with a normal or low BUN, water retention has occurred either because of an elevated ADH (appropriate or inappropriate) or because of hypotonic water intake that exceeded the kidney's ability to excrete the excess. Such a patient is not dehydrated, and the treatment is water restriction, not extra fluids. In assessing the hypernatremic patient, if the hypernatremia is present in a patient who has signs of fluid overload, fluid restriction and/or dialysis may be indicated. In addition, that patient is not dehydrated.

CLINICAL PRESENTATION

As dehydration progresses, its effects on the extracellular volume, such as absence of tears, dry mucous membranes, or a sunken fontanel, can be seen. Its presence and evolution can also be inferred because of compensatory changes occurring in the patient. Tachycardia, prolonged capillary refill, and narrowed pulse pressure indicate a more advanced degree of dehydration. In children, hypotension is a late finding indicative of severe dehydration, and its presence requires urgent fluid resuscitation.

Mild dehydration may produce only minimal clinically detectable changes, and its diagnosis may have to be based primarily on a history of fluid loss exceeding intake. There may be dryness of mucous membranes, decreased frequency of urination, and tachycardia, but capillary refill time and blood pressure are still normal. By the time moderate dehydration has developed, signs of early shock begin to appear: the capillary refill time exceeds two seconds and the pulse pressure is narrowed. Hypotension is a reflection of severe dehydration, and vascular collapse may be imminent.

DIFFERENTIAL DIAGNOSIS

The differential diagnosis can be approached in steps:

1. Is the total body water decreased, normal or increased?
2. What is the osmolar status of the extracellular fluids?
3. Are the kidneys contributing to, compensating for, or damaged by the process under consideration?

The first question is answered by correlating historical and physical examination data. The second and third questions require laboratory information. Figure 25.1 classifies etiologies of disturbances in fluid and electrolyte balance suggested by answers to these questions.

LABORATORY EVALUATION

Essential information needed from the laboratory to guide management of fluid and electrolyte disorders include

1. Serum Ph, Na+, K+, Cl−, CO_2, BUN, Cr, and glucose
2. Urine volume in amount/kg/h
3. Random urine specific gravity or osmolality and Cr, Na+, Cl−, and K+

The serum sodium is a major determinant of distribution of fluids within fluid compartments. The BUN and Cr reflect adequacy of renal perfusion. The serum pH and CO_2 provide insight into the possible etiology of the dehydration as well as into the effect the dehydration has had on physiologic compensation for the illness. If the fluid loss is from the gastrointestinal (GI) tract distal to the pylorus, a metabolic acidosis ensues; fluid and electrolyte loss from above the pylorus or from hypertonic sweat (for example, cystic fibrosis) results in a metabolic alkalosis. Metabolic acidosis that develops from uncomplicated dehydration has a normal anion gap. An increase in the anion gap should stimulate the clinician to investigate the possibility of drug ingestions, metabolic diseases or development of renal failure. Another fairly simple method of assuring an uncomplicated metabolic acidosis is to note the relationship between the pH and the total CO_2 in the patient. In uncomplicated metabolic acidosis, which has normal respiratory compensation, the digits to the right of the decimal point in the venous pH should approximate the value of the total CO_2. Thus, a total CO_2 of 18 would be found in the dehydrated patient with a pH of 7.18 if no mitigating factors effect the acid base balance.

Determination of the potassium loss that invariably occurs with dehydration cannot be recognized from the serum K+ value alone. Potassium shifts into the intracellular space at a rate of 1 mEq/l for each 0.2 increase in pH. Total body potassium deficit should be suspected in the patient who has a low (less than 10mEq/l) urinary potassium concentration, and should be considered in selecting treatment for dehydrated children.

Dehydration and Electrolyte Problems | 289

MANAGEMENT

Management of dehydration can be divided into six stages (Figure 25.2):

1. Assessment of the need to treat shock or significant intravascular volume depletion
2. Calculation of the amount of calories, water, and electrolytes needed to maintain normal cellular metabolism

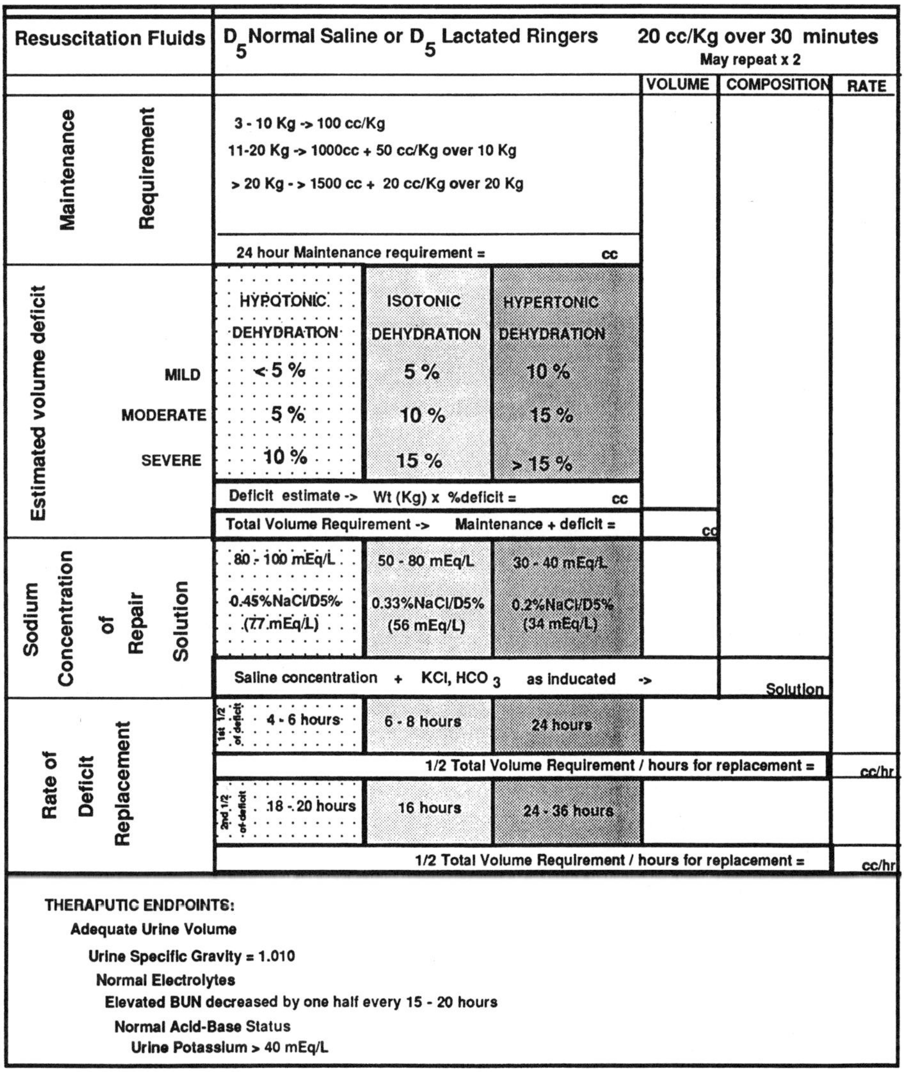

						VOLUME	COMPOSITION	RATE
Resuscitation Fluids		D_5 Normal Saline or D_5 Lactated Ringers				20 cc/Kg over 30 minutes May repeat x 2		
Maintenance	**Requirement**	3 - 10 Kg -> 100 cc/Kg 11-20 Kg -> 1000cc + 50 cc/Kg over 10 Kg > 20 Kg -> 1500 cc + 20 cc/Kg over 20 Kg						
		24 hour Maintenance requirement =			cc			
Estimated volume deficit			HYPOTONIC DEHYDRATION	ISOTONIC DEHYDRATION	HYPERTONIC DEHYDRATION			
		MILD	< 5 %	5 %	10 %			
		MODERATE	5 %	10 %	15 %			
		SEVERE	10 %	15 %	> 15 %			
		Deficit estimate -> Wt (Kg) x %deficit =			cc			
		Total Volume Requirement -> Maintenance + deficit =				cc		
Sodium Concentration of Repair Solution		80 - 100 mEq/L	50 - 80 mEq/L	30 - 40 mEq/L				
		0.45%NaCl/D5% (77 mEq/L)	0.33%NaCl/D5% (56 mEq/L)	0.2%NaCl/D5% (34 mEq/L)				
		Saline concentration + KCl, HCO$_3$ as inducted ->					Solution	
Rate of Deficit Replacement		1st 1/2 of deficit	4 - 6 hours	6 - 8 hours	24 hours			
		1/2 Total Volume Requirement / hours for replacement =						cc/hr
		2nd 1/2 of deficit	18 - 20 hours	16 hours	24 - 36 hours			
		1/2 Total Volume Requirement / hours for replacement =						cc/hr

THERAPUTIC ENDPOINTS:
  Adequate Urine Volume
    Urine Specific Gravity = 1.010
      Normal Electrolytes
        Elevated BUN decreased by one half every 15 - 20 hours
          Normal Acid-Base Status
            Urine Potassium > 40 mEq/L

Figure 25.2

3. Estimation of the degree of volume deficit that has occurred
4. Selection of a fluid composition that should correct accrued deficits and provide ongoing maintenance needs
5. Estimation of the optimal time necessary to correct the fluid and electrolyte imbalance most safely
6. Use of therapeutic endpoints to monitor needs to alter the initial plan

Resuscitation Fluids

If shock is present, an initial bolus of isotonic crystalloid should be given. Either normal saline or lactated Ringer's solution (20 mls/kg over 5 minutes) is appropriate. Since many conditions that lead to dehydration in children also result in starvation, most children also benefit from the addition of 5 percent glucose to the replacement fluid. Whether it should be added immediately or later can be assessed by a dextrostix glucose determination if there is doubt. Giving the resuscitation fluids in measured boluses, instead of as a steady infusion, aids in evaluating the response to the bolus. The response to the bolus then can be used to assess whether the original estimate of the degree of dehydration was accurate and to detect renal failure should dehydration develop.

Maintenance Fluids

After resuscitation needs have been addressed, the clinician can calculate the expected maintenance fluid volume. The maintenance fluid and electrolytes are those needed to maintain normal cellular function. In treating dehydration, the maintenance requirement of fluid and electrolytes is added to that required to replace accrued deficits. The type of dehydration being treated determines the optimal safe rate of the fluid to be replaced because the clinician must take into account fluid shifts that can occur as a result of the treatment. As will be seen in the next section of this chapter, the deficit fluid requirement is divided into halves, each half to be given over a time period dictated by the type of dehydration present. Therefore it is more convenient to use the number of cc/hr than to use the total 24-hour volume of maintenance fluid for determining how much maintenance volume to add to the anticipated deficit replacement volume. By using 4 cc/kg for the first 10 kg of the patient and by adding 2 cc/kg for the next 10 kg and 1 cc/kg for each kg over 20 kg, the cc/hr needed for maintenance can be arrived at. Ongoing fluid losses require addition to this maintenance requirement, and oliguria or anuria require its reduction. To verify that the estimates were correct, properly hydrated children who are not being fed should lose between ½ and 1 percent of their body weight per day.

Volume Deficit Estimation

While an initial estimate of the volume of fluid deficit that will need to be replaced can be based on a diagnosis of mild, moderate, or severe dehydration, this estimate may need to be adjusted if it is found that the patient is hyper- or hyponatremic. As has already been mentioned, hypertonic dehydration will require more fluid to replace the deficit than expected on the basis of an initial clinical assessment (that is, mild, moderate, or severe dehydration), and hypotonic dehydration will require less such fluid. The type of dehydration will also determine the time period over which the initial one-half of the volume deficit should be given.

Electrolyte Composition of Replacement Fluid

In the emergency department, it is not necessary to make meticulous calculations of electrolyte replacement needs. Discussions of the derivation of replacement fluid compositions are given in many other books (see Suggested Reading) and can be summarized here as NS (normal saline)

If the dehydration is	Use
Hypotonic	½ to ¾ NS
Isotonic	⅓ to ½ NS
Hypertonic	¼ NS

If these fluid concentrations are given over the time periods recommended for the type of dehydration, they should safely provide requirements of both maintenance and deficits present. Other more detailed calculations can be found, but after adding together all the components, the final fluid composition will still fall within these ranges. The volume of the selected fluid needed equals that needed to replace the estimated deficit plus that required for maintenance.

Time Allowances for Safe Replacement of Deficit

As a rule of thumb, hypotonic dehydration should be corrected over a few hours, whereas hypertonic dehydration should be corrected over a few days. After selecting a replacement fluid and electrolyte volume and composition based on the severity and type of dehydration, one can identify another time period for giving the first half and another time period for giving the second half of that volume. These time periods are based on the type of dehydration present and are conveniently listed as:

Type of Dehydration	First ½	Second ½
Hypotonic	4–6 hours	20–18 hours
Isotonic	6–8 hours	18–16 hours
Hypertonic	24 hours	24 hours

These guidelines may need to be modified in patients at either extreme of the type of dehydration, that is, the hypotonic patient with a serum sodium less than 120 mEq/l or the hypernatremic patient whose serum sodium exceeds 180 mEq/l. The acutely and severely hyponatremic child who is symptomatic (that is, has seizures) may benefit from receiving enough hypertonic saline to raise the serum sodium level 10 mEq/l. This can be achieved by giving 10 to 12 cc/kg of 3 percent sodium chloride (0.5 mEq/cc). The severely hypernatremic child may require dialysis in addition to fluid replacement.

Therapeutic Endpoints

Treatment is begun based on an estimate of safe ranges both of composition of the replacement fluid and electrolytes and of the rate at which it is given. The patients' response to that treatment dictates subsequent modifications to the treatment. An adequate urine output (at least 1 cc/kg/hr) should be apparent within the first few hours of treatment, and electrolyte imbalances should be corrected. With restoration of normal renal function, any elevation of BUN should decrease by one-half every 15 to 20 hours. Metabolic acidosis due to dehydration should resolve within a couple days. Replenishment of total body potassium deficits may require several days.

SUGGESTED READING

1. Barkin RM. Problems in the management of vomiting, diarrhea and dehydration. In Luten RC, ed. Problems in pediatric emergency medicine. New York: Churchill Livingstone, 1988.
2. Finberg L, Kravath RE, Fleishman AR. Water and electrolytes in pediatrics. Philadelphia: Saunders, 1982.
3. Kallen RJ. Diarrheal dehydration in infants. Pediatr Clin North Am 1990;37(2):265–286.
4. Perkins RM, Levin DL. Common fluid and electrolyte problems in the pediatric intensive care unit. Pediatr Clin North Am 1980;27(3):567–586.
5. Winters RW. Principles of pediatric fluid therapy. 2nd ed. Boston: Little, Brown, 1982.

26

Acute Scrotum

J. Stephen Archer
Philip L. Jones

The acute scrotum presents a clinical problem that usually is secondary to infection, trauma, vascular compromise of the testes, appendages of the testes, or herniation of intra-abdominal contents into the scrotum. The differentiation of the etiologies of acute scrotal pain and swelling can be difficult and often requires surgical exploration for definitive diagnosis. The challenge for the clinician in the emergency department setting is to distinguish quickly and accurately surgical from medical conditions of the scrotum. It must also be remembered that a missed testicular torsion or strangulated hernia is much worse than a negative scrotal exploration. This chapter emphasizes various entities causing acute red painful scrotum by describing the pathogenesis, clinical presentation, and therapy for each of these conditions.

TESTICULAR TORSION

One of the most common causes of sudden scrotal pain and swelling in boys or adolescent males is testicular torsion. The clinician should maintain a high index of suspicion because torsion must be diagnosed and treated rapidly if the testicle is to be spared.

Torsion of the testis is surprisingly common and the incidence may be as high as 1 in 160 males (1). If the testicle is completely enveloped by the tunica vaginalis (bell clapper anomaly), it is not appropriately fixed to the scrotal wall, which allows twisting and resultant ischemia or infarction. If blood flow can be restored within six hours, the testis will remain viable in 80 percent to 100 percent of cases. Salvage rates drop quickly with each hour that passes after the initial six-hour period. When surgical exploration and detorsion are accomplished, simultaneous fixation of the contralateral testis should be performed because bilaterality of the bell clapper deformity is common (2).

Torsion classically presents with sudden, severe scrotal pain that radiates to the groin. Swelling quickly develops initially in the epididymis followed by more global swelling of the testicle. Finally scrotal wall edema and erythema develop. The torsed testicle is usually found high in the scrotum. The lie or orientation of the testis may be grossly abnormal. Pyuria is usually absent but has been documented in up to 30 percent of cases. The well-known Prehn's sign (diminution of pain when the testicle is elevated) is clinically unreliable in distinguishing inflammatory processes from torsion (2). Patients that present with severe pain and swelling within hours of presentation should be treated as highly suspicious for torsion, and urgent urologic consultation should be obtained.

Radionuclide scrotal scanning can distinguish testicular torsion from inflammatory conditions involving the testis and epididymis (3). The diagnosis of torsion is based on assessment of blood flow to the scrotal contents. With acute testicular torsion, the most reliable finding is a photogenic region corresponding to the testes in the symptomatic hemiscrotum (Figure 26.1). With inflammatory processes there is increased blood flow present in contrast to the normal hemiscrotum. Studies indicate that the sensitivity and specificity of this technique exceed 90 percent.

Recent reports have encouraged the use of color Doppler ultrasonography in evaluation of the acute scrotum (4). Color flow imaging with use of a duplex Doppler generally shows increased flow throughout the epididymis or testicle in acute inflammatory processes. In acute torsion, color Doppler imaging will reveal a relatively isoechoic testis with minimal or no flow to the testicular artery and its branches (Figures 26.2, 26.3, and 26.4). Timely access to these studies as well as availability of experienced personnel to interpret findings may limit their usefulness in the evaluation of the acute scrotum.

EPIDIDYMITIS

Inflammation of the epididymis secondary to bacterial infection is the most common cause of scrotal pain and swelling in the sexually active male, but it has been historically thought to be rare in boys without urologic anomalies. Although epididymitis in boys is still considered a warning of underlying abnormalities, it is a common cause (up to 40 percent) of acute scrotal pain and swelling in boys and adolescent males seen in the emergency room (5).

The pathogenesis of epididymitis in prepubertal males is more complex and is poorly understood when compared to epididymitis in sexually active males. Although typical gram-negative organisms are frequently cultured, a high percentage of nonspecific or idiopathic cases are encountered.

The onset of pain and swelling with epididymitis is classically insidious or gradual in onset. Testicular pain and swelling can be impressive on presentation and cannot be uniformly characterized as less severe than that of testicular torsion.

The epididymis is classically more tender than the testis or scrotal wall. Tenderness usually involves the cord and may extend to the external ring. Commonly the epididymis is not distinct from the testis by palpation. Pain, anxiety, and scrotal wall edema may preclude accurate examination of scrotal contents.

Pyuria is noted in up to 30 percent of patients, but cultures are positive in less than half of these children. Leukocytosis, although common, is not a specific diagnostic sign (5).

Doppler ultrasound and nuclear imaging may aid in the diagnosis by demonstrating increased blood flow to the inflamed epididymis and testis (3,4).

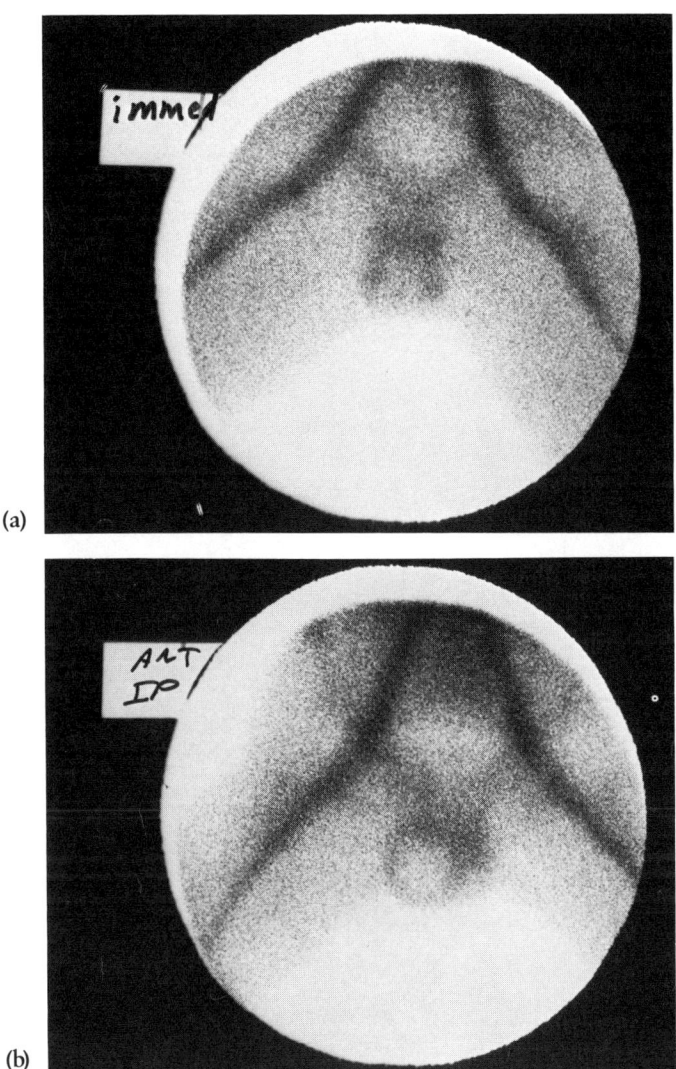

Figure 26.1 Nuclear scrotal scans demonstrating decreased flow ("halo sign") of the right testis in a child with a missed torsion. Scan (b) is normal. (Reprinted courtesy of Dr. Joe Leonard, Oklahoma Childrens' Memorial Hospital.)

Treatment involves scrotal elevation, bed rest, and application of cold compresses as well as antimicrobials and analgesics. Cultures, when they are positive, help direct the choice of antibiotics, but they are commonly not helpful as was mentioned previously. Empiric antibiotic therapy is based on treating epididymitis as a sexually transmitted disease in adolescent patients at risk, or as a gramnegative urinary tract infection in children when sexual activity can be ruled out.

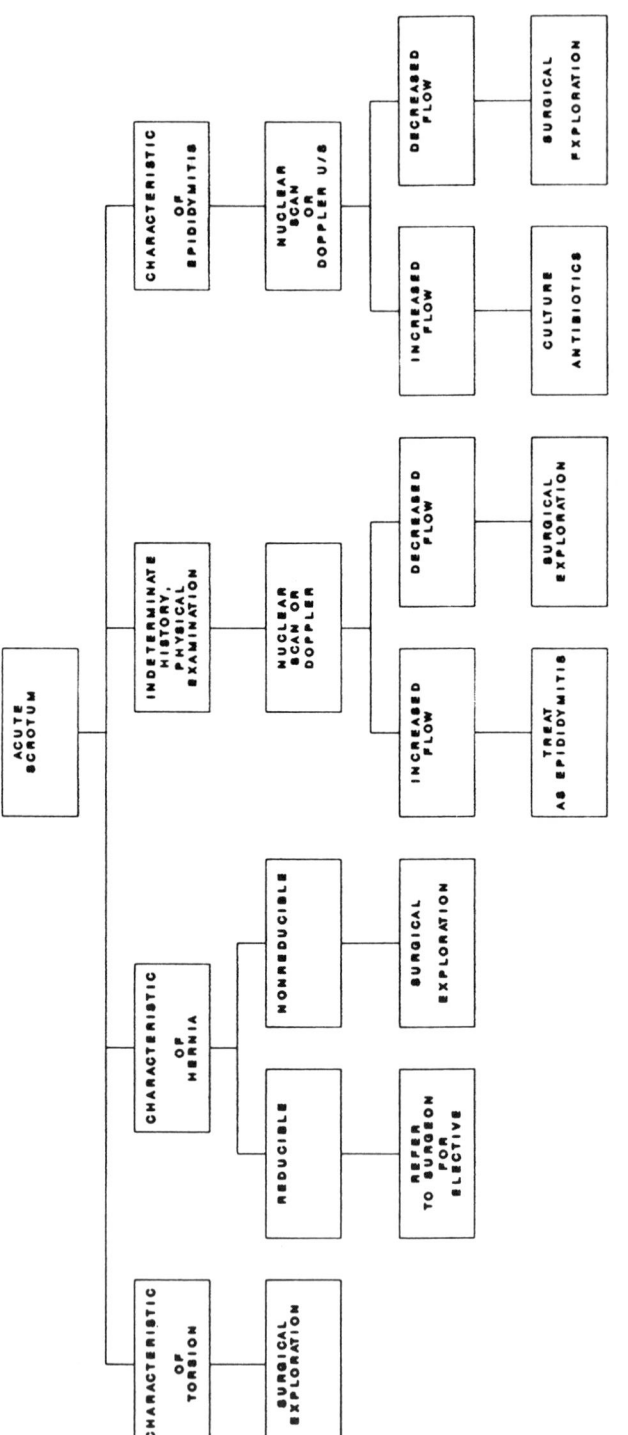

Figure 26.2 Algorithm of the management of the acute scrotum in childen and infants.

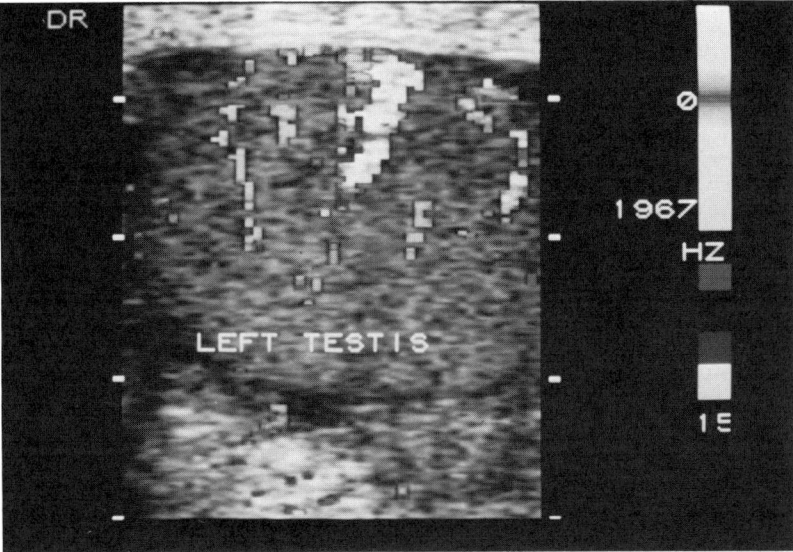

Figure 26.3 Normal left testes indicating good blood flow (Doppler sonography).

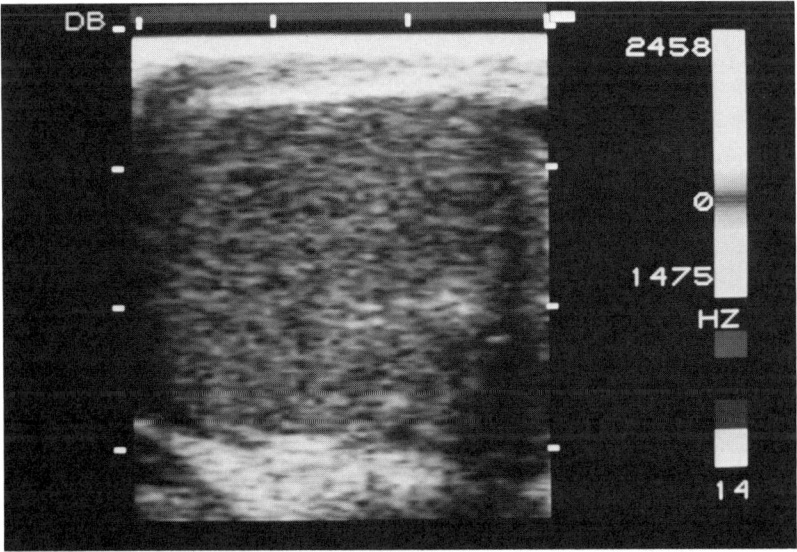

Figure 26.4 Acute testicular Doppler sonography (torsion) showing no blood flow. This was the symptomatic (painful) testes.

TORSION OF THE TESTICULAR APPENDAGES

Torsion of the appendix testis or appendix epididymis may be more common than testicular torsion (6). The presentation of torsion of the testicular appendages is usually less dramatic. Patients typically present with a longer duration of symptoms than those with torsion of the testis, and pain may be somewhat less severe. Ideally the diagnosis is made by identification of a tender nodule at the upper pole of the testis. The "blue dot" sign is the pathognomonic feature of this condition representing the cyanotic torsed appendage seen through the scrotal skin. The diagnosis of torsion of the appendages is difficult, and emergency surgical consultation is advisable. Conservative management (scrotal support, oral analgesics) may be appropriate but only after consultation by an urologist or surgeon. Surgical intervention is not necessarily essential in the management of this disorder. Again it is important to note that, if testicular torsion is not ruled out clinically, scrotal exploration is indicated.

INGUINAL HERNIA

Inguinal hernia is a common condition of infancy and childhood (7). Incarceration or strangulation of inguinal hernias may present as an acutely red, swollen, and painful scrotum and require prompt diagnosis and initiation of treatment. These potentially catastrophic complications of inguinal hernias require immediate surgical attention.

Most infantile hernias occur within the first year of life with the diagnosis usually made in the first month. The overall incidence is reported as from 1.0 to 4.4 percent. Prematurity and low birth weight may raise the incidence to as high as 17 percent. The condition occurs in boys from six to nine times as frequently as it does in girls (7).

Inguinal hernias occur because the processus vaginalis remains open after birth, allowing abdominal contents to traverse the passage. The processus develops as a result of testicular migration from the abdomen to the scrotum. By the seventh month, the testis has usually completed its descent, and the processus or peritoneal investment begins to obliterate. Patency persists in 80 percent to 90 percent of newborns and decreases to 10 percent to 20 percent in the adult. Many of the adults with patent processes are not clinically evident and persist undetected.

Clinical features of an inguinal hernia include a bulge in the groin that increases in size with crying or straining. The diagnosis may be very easy or quite difficult. The bulge may be obvious or hard to reproduce. Stretching an infant with arms and legs extended will usually cause the infant to strain, which may define the defect. Older children can be asked to cough or to blow up a balloon, which may reproduce the bulge. If these maneuvers fail, a second examination may be indicated rather than prompt surgical exploration.

The position of the testicle requires note since up to 6 percent of congenital hernias are associated with incomplete descent. Bowels within hernias may transilluminate and can be confused with hydroceles if they occupy space within the scrotum.

Inguinal hernias will not resolve spontaneously. Repair is indicated to eliminate the risk of incarceration that occurs when the contents of the sac cannot be reduced into the abdominal cavity.

Strangulation occurs when the contents of the sac becomes ischemic or gangrenous. Abdominal pain and vomiting may be present with strangulation. Examination reveals a tense, painful, and potentially discolored bulge in the groin or scrotum. Symptoms intensify as ischemia occurs. Bloody stools or signs of bowel obstruction may be found. Emergent surgical exploration is indicated if nonoperative reduction fails. Sedation and elevation of the lower extremities with manipulation of the bulge may reduce the hernia, allowing elective repair after the edema resolves.

HYDROCELE

Hydroceles occur because abdominal fluid passes through the patent processus into the tunica vaginalis (7). They generally present as painless swellings of the scrotum that surrounds the testis and transilluminate easily. Hydroceles are generally confined to the scrotum, which distinguishes them from hernias. Their size may vary with activity as long as the processus is patent. Closure of the processus usually results in reabsorption of the hydrocele within the first 12 to 18 months of life. Persistence of a hydrocele after 2 years requires surgical repair. Although needle aspiration is used in treatment of adult hydroceles, it has no role in the evaluation or treatment of pediatric scrotal abnormalities.

Scrotal trauma may produce changes consistent with an acute hydrocele or hematocele. Blood within the tunica vaginalis will not transilluminate and requires emergency surgical consultation and repair.

ORCHITIS

Acute bacterial infection involving only the testis is rare as compared to epididimorchitis, which is thought to be a consequence of severe epididymitis. Mumps orchitis is fairly common, effecting 20 to 30 percent of patients with parotitis. Mumps orchitis is usually unilateral and clinically similar to acute infective orchitis except that it usually occurs four to six days after the parotitis. Mumps orchitis is managed with conservative, supportive treatments including scrotal support and oral analgesics.

OTHER CAUSES OF ACUTE SCROTUM

Henoch-Schonlein syndrome is an acute vasculitis characterized by skin rash, joint edema, and involvement of the renal and gastrointestinal (GI) systems. Fifteen to 20 percent of cases involve pain or scrotal swelling. The use of Doppler ultrasound or nuclear imaging may help avoid surgical exploration in these cases.

Acute idiopathic scrotal edema is an unusual condition that may mimic signs of an acute scrotum. Some authors have described it as the causative factor in a significant number of scrotal disorders. The pathogenesis of this process is poorly understood but infectious as well as immunologic theories have been proposed. Age of presentation varies and condition is not limited to the infant or pediatric population. The scrotum may display features typical of acute inflammation. Examination almost always reveals an absence of pain or fever. Palpation reveals a normal testis and epididymis. Lymphadenopathy is not common. Cultures are uniformly negative with laboratory evaluation showing eosinophilia in some cases. Evaluation should include Doppler ultrasound or nuclear imaging to rule out a surgical entity. Treatment recommendations vary, but spontaneous resolution usually occurs within a matter of days.

Tumors of the scrotal contents are rare in infants and children (8). They represent only 2 percent of solid childhood tumors. Seventy-five percent of childhood testicular tumors are germ cell in origin with most being yolk sac carcinomas or teratomas. The nongerminal tumors are generally benign with the exception of rhabdomyosarcoma and comprise the remaining 25 percent of scrotal tumors. Painless unilateral testicular enlargement is the most common presentation of a childhood testicular tumor. The mass is usually firm and nontender and does not transilluminate.

Hernia, hematocele, or infarction from torsion may be difficult to differentiate from tumor. Inguinal exploration with tourniquet compression of the cord prior to testicular delivery into the wound is mandatory if tumor is considered a possibility (8).

CONCLUSION

The acute scrotum in the infant pediatric population requires prompt and accurate diagnosis and treatment. Although a wide variety of conditions can produce the acute scrotum, the inability to distinguish these should lead to surgical exploration. Patients with signs and symptoms that are suspicious for testicular torsion or strangulated inguinal hernia should undergo immediate surgical exploration.

REFERENCES

1. Haynes BE, Bessen HA, Haynes VE. The diagnosis of testicular torsion. JAMA 1983;249(18):2522–2527.
2. O'Brien WM, Lynch JH. The acute scrotum. AFP 1988;37(3):239–247.
3. Eshghi M, Silver L, Smith AD. Technetium 99M scan in acute scrotal lesions. Urology 1987;30(6):588–593.
4. Middleton WD, Siegel BA, Melson GL. Acute scrotal disorders: Prospective comparison of color Doppler US and testicular scintigraphy. Radiology 1990;177(1):177–181.
5. Jayanthi VR, Bennett AH, Cromie WJ. Acute epididymitis in the prepubertal male. Infections in Urology 1991;4:3.
6. Hastie KJ, Charlton CAC. Indications for conservative management of acute scrotal pain in children. Br J Surg 1990;77(3):309–311.
7. Nakayama DK, Rowe MI. Inguinal hernia and the acute scrotum in infants and children. Pediatrics in Review 1989;11:3.
8. Brosman SA. Testicular tumors in prepubertal children. Urology 1979;13(6):581–588.

PART IX

Metabolic/Endocrine

27

Diabetic Ketoacidosis

Pierce R. Blackett
Adolfo D. Garnica
David B. Domek

The changing epidemiology of Type I diabetes appears to indicate an increase in newly diagnosed cases, particularly in Britain where the prevalence appears to be doubling every decade (1). The onset of diabetes is fairly frequent in early childhood with an increasing number of cases presenting with diabetic ketoacidosis (DKA) in late childhood and early adolescence. Hyperglycemia of varying severity precedes the onset of ketoacidosis as indicated by a wide range of glycosylated hemoglobin results at the time of presentation (2).

The treatment of DKA may be associated with serious complications, especially in relation to fluid shifts that cause cerebral edema and potassium deficits that can result in cardiac arrest. Less than 15 percent of patients are comatose at the onset, and this group is particularly at risk for cerebral edema. Although optimal management of these situations has been reviewed extensively, a workable approach to therapy with a strategy should be based on the pathophysiology and severity of initial presentation.

PATHOPHYSIOLOGY

Frequent presentation of new cases during the winter months reflects a weak association with seasonal viruses. The viruses may cause decompensation of normal glucose homeostasis following a long period of autoimmune islet cell damage that is known to cause as much as 90 percent loss of the beta cell mass (2). All too often, the diagnosis is preceded by a two to three week period of polydipsia and progressive dehydration. The progression to life-threatening metabolic imbalance could have been averted by earlier recognition of this problem. Already diagnosed insulin-treated cases may also present with serious DKA, especially during adolescence, particularly cases with labile counterhormonal fluxes. Omission of insulin doses and intercurrent viral illnesses are also frequent precipitating factors.

With relative insulin insufficiency, the passage of glucose into cells is impaired, and the mobilization of free fatty acids from adipose tissue rapidly follows. This process is enhanced by the lipolytic and hyperglycemic actions of stress-induced release of glucagon, norepinephrine, corticosteroids, and growth hormone. Glucagon enhances both ketosis and hepatic glucose production by modulating serum glucose in a state of relative insulin deficiency. All these hormones promote fatty acid mobilization, beta-oxidation in hepatic mitochondria, and the formation of ketone bodies. As a consequence, accumulation of the major ketone bodies, acetoacetic acid and beta-hydroxybutyric acid results in metabolic acidosis. Intracellular potassium exchanges for the hydrogen ions and passes out into the plasma and urine as a ketone salt, resulting in total body potassium depletion without necessarily lowering plasma levels.

Osmotic diuresis results when glucose concentration in the glomerular filtrate exceeds the reabsorptive capacity of the renal tubule. The consequence is a water deficit. The formation of ketone salts results in relatively less urine chloride loss than in nonketotic states, but vomiting may offset this effect and often may be associated with sodium, potassium, and chloride losses. Phosphate reabsorption in the proximal tubule is inhibited by glucose accounting for phosphate losses.

The administration of excessive insulin may cause hypoglycemia followed by rebound hyperglycemia and ketosis (3,4). This effect, known as the *Somogyi phenomenon*, occurs in response to insulin-induced hypoglycemia, which is followed by a counterhormonal response and an enhancement of glycolysis and fatty acid mobilization. This offers an explanation for the susceptibility of poorly controlled subjects. The Somogyi phenomenon is most often observed in noncompliant patients with chronically unstable blood glucose control, for which excessive doses of insulin have been inappropriately prescribed or in younger children with greater sensitivity to insulin in the summer months. Many cases with poor control have labile counterhormones as illustrated by Tamborlane and associates in a group of adolescents studied before and after improved control using continuous subcutaneous insulin infusion (5). Two weeks of improved control with an insulin pump resulted in a significant reduction in the counterhormonal responses to a standardized exercise test.

CLINICAL PRESENTATION

A family history of diabetes or other autoimmune diseases may often be elicited but Type I diabetes does not follow a Mendelian pattern of inheritance. The incidence only ranges from two percent to six percent in first-degree relatives. The child with previously diagnosed diabetes mellitus will frequently be wearing a medical identification necklace or bracelet, indicating the diagnosis. This is important time saving information when parents are not available.

A recognizable sequence of clinical events correlates with underlying physiological processes and precedes the onset of severe acidosis and hyperglycemia (Figure 27.1). Polyuria and polydipsia of a few days or weeks duration results from the glucose-induced osmotic diuresis. An associated weight loss is secondary to dehydration and tissue catabolism. Appetite is increased representing the third component of the classical triad of polyuria, polydipsia, and polyphagia (PPP). The severity of these abnormalities at the time of presentation determine their rate of correction. Accordingly each case requires individual assessment and therapeutic strategy.

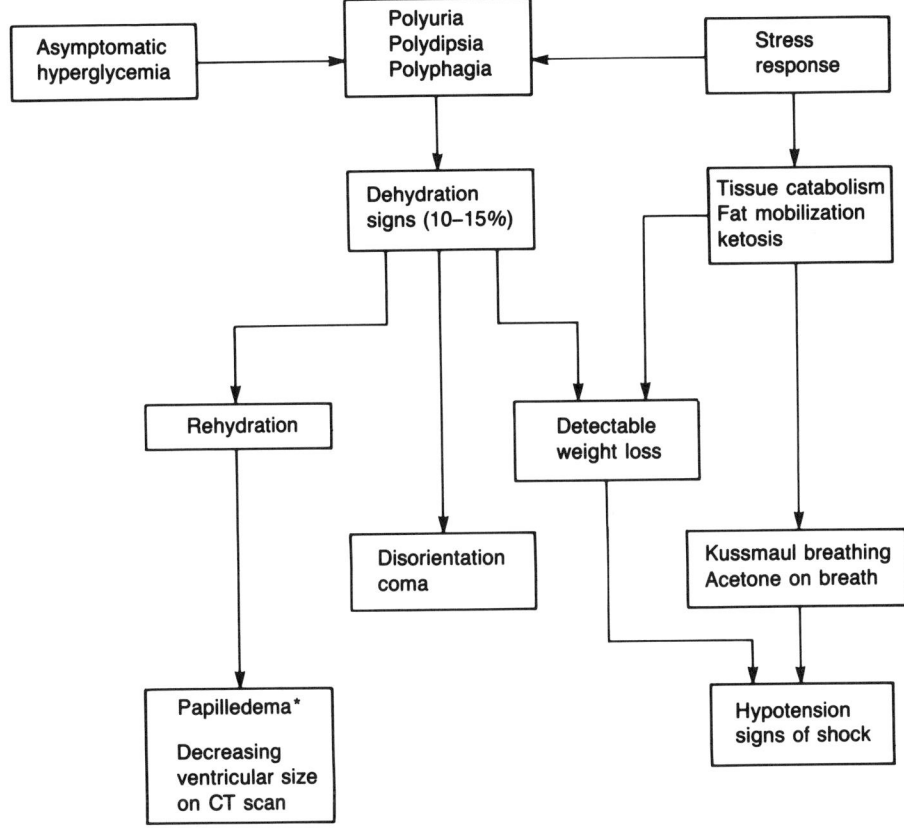

*Occurs during rehydration

Figure 27.1 Clinical presentation.

In severe ketoacidosis, there is always an associated dehydration manifested by sunken eyes, dry mouth, and decreased tissue turgor. Progression to hypotension and shock is imminent. Progression to coma is unpredictable, and there does not appear to be a relationship to the plasma biochemistry. Characteristic rapid, deep breathing (Kussmaul respiration) is a feature of acidosis, and the sweet odor of acetone may frequently be detected on the child's breath. In many cases, abdominal pain, which is attributed to stress-induced gastrointestinal (GI) spasm, occurs and is often associated with vomiting. The pain usually subsides with treatment; tenderness and occasional guarding may be present, however.

An attempt should be made to identify the circumstances primarily responsible for the development of the ketoacidosis. These include: (1) A missed insulin dose, (2) progressive deterioration in control associated with a decline in compliance with the management routine, (3) chronic overinsulinization, (4) psychosocial stress, (5) drugs and alcohol, (6) infections or a secondary illness, and (7) trauma.

Infants and toddlers are prone to present with severe hyperglycemia and relatively little of the ketosis, a condition known as hyperglycemic nonketotic coma (6). The extreme hyperosmolality associated with glucose levels in excess of 1000 mg/dl is very responsive to small doses of insulin and often results in coma due to cerebral fluid shifts. This condition has a higher mortality rate than does DKA, which may relate to the greater predisposition to fluid shifts into the brain. Although it is more frequently seen in the elderly, young children develop this metabolic sequela of insulin deficiency in which relatively normal levels of growth hormone and cortisol may account for normal plasma-free fatty acids and the absence of ketone bodies.

The metabolic derangements of ketoacidosis lead to two significant and potentially fatal complications: cerebral edema caused by fluid shifts into the brain and cardiac arrest caused by potassium deficiency.

Cerebral edema occurs in some apparently predisposed cases during the first 24 hours of therapy and when the patient is improving clinically (7). Factors such as the rate of fall of glucose or the degree of hyponatremia fail to correlate with its development indicating that the gradient for water passage into the brain appears to be predetermined. Intracerebral osmole formation may result from disruption of intracerebral metabolism. The formation of osmoles is thought to be derived from protein breakdown products, released anions, and possibly sorbitol formation. Harris and associates have identified risk factors that predispose children to cerebral edema. These include an extended history of poor metabolic control, acidosis with a pH less than 7.2, an initial corrected sodium value in the hypernatremic range, a decrease in serum sodium during treatment, and the development of early symptoms of increased intracranial pressure during therapy. The corrected sodium can be calculated by adding the measured serum sodium (2.75 mEq/l) for each 100 mg/dl of plasma glucose over 100 mg/dl (8).

Cardiac arrest, on the other hand, is related to the intracellular potassium status. A total body depletion of potassium occurs during prolonged acidosis, and at the time of presentation in DKA, cardiac stores of potassium are dangerously low. Correction of the acidosis results in restoration of the intracellular deficit and rapid depletion of plasma potassium, which requires replacement to offset arrythmias and the danger of cardiac arrest.

DIFFERENTIAL DIAGNOSIS

The unconscious, insulin-treated child may have hypoglycemia, which is rapidly diagnosed using a glucose meter. The clinical history is of shorter duration than it is in diabetic ketoacidosis, and there is no dehydration or Kussmaul breathing. Hypothermia may be striking, and seizures are likely to occur. Dextrose, 1 ml/kg of a 50 percent solution or 2 ml/kg of a 25 percent solution, may be given intravenously for acute hypoglycemia. Alternatively, glucagon 1 mg intramuscular (IM) may be given in an emergency situation and is preferable to an intravenous (IV) dextrose infusion. If the index of suspicion for hypoglycemia is high, dextrose or glucagon may be given after a blood sample for glucose has been obtained.

Other causes of coma must be considered, bearing in mind that the diabetic may also be more likely to have accidents. Head injuries may be excluded by careful examination and possibly by investigation with a computerized tomography (CT) scan of the head. Alcohol is known to block gluconeogenesis and glycogenolysis resulting in a predisposition to hypoglycemia, especially if caloric intake has been insufficient. Excessive alcohol may accentuate dehydration, precipitate ketosis, and contribute to a comatose state, however. Drug addiction is not an improbable association in the adolescent diabetic, and recent drug overdosing may also be responsible for neurological impairment.

Metabolic acidosis secondary to inherited enzyme deficiencies are more likely to present with seizures and vomiting in infancy in contrast to diabetes, which seldom presents before one year of age. Salicylate toxicity, however, can mimic ketoacidosis even though it results in a lactic acidosis associated with hypoglycemia due to metabolic blocks in gluconeogenesis and glycogenolysis; occasionally stress-induced hyperglycemia accompanies the acidosis. Profound acidosis can be a consequence of diarrheal dehydration, and low pHs can be associated with Kussmaul breathing. Acute illness or trauma in childhood can result in a significant stress response characterized by hyperglycemia and minimal ketosis, which is rapidly correctable during rehydration alone without the need for insulin. Extensive burns, hypothermia, heat stroke, febrile illnesses, corticosteroid therapy, hemodialysis, IV hyperalimentation, and cancer chemotherapy may all be predisposing.

Occasionally such children may present with early manifestations of diabetes. The additional information such as family history or the presence of islet cell antibodies will predict Type I diabetes and serve to prevent presentation in ketoacidosis by heeding the early warning signs.

LABORATORY EVALUATION

A recent weight, if taken under conditions of good control, will aid in estimating the percentage dehydration, which is at least 10 percent, bearing in mind that tissue catabolism contributes to the weight loss.

Laboratory results should be charted on a flow sheet to aid rapid assessment of progress. A blood sample is taken for glucose, electrolytes, phosphate, ionized calcium, venous pH, bicarbonate, serum acetone, and a complete blood count (CBC). A drop of the venous blood sample is placed on a reagent strip for an immediate reading with a glucose meter to provide early information. The glucose concentration does not correlate with the severity of the acidosis (9) and may range from over 1000 mg/dl to under 300 mg/dl, reflecting the contribution of hepatic glucose production and the independence of two metabolic processes: glucose production and ketone formation. A glycosylated hemoglobin result at the outset provides information about preceding glucose concentrations. Transient, stress-induced hyperglycemia is associated with a normal glycosylated hemoglobin, whereas diabetic patients have higher results indicative of chronic hyperglycemia.

Hyponatremia is common, often due to dilution of the intravascular space with body water drawn from the interstitial and cellular spaces by osmotic attraction. Urine sodium loss as ketoacid salts contributes to hyponatremia. In a few cases, bicarbonate loss leads to hyperchloremia, which requires correction (10).

A factitious lowering of all the serum values, including sodium, occurs in patients with hypertriglyceridemia as a consequence of the displacement of the aqueous phase with plasma lipids. In this situation, the aqueous infranate should be measured after ultracentrifugation (11), which can be conveniently done using a tabletop ultracentrifuge (Airfuge, Beckman Co.). An alternative method is to extract the lipid with a solvent prior to serum analysis.

When the osmotic diuresis continues until water losses are maximal, the serum sodium increases in association with hemoconcentration. When this occurs, reserves of body water from the interstitial and intracellular spaces ("third space") have become depleted to the point that further passage of water into the intravascular space is markedly reduced. This situation is usually associated with severe acidosis and impending shock.

Potassium concentrations may be increased, normal, or, rarely, decreased at the onset of ketoacidosis, depending on factors such as tissue catabolism, acidosis, tissue uptake, and renal excretion. Increased aldosterone secretion in response to hypovolemia may contribute to lowering the serum potassium concentration.

Low arterial or venous pH and decreased plasma bicarbonate are typical findings in ketoacidosis and reflect a metabolic acidosis with an increased anion gap due to increased endogenous acid production, primarily in the form of ketones.

Severe and prolonged ketosis predisposes to infection because of disturbed polymorphonuclear phagocytosis, thus a blood culture, a urine culture and a chest X-ray should be considered, particularly in new cases. Other laboratory findings include a characteristic leukocytosis due to stress and splenic contraction; hemoconcentration with an increased blood urea nitrogen (BUN) occurs secondary to the osmotic diuresis.

MANAGEMENT

Figure 27.2 outlines the management sequence.

Airway, Breathing, Circulation (ABCs)

Initially, establishing a good airway and stabilizing the hemodynamics are priorities. Vomiting and aspiration may be avoided by inserting a nasogastric tube.

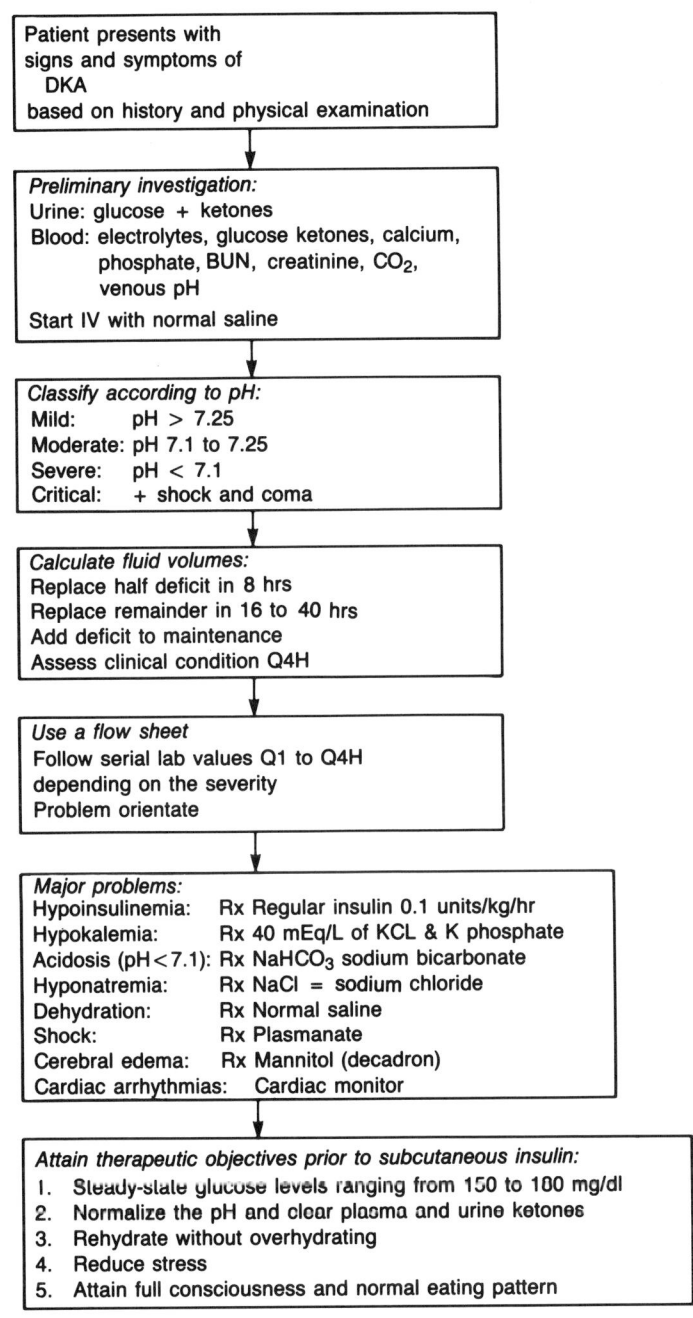

Figure 27.2 Management sequence.

Fluids and Electrolytes

Immediate treatment of dehydration usually consists of IV infusion with normal saline to expand the intravascular volume and to increase peripheral flow while replacing sodium lost during the osmotic diuresis. The infusion rate should be 10 ml/kg or more for the first hour. Half the estimated initial deficit, in addition to maintenance requirements, should be given during the first 8 to 12 hours. The remaining deficit, plus maintenance requirements, are given in the subsequent 24 hours or over a longer period of up to 48 hours if necessary, depending on the clinical state of hydration. Conventional calculation of the maintenance fluids will suffice provided the blood glucose is not in excess of the renal threshold for longer than 3 hours. If prolonged hyperglycemia occurs, maintenance fluid requirements may be calculated as the sum of the ongoing losses in the urine and the insensible water loss. Fluid balance, as indicated by the difference between fluid intake and output, should be retrospectively assessed at least every 4 hours and corresponding adjustments should be made in the infusion rate. The 24-hour fluid total should never exceed 3 $l/m^2/day$ since volume loading with large amounts of crystalloid solution results in a hyperoncotic load that may contribute to the development of subclinical or overt cerebral edema (12,13,14). Rapid glucose lowering (>90 mg/dl/hr), with associated loss of osmoles from the vascular space or infusion of hypotonic solutions, may also increase the risk of cerebral edema. An etiologic role for the rate of blood glucose lowering or fluid infusion rate, however, is controversial (15,16).

Insulin

In order to reduce hyperglycemia and to reestablish the antilipolytic and antiketogenic effect of insulin, it is necessary to maintain consistent insulinization. To achieve this goal, the most effective regimen has been found to be continuous IV infusion of low-dose regular human insulin (17). This route is preferable because complete absorption of subcutaneous insulin may not occur until rehydration is underway. The dose administered should achieve serum insulin levels within a therapeutic range (20 to 200 microunits/ml) so that there will be sufficient circulating insulin to saturate cellular receptor sites and achieve the necessary metabolic effects.

Efficacy and convenience support the use of a low-dose insulin infusion if biochemical criteria of sufficient severity, such as a blood glucose greater than 300 mg/dl or venous pH less than 7.25 with a bicarbonate less than 15 mEq/l are met. Under these conditions, the serum acetone is usually positive in a 1:2 dilution or greater. Usually an initial dose of 0.1 units of insulin/kg is given as an IV bolus followed by an infusion dose of 0.1 kg/hr. The latter is administered by diluting the insulin with normal saline to a concentration of 0.1 unit of regular insulin/ml. The insulin is conveniently mixed in a 250 ml bag of normal saline by adding 25 units of regular human insulin. This should be checked by a colleague or team member. The insulin should be remixed every 12 hours. The insulin should then be infused via a Y connection, the other arm of the Y being connected to the replacement fluids. The drip rates of the infusions should be monitored mechanically. Before running the insulin infusion, about the first 20 ml is discarded, allowing the insulin to saturate the plastic tubing and avoid an initial insulin deficit due to its binding to the plastic.

In exceptional patients with extreme salt and water depletion associated with hypovolemia, the intravascular volume is partially maintained by a high blood glucose concentration, which osmotically draws fluid from intracellular and interstitial spaces. A decrease in blood glucose under these circumstances might precipitate severe shock. It is advisable, therefore to withold the insulin for 15 to 30 minutes or to administer a sufficiently low dose to inhibit ketogenesis without significantly decreasing the blood glucose. Cases presenting initially with hypotension should be treated with colloid infusion in the form of plasmanate or human albumin infusion (20 ml/kg) over 20 minutes. Central venous pressure monitoring is indicated to ensure that the pressure is increased above 5 mm Hg by the colloid infusion.

In the usual case, the decrease in blood sugar over the first few hours is predictable and should occur at a rate of 60 to 90 mg/dl/hr. The infusion rate of insulin may be increased or decreased according to the rate of glucose decline. Usually infants and children below age five years are very sensitive to insulin and require a half to quarter of the usual 0.1 unit/kg/hr infusion dose. To prevent an excessive decrease in blood glucose, 5 percent dextrose is added to the infusion solution when the blood glucose decreases to below 250 mg/dl.

Circulating insulin levels are maintained by continuing the insulin infusion until the pH is above 7.3. The continuation of the insulin infusion will facilitate the correction of the acidosis that often lags behind changes in blood glucose. A subcutaneous injection of regular- or intermediate-acting insulin should be given at least an hour before discontinuing the insulin infusion. This avoids a potential gap in insulin supply and prevents counterhormone induced lipolysis and ketosis.

Potassium

In the insulin-deficient state, progressive intracellular depletion of potassium is associated with a period of protein, glycogen, and fat catabolism during the days or weeks prior to the onset of ketoacidosis. A total body potassium deficit exists even though normal or high serum concentrations are recorded. After insulin treatment, a fall in the serum level is inevitable, concurrent with the intracellular diffusion of glucose and the correction of the acidosis. Potassium should be infused shortly after the IV insulin infusion is started because of the immediate action of insulin and/or bicarbonate therapy on the intracellular passage of potassium. If potassium is not replaced early, cardiac function will be endangered. Good peripheral perfusion is essential prior to the infusion of potassium because the administration of potassium to a shocked and dehydrated patient with low urine output could induce dangerous hyperkalemia.

A dose of 30 to 40 mEq of potassium is added to each liter of the IV solution. Larger doses may be necessary in the treatment of severely acidotic potassium-depleted patients. It is recommended that the potassium should be given as a mixture of buffered potassium phosphate and potassium chloride. The potassium deficit is calculated as 5 mEq/kg and the phosphate deficit as 3 mEq/kg. Replacement of the phosphate deficit improves oxygen delivery to tissues by repleting red blood cell 2,3-diphosphoglycerate so that impaired brain and myocardial oxygenation is avoided (18). Determination of an initial ionized calcium is also advisable since excessive phosphate may precipitate with calcium and decrease the serum calcium level.

When in doubt about serum potassium, immediate information may be obtained from an electrocardiogram (EKG). If hypokalemia is present, prolongation of the QT interval with wide, low amplitude T waves will be seen.

Bicarbonate

A major concern is whether to treat the acidosis with bicarbonate. It has been observed that the administration of bicarbonate to patients with severe ketoacidosis does not affect recovery, and the consensus is to use bicarbonate sparingly because of possible unfavorable effects when it is used in excess. The theory, based on limited experimental evidence (19), is that bicarbonate is converted to carbon dioxide that crosses the blood-brain barrier and causes intracerebral acidosis. This would be undesirable if the level of consciousness is already impaired. The advantages of bicarbonate use must be weighed against possible disadvantages such as promotion of intracerebral acidosis resulting in a shift of the oxygen dissociation curve to the left and decreased oxygen delivery to tissues. Correction of acidosis also results in accelerated potassium entry into the intracellular space. It is known that depressive effects of acidosis on the respiratory minute volume and myocardial contractility occur below a blood pH of 7.1 (20). Thus when the pH is less than 7.1 or when the bicarbonate is below 10 mEq/l, the administration of bicarbonate is recommended to preserve optimal cardiac function. The bicarbonate dose is calculated to attain partial correction to an actual concentration of 15 mEq/l:

$$\text{Correction dose (mEq)} = \text{body weight (kg)} \times 0.6 \times 15\text{-measured bicarbonate (mEq)}.$$

Alternatively, a dose calculated as 2 mEq/kg is a conservative estimate. The bicarbonate should not be given as a bolus that represents a significantly high osmotic load, and the concentration should not exceed 80 mEq/l. Half the calculated amount given by slow IV infusion over 30 minutes and the remainder given over four to six hours is appropriate. When the pH exceeds 7.25, additional bicarbonate is no longer necessary.

Conversion of ketoacids to bicarbonate, a process enhanced by insulin administration, contributes to the correction and further supports the argument for calculating only partial correction of the bicarbonate deficit. Some allowance should be made, however, for patients with hyperchloremic acidosis who tend to recover more slowly although they have less of an anion gap (10). It should be remembered that testing for ketones with nitroprusside reagents (strips or tablets) may be misleading because most of the ketones will initially be in the form of beta-hydroxybutyric acid, which does not react with nitroprusside, whereas acetoacetic acid will. During effective therapy, beta-hydroxybutyric acid is converted to acetoacetic acid. Thus the ketones may appear to increase during the recovery period when they are tested with these reagents although the level of beta-hydroxybutyric acid decreases substantially.

Recovery

There should be no ingestion of food or fluids during severe acidosis to prevent aspiration of gastric contents in the event of vomiting. Appetite usually returns when the acidosis is corrected, and a normal diet can be introduced gradually. When the electrolytes are normal and when the serum pH is above 7.3, it is safe to allow the child a liquid diet with the provision that large volumes of hypotonic fluid, which could precipitate cerebral edema, are avoided. Careful recording of fluid intake and output should continue until complete correction is attained, which is usually within a 48-hour period.

It is necessary to begin with a dose of subcutaneous insulin the morning following initial IV correction or at another convenient starting point. Estimation of the dose is a question of judgment based on the response to insulin observed during correction, previous insulin dosages in diagnosed cases, and age. Infants and young children are insulin-sensitive and may require no more than 0.25 units/kg/day given as a single daily dose of intermediate-acting insulin. Older children and adolescents require a total dose of 0.5 to 1.5 units/kg/day given as combined doses of intermediate- and short-acting insulins before breakfast and supper. About a third of the total dose is generally given in the evening due to lower requirements for the night hours and increased sensitivity to insulin.

During the ensuing months, the newly diagnosed case may transiently require less insulin after which a decline in endogenous insulin reserves leads to increased dose requirements. Somatic growth, increases in counterhormonal responses, and stresses of adolescence may contribute to an increased insulin demand. Excessive insulin may lead to repeated hypoglycemia associated with corresponding counterhormonal responses, leading to repeated fluctuations in blood glucose and a predisposition to ketoacidosis.

In order to determine an approximate dose requirement, most children will need a short period of in-hospital adjustment during which blood sugars are monitored under conditions that simulate the home environment with respect to diet and activity. The initial period after diagnosis is an important phase of therapy that involves education and encouragement of both parents and child. At this time factors such as age, level of education, maturity, and acceptance of diabetes should be taken into consideration.

Successful prevention of DKA and long-term complications depend on good communication with a health care team consisting of a physician, a diabetes nurse educator, and a dietitian with additional availability of social workers and psychologists. Following discharge, good telephone contact should be insured so that decisions on dose, diet, and activity changes can be discussed between clinic visits. If possible, other members of the family should be progressively involved in the education process so that a strong support system is developed between the patient and the family with sufficient confidence to manage the diabetes during future years.

REFERENCES

1. Stewart-Brown S, Haslum M, Butler N. Evidence for increasing prevalence of diabetes mellitus in childhood. Br Med J 1983;286:1855.
2. Blackett PR, Lera T Jr., Garnica A, et al. Diabetic ketoacidosis at Children's Hospital of Oklahoma: A review on presentation and management. J Oklahoma State Med Assoc 1990;83:594.
3. Bolli G, Gottesman I, Campbell P, et al. Glucose counterregulation and waning of insulin in the Somogyi phenomenon (posthypoglycemic hyperglycemia). N Engl J Med 1984;311:1214.
4. Somogyi M. Exacerbation of diabetes by excess insulin action. Am J Med 1959;26:169.
5. Tamborlane WV, Sherwin RS, Koivisto V, et al. Normalization of the growth hormone and catecholamine response to exercise in juvenile-onset diabetic subjects treated with a portable insulin infusion pump. Diabetes 1979;28:785.
6. Yamashiro Y, Yamamoto T, Mayama H. Nonketotic hyperosmolar coma in two diabetic children. Acta Paediatr Scand 1981;70:337.
7. Rosenbloom AL, Riley WJ, Weber FT. Cerebral edema complicating diabetic ketoacidosis in childhood. J Pediatr 1980;96:357.
8. Harris GD, Fiordalisi I, Finberg L. Safe management of diabetic ketoacidemia. J Pediatr 1988;113:65.
9. Brandt KR, Miles JM. Relationship between severity of hyperglycemia and metabolic acidosis in diabetic ketoacidosis. Mayo Clin Proc 1988;63:1071.
10. Adrogue HJ, Wilson H, Boyd AE, et al. Plasma acid-base patterns in diabetic ketoacidosis. N Engl J Med 1982;307:1603.
11. Blackett PR, Holcombe JH, Alaupovic P, et al. Case report: Plasma lipids and apolipoproteins in a 13-year-old boy with diabetic ketoacidosis and extreme hyperlipidemia. Am J Med Sci 1986;291:342.
12. Fein IA, Rackow EC, Sprung CL, et al. Relation of colloid osmotic pressure to arterial hypoxemia and cerebral edema during crystalloid volume loading of patients with diabetic ketoacidosis. Ann Intern Med 1982;96:570.
13. Krane EJ, Rockoff MA, Wallman JK, et al. Subclinical brain swelling in children during treatment of diabetic ketoacidosis. N Engl J Med 1985;312:1147.
14. Duck SC, Weldon VV, Pagliara AS, et al. Cerebral edema complicating therapy for diabetic ketoacidosis. Diabetes 1976;25:111.
15. Duck SC, Wyatt DR. Factors associated with brain herniation in the treatment of diabetic ketoacidosis. J Pediatr 1988;113:10.
16. Rosenbloom AL, Riley WJ, Weber FT, et al. Cerebral edema complicating diabetic ketoacidosis in childhood. J Pediatr 1980;96:357.
17. Martin MM, Martin ALA. Continuous low-dose infusion of insulin in the treatment of diabetic ketoacidosis in children. J Pediatr 1976;89:560.
18. Ditzel J. Importance of plasma inorganic phosphate on tissue oxygenation during recovery from diabetic ketoacidosis. Horm Metab Res 1973;5:471.
19. Posner J, Plum F. Spinal fluid pH and neurological symptoms in systemic acidosis. N Engl J Med 1967;277:605.
20. Opie LH. Cardiac metabolism: The effect of some physiologic, pharmacologic, and pathologic influences. Am Heart J 1965;69:401.

28

Acute Adrenal Insufficiency/Crisis

Adolfo D. Garnica
Pierce R. Blackett

Although adrenal crisis occurs infrequently since effective antimicrobial therapy and public health measures have significantly reduced the prevalence of tuberculosis, it remains a serious, potentially fatal, medical emergency. Most often the adrenal crisis presents as circulatory collapse associated with electrolyte imbalance and hypoglycemia. Early recognition and treatment is essential to reduce morbidity and the risk of death. The clinical manifestations are best understood and recognized in the context of the normal production, regulation, secretion, and biological function of the adrenocortical hormones.

PATHOPHYSIOLOGY

The adrenocortical hormones are steroids synthesized and released by the zonae fasciculata and reticularis of the adrenal cortex (1,2,3,4). The three groups of biologically active adrenocorticoids include the glucocorticoids, the mineralocorticoids, and the adrenal sex hormones. The major glucocorticoid is cortisol; cortisone, a metabolite of cortisol, and corticosterone, a precursor of the mineralocorticoids, possess relatively less biological activity.

The hypothalamic-pituitary-adrenal axis constitutes a regulatory system (1,2,3). The pituitary controls adrenal steroidogenesis through the secretion of adrenocorticotropin (ACTH), which stimulates corticosteroid synthesis by increasing the conversion of cholesterol to pregnenolone, which is the major substrate for the steroidogenic pathways. The release of ACTH from the pituitary, its diurnal variation, and its increase during stress are mediated by the central nervous system (CNS) through the pulsatile secretion of hypothalamic corticotropin-releasing hormone (CRH) in response to variation in the plasma concentration of unbound cortisol (1,2,3,4,5). Decreasing concentrations of circulating cortisol result in increased secretion of ACTH and a corresponding increase in cortisol level; conversely, high cortisol concentrations directly inhibit the release of ACTH.

The biological activity of the glucocorticoids primarily affects the metabolism of glucose and protein (1,2,3). Their effects in the liver are anabolic, facilitating protein synthesis while increasing glucose production and glycogen storage. In peripheral tissues other than the nervous system, glucocorticoid effects are catabolic, reducing glucose uptake and use, decreasing amino acid incorporation, and increasing the enzymatic degradation of proteins. The resulting liberation of amino acids promotes hepatic gluconeogenesis and, together with reduced glucose use, raises the blood glucose concentration.

The mineralocorticoids are produced in the zona glomerulosa (1,2,3). The principal mineralocorticoid is aldosterone; its precursors are desoxycorticosterone, corticosterone, and 18-hydroxycorticosterone. Aldosterone acts primarily in the kidneys, increasing sodium reabsorption and potassium excretion in the ascending limb of the loop of Henle and the distal convoluted tubule.

Destruction of the adrenal cortex, regardless of etiology, results in primary adrenocortical insufficiency. The adrenal cortex normally responds to stress with a marked increase in cortisol secretion (1,2,3,5); in patients with adrenal insufficiency, the stress response does not occur. The clinical manifestations are a consequence of cortisol deficiency with or without aldosterone deficiency.

CLINICAL MANIFESTATIONS

The clinical symptoms and signs of adrenal insufficiency usually do not become apparent until more than 90 percent of the cortex has been destroyed (6,7). Primary dysfunction of the adrenal cortex is the most common cause of adrenocortical insufficiency; secondary insufficiency resulting from decreased ACTH secretion occurs less frequently.

The onset of symptoms may be gradual or sudden. An acute presentation with classical adrenal crisis may be seen in association with conditions like adrenal hemorrhage or congenital adrenal aplasia (2,3,6,7). An apparent acute presentation may, however, also represent the final decompensation following a gradual deterioration in function the subtle, early signs of which were not recognized (6,7,8,9).

The age of onset and clinical manifestations are determined by the etiology of the dysfunction (2,3,7). In infants, the presentation is difficult to differentiate from that of overwhelming sepsis, intracranial hemorrhage, or severe pneumonia. Symptoms and signs of salt loss beginning shortly after birth are the most prominent manifestations in primary adrenal aplasia or congenital adrenal hyperplasia. Other clinical features include poor feeding; occasional vomiting; poor weight gain or weight loss; intermittent fever; dehydration associated with hyponatremia, hyperkalemia, and acidosis; and hypoglycemia. Particularly in neonates with primary adrenal aplasia, circulatory collapse may occur terminally. Congenital adrenal hyperplasia must be suspected in any newborn with ambiguous genitalia.

The clinical onset of acute adrenocortical insufficiency in older children is usually gradual, and the absence of specific clinical manifestations may delay diagnosis. The presenting manifestations are predominantly gastrointestinal: anorexia, abdominal pain, intractable vomiting, and diarrhea followed by dehydration and hypotension (2,3,7,13). Less frequently headaches, psychological disturbances, or convulsions may be the first symptoms. A failure to recognize, accurately diagnose, and appropriately treat may result in adrenal crisis and signs of imminent cardiovascular collapse (12). The features include the sudden development of cyanosis and cool skin, weak and rapid pulse, decreased blood pressure, and rapid and labored respirations. Without immediate, appropriate therapy, there is significant risk of sudden death.

Symptoms of acute adrenal insufficiency, beginning under conditions of medical or traumatic stress, may be the first indication of previously undiagnosed chronic adrenocortical insufficiency (9,10,11,12). Acute decompensation is more easily identified when the suggestive pattern of nonspecific, early clinical features is recognized, especially in the presence of hyperpigmentation (2,3,7,12,13). A typical early complaint in patients with chronic insufficiency is a sense of weakness with undue fatigue, although this symptom is difficult to elicit in young children. Approximately 90 percent of patients complain of anorexia with mild nausea; abdominal pain may mimic an acute abdomen. Otherwise the most common early symptoms include lassitude, weight loss, general wasting, irritability, periods of depression, and hypotension. All patients complain of increased sensitivity to the taste of salt, sucrose, and other substances; approximately 15 percent relate a history of craving salty foods. Virtually all patients demonstrate cutaneous hyperpigmentation and hypotension.

Cutaneous hyperpigmentation is a common finding under conditions where prolonged cortisol deficiency results in compensatory ACTH hypersecretion, and it should always raise the possibility of chronic adrenocortical insufficiency. Hyperpigmentation may begin so subtly that it is mistaken for suntan: darkening of the palmar creases is specific; pigmentation is usually exaggerated over areas exposed to trauma or pressure such as knuckles, knees, and intertriginous folds; and the axillae, perineum, nipples, and mucous membranes hyperpigmented. The pigment may deposit as small, circumscribed, dark, freckle-like macules or as longitudinal streaks in the nails.

Hypotension may at first be only orthostatic, but in more advanced cases, the blood pressure may be low even when the child is recumbent (2,3,7). Hypoglycemia occurs in about half the patients. Central nervous dysfunction, reflected in uniformly abnormal electroencephalogram (EEG), is present in nearly all patients; chronic hyperkalemia may rarely produce a neuromyopathy.

DIFFERENTIAL DIAGNOSIS

Acute adrenocortical insufficiency is most often precipitated by an identifiable stress although it may occur spontaneously (8). The diagnosis is not difficult in a child with documented chronic adrenal insufficiency who presents with characteristic clinical features after being exposed to obvious stress (6,9). In most cases, however, there is no history of chronic adrenal insufficiency or only a history of nonspecific symptoms.

Congenital adrenal hyperplasia (CAH) refers to histologic alterations in adrenocortical tissue that occur as a consequence of chronically elevated circulating ACTH levels (2,3). CAH comprises a group of inborn errors of adrenocortical hormone biosynthesis resulting from specific deficiencies in the activity of one of the enzymes involved in cortisol synthesis; a reduction in cortisol production leads to a corresponding increase in ACTH secretion. Each enzyme deficiency produces specific, recognizable alterations in concentrations of serum adrenal steroid hormones and their precursors. The particular hormone imbalances in each case may cause abnormalities in fetal genital development, along with characteristic metabolic and chemical disturbances.

CAH most commonly presents with a salt-wasting syndrome during the newborn period (2,3). All infants with lipoid adrenal hyperplasia (20,22-desmolase deficiency), most infants with 3-β-hydroxysteroid dehydrogenase deficiency, and approximately half of those with 21-hydroxylase deficiency present with symptoms of salt loss during the newborn period. The 21-hydroxylase block in cortisol synthesis causes channeling of precursor steroids into androgenic pathways, resulting in hyperandrogenic effects in both sexes that is expressed as pseudohermaphroditism in females. The 3-β-hydroxysteroid dehydrogenase deficiency may be associated with virilization in females and pseudohermaphroditism in males, In 20,22-desmolase deficiencies, defective synthesis of adrenal androgen precursors causes pseudohermaphroditism in males.

Acute Adrenal Crisis of Infection

Acute adrenal insufficiency accompanying overwhelming infection has been well documented (14). The dominant features include fever, rash, and meningitis. Overwhelming meningococcemia, cutaneous purpura, and bilateral adrenal hemorrhage progress rapidly to shock, coma, and death (14,15). Approximately 50 percent of patients develop petechiae or purpura, usually on the chest, upper arms, and axillae; a petechial rash extends rapidly and coalesces, forming large ecchymoses; a maculopapular rash may also be present even in the absence of petechiae. In the fulminant form, meningitis may be absent, but signs of cardiovascular collapse and septic shock may progress rapidly and lead to death within a few hours. Children with overwhelming septicemia and bilateral adrenal hemorrhage are incapable of normal stress cortisol release; circulatory collapse has been attributed to impaired adrenocortical function, but the serum cortisol is appropriately elevated in many patients (14). Although the syndrome has been associated most commonly with overwhelming meningococcemia, similar crises have been observed less frequently with overwhelming pneumococcal, streptococcal, and diphtheritic infections.

Adrenal hemorrhage presents with acute shock as a consequence of blood loss and adrenal insufficiency (15,16). During infancy, this disorder occurs most commonly in large newborn males after traumatic delivery, and it is usually associated with a palpable flank mass. Adrenal hemorrhage in the newborn may also be associated with hypoxia, hemorrhagic disease, infection, and shock. Chemical evidence of adrenal insufficiency may be attributed to intercurrent illness. In older children, signs of bilateral adrenal hemorrhage are nonspecific: chest, back, flank, and abdominal pain associated with fever are common; hypotension may be a preterminal event. Children with unilateral hemorrhage do not demonstrate signs of acute adrenal insufficiency but may show signs of hypovolemia secondary to blood loss. Adrenal hemorrhage is associated with microscopic hematuria and normal excretion of contrast on intravenous (IV) urography. In infants, it is to be differentiated from renal vein thrombosis, which shows gross hematuria and no excretion of contrast on the involved side. Early diagnosis of bilateral adrenal hemorrhage requires prompt identification of patients at risk and recognition of the manifestations of acute adrenal insufficiency. Once the diagnosis is suspected, emergency corticosteroid replacement can be instituted while the anatomical diagnosis is confirmed by computed tomography (CT) of the adrenals (17). Adrenal hemorrhage may initially be asymptomatic, and it may be recognized only later by the incidental finding of calcification. Rarely gradual deterioration in function following adrenal hemorrhage may evolve into adrenocortical insufficiency which presents later in infancy or childhood.

Idiopathic Autoimmune Adrenalitis

Destructive processes involving the adrenal glands are the most common cause of chronic adrenal insufficiency in older children. Formerly tuberculosis was the most common etiology agent, but now it accounts for less than 20 percent of cases (2,3,7). Currently the major cause of insidious chronic adrenocortical insufficiency is primary autoimmune adrenalitis, or idiopathic atrophy, which apparently represents the end result of a destructive autoimmune process. The majority of affected individuals have antibodies against adrenal tissue (9,10,11). A number of conditions believed to be of autoimmune origin show a high association with idiopathic adrenal insufficiency (2,3,7,18).

Secondary adrenocortical insufficiency results from pituitary ACTH deficiency. Conditions that compromise hypothalamic or pituitary integrity and, as a consequence, impair pituitary ACTH secretion include pituitary or parasellar tumors, hypothalamic tumors, inflammatory or infiltrative processes, infarction, hemorrhage, or head trauma (6,19,20). Approximately 50 percent of patients with secondary insufficiency are capable of maintaining normal basal cortisol secretion but are not able to sustain a normal response during stress. Hypoglycemia may occur but salt-losing is uncommon, presumably because of residual ability of the adrenal to secrete aldosterone. Patients with adrenocortical insufficiency as a consequence of ACTH deficiency or panhypopituitarism do not develop cutaneous hyperpigmentation.

The most common cause of secondary adrenocortical insufficiency is chronic suppression of the hypothalamic-pituitary-adrenal axis by exogenous glucocorticoids (21,22). Clinically apparent adrenal insufficiency develops either when maintenance corticosteroids are not increased during times of stress or when chronically administered steroids are withdrawn too rapidly. Children who have received chronic glucocorticoid therapy may have prolonged suppression of the hypothalamic pituitary-adrenal axis and recovery may require as long as 12 to 16 months following withdrawal of treatment (23). In patients with inadequately treated chronic adrenal insufficiency, crises may be precipitated by infection, trauma, excessive fatigue, or drugs such as morphine, barbiturates, laxatives, thyroid hormone, or insulin.

There are a number of rare, genetically determined disorders that affect either adrenocorticosteroid production or function. Congenital aplasia or hypoplasia of the adrenals and the adrenoleukodystrophies present with features of cortisol and aldosterone deficiency (24,25). ACTH unresponsiveness and familial glucocorticoid deficiency demonstrate findings of cortisol deficiency (26,27), while the inborn errors of aldosterone synthesis and pseudohypoaldosteronism present with symptoms of salt-wasting (28–30).

DIAGNOSIS

Adrenocortical insufficiency can occur either as a consequence of a primary disorder involving the adrenal glands or secondary to disease of the hypothalamus-pituitary. Children with suspected acute adrenal insufficiency should have a careful history and a thorough physical examination (2,3,6,8,13). The emergency evaluation must include a careful history to elicit early symptoms as well as precipitating factors such as infection, sepsis, and trauma. Adrenal insufficiency must be considered in any child with a history of rapid, nonspecific clinical deterioration with no apparent underlying etiology (6,31). Important suggestive features include abnormal mental status, fever, signs of dehydration, and cutaneous hyperpigmentation; vital signs may demonstrate hypotension and tachycardia as well as orthostatic changes in the heart rate and blood pressure.

Congenital adrenal hyperplasia must be suspected in any infant born with ambiguous genitalia (2,3). Diagnosis involves definition of the specific metabolic disorder and determination of the genetic sex; the diagnosis must be made as quickly as possible in order to institute the therapy necessary to avoid adrenal crisis and arrest the clinical effects of the metabolic abnormalities. Chromosome analysis is essential to establish genetic sex; furthermore each form of congenital adrenal hyperplasia has its own unique serum corticosteroid profile (3). Reliable radioimmunoassays for circulating adrenal steroids now permit direct measurement of accumulated adrenal steroid precursors in serum, and hormone profiles diagnostic of different forms of CAH have been established.

The diagnosis of a child with suspected acute adrenocorticosteroid insufficiency involves defining the nature and etiology of the physiological abnormality as well as establishing a presumptive diagnosis. The laboratory evaluation includes (1) routine chemical measurements suggestive of adrenal insufficiency and (2) definitive diagnostic studies. Important chemical findings include reduced serum sodium and chloride concentrations along with persistent urinary sodium loss; sodium can be measured in random urine specimens as diagnosis should not be delayed by waiting for timed collections. Serum potassium concentration is consistently high; acidosis, hypoglycemia, and azotemia are frequently observed. Serum calcium may be elevated, but ionized calcium and parathormone concentrations are usually normal.

The diagnosis of adrenocortical insufficiency requires a demonstration of decreased cortisol production or diminished pituitary ACTH reserve. When adrenal insufficiency is suspected, whether primary or secondary, the response to ACTH stimulation should be evaluated. A random measurement of plasma or urine corticosteroids is not sufficient since a single determination may be normal; a presumptive diagnosis can be made, however, if a low serum cortisol concentration is found to be associated with a high ACTH.

The short ACTH test can be performed concurrent with treatment of adrenal insufficiency if it is necessary to evaluate a patient previously started on treatment in whom the interruption of therapy might be dangerous (3,32).

TREATMENT, ACUTE ADRENAL INSUFFICIENCY

Adrenocortical insufficiency involves deficiencies of both cortisol and aldosterone that results in marked dehydration, hyponatremia, hyperkalemia, and acidosis. The most important elements of successful treatment include the restoration of intravascular volume and the administration of corticosteroids. Patients should be placed on monitors, and vital signs should be recorded frequently during replacement therapy.

During the newborn period, an infant can usually be maintained with fluid and electrolyte replacement while urine specimens and blood samples are collected for diagnosis. During the first hour, 20 ml/kg of a 5 percent dextrose solution containing either 0.85 percent sodium chloride (isotonic saline) or Ringer lactate should be infused. If the blood pressure is satisfactory and the vital signs are stable at the end of the first hour, the IV solution should be continued to deliver appropriate replacement fluid and electrolytes over the next 24 to 48 hours. The 24-hour fluid requirement is 80 to 120 ml/kg body weight. In the newborn period, this regimen is usually sufficient for the treatment of acute crises. Therapy must be guided by serial evaluation of circulatory and hydrational status as well as serum electrolytes.

If the infant has not improved clinically by the end of the first hour and the blood chemistries have not changed, hydrocortisone sodium succinate (Solu-Cortef) may be given, a 50 mg dose initially followed by 25 mg added to the 24-hour IV maintenance solutions. Glucocorticoids are administered intravenously. Although both cortisol and aldosterone may be deficient, only cortisol is necessary during acute therapy (33). Corticosteroids with negligible mineralocorticoid activity such as dexamethasone (Decadron) should be avoided during initial treatment (6). If further decompensation occurs, plasma (10 ml/kg) may be used instead of other IV fluids. Once enteral medication is established, mineralocorticoid replacement with 9a-fluorocortisone (Florinef), 0.05 to 0.10 mg twice daily, may be initiated.

In the older children, fluid and electrolyte therapy consists of 5 percent dextrose-isotonic saline or Ringer lactate, 120 to 150 ml/kg/day; half is given within the first 3 hours (3). In children weighing more than 25 kg, the hydrocortisone dose is based on body weight. The initial dose is hydrocortisone sodium succinate (Solu-Cortef), 2.0 mg/kg, administered intravenously. This is followed by 5 mg/kg over the first 3 hours; hydrocortisone sodium succinate (Solu-Cortef), 5 to 10 mg/kg/day, is then added to the 24-hour maintenance IV solutions. The dose of 9a-fluorocortisone (Florinef) is 0.05–0.10 mg twice daily as it is in infants.

With appropriate volume replacement, the acute phase of treatment for adrenocortical insufficiency requires 24 to 48 hours. IV steroids should be continued for

24 hours after recovery from the acute crisis (22). When the child is hemodynamically stable, oral glucocorticoids in doses 3 to 4 times maintenance (maintenance: equivalent of cortisol, 12 mg/m^2 body surface area daily) can be started on a three times daily schedule and then gradually reduced to maintenance (2,3,4,6). The maintenance doses of 9a-fluorocortisone (Florinef), 0.05–0.10 mg twice daily, may be started once enteral intake has been established. The treatment of secondary adrenal insufficiency differs from that for primary hypoadrenocorticism only in that the deficiency of salt-active hormone is usually negligible so that 9a-fluorocortisone (Florinef) is usually not required.

CONCLUSION

Acute adrenal insufficiency of childhood is a life-threatening condition that commonly presents with atypical manifestations. Early manifestations may be subtle, especially in older children. Hyperpigmentation is not found in children with primary acute adrenal insufficiency of recent onset and is not a feature of secondary adrenal insufficiency.

Acute assessment and management are based on principles that take into account the electrolyte composition of the predominant fluids lost and the need to replace the deficient adrenal hormones. The differential diagnosis provides a challenge initially in distinguishing other hypovolemic conditions and subsequently in defining the precise adrenal disorder. Long-term measures involve an emphasis on compliance with maintenance corticosteroid replacement, glucocorticoid supplementation for stress, and a high index of suspicion for subtle symptoms and signs of impending adrenal insufficiency.

REFERENCES

1. Simpson ER, Waterman MR. Steroid hormone biosynthesis in the adrenal cortex and its regulation by adrenocorticotropin. In DeGroot LJ, ed. Endocrinology. Philadelphia: Saunders, 1989.
2. Job J-C, Chaussain J-L. The adrenals. In Job J-C, Pierson M, eds. Pediatric endocrinology. New York: Wiley, 1981.
3. New MI, del Balzo P, Crawford C, et al. The adrenal cortex. In Kaplan SA, ed. Clinical pediatric endocrinology. Philadelphia: Saunders, 1990.
4. Kenny FM, Richards C, Taylor FH. Reference standards for cortisol production and 17-hydroxycorticosteroid excretion during growth: Variation in the pattern of excretion of radiolabeled cortisol metabolites. Metabolism 1970;19:280.
5. Parker LN, Levin ER, Lifrak ET. Evidence for adrenocortical adaption to severe illness. J Clin Endocrinol Metab 1985;60:947.
6. Rusnak RA. Adrenal and pituitary emergencies. Emerg Med Clin NA 1989;77(4):903.
7. Bethune JE. The diagnosis and treatment of adrenal insufficiency. In DeGroot LJ, ed. Endocrinology. Philadelphia: Saunders, 1989.
8. Jordan RM. Endocrine emergencies. Med Clin NA 1983;67:1193.
9. Nerup J. Addison's disease—clinical studies: A report of 108 cases. Acta Endocrinol 1974;76:127.
10. Ketchum CH, Riley WJ, McLaren NK. Adrenal dysfunction in asymptomatic patients with adrenocortical autoantibodies. J Clin Endocrinol Metab 1984;58:1166.

11. Betterle C, Zanette F, Zanchetta R, et al. Complement-fixing adrenal autoantibodies as a marker for predicting onset of idiopathic Addison's disease. Lancet 1983;1:1238.
12. Hubay CA, Weckesser EC, Levy RP. Occult adrenal insufficiency in surgical patients. Ann Surg 1975;181(3):325.
13. Leshin M. Acute adrenal insufficiency: Recognition, management, and prevention. Urol Clin North Amer 1982;9:229.
14. Hodes HL, Moloshok RE, Markowitz M. Fulminating meningococcemia treated with cortisone: Use of blood eosinophil count as a guide to prognosis and treatment. Pediatrics 1952;10:138.
15. Black J, Williams DI. Natural history of adrenal hemorrhage in the newborn. Arch Dis Child 1973;48:183.
16. Goldzieher MA, Gordon MB. The syndrome of adrenal hemorrhage in the newborn. Endocrinol 1932;16:165.
17. Liu L, Haskin ME, Rose LI, et al. Diagnosis of bilateral adrenocortical hemorrhage by computed tomography. Ann Int Med 1982;97:720.
18. Leshin M. Polyglandular autoimmune syndromes. Am J Med Sci 1985;290:77.
19. Baxter JD, Tyrell B. The adrenal cortex. In Felig P, Baxter JD, Broadus AE, et al, eds. Endocrinology and metabolism. New York: McGraw-Hill, 1987.
20. Klibanski A. Non-secreting pituitary tumors. Endocrinol Metab Clin North Am 1987;16:793.
21. Melby JC. Drug spotlight program: Systemic corticosteroid therapy: Pharmacology and endocrinologic considerations. Ann Intern Med 1974;81:505.
22. Bagdade JD. Endocrine emergencies. Med Clin North Amer 1986;70:1111.
23. Chamberlain P, Meyer WJ. Management of pituitary-adrenal suppression secondary to corticosteroid therapy. Pediatrics 1981;67:245.
24. Petersen KE, Bille T, Jacobsen BB, et al. X-linked congenital adrenal hypoplasia: Study of five generations of Greenlandic family. Acta Pediatr Scand 1982;71:947.
25. Benke PJ, Reyes PF, Parker JC. New form of adrenoleukodystrophy. Hum Genet 1981;58:204.
26. Franks RC, Nance WE. Hereditary adrenocortical unresponsiveness to ACTH. Pediatrics 1970;45:43.
27. Allgrove J, Clayden GS, Grant DB, et al. Familial glucocorticoid deficiency with achalasia of the cardia and deficient tear production. Lancet 1978;1:1284.
28. Visser HKA, Cost WS. A new hereditary defect in the biosynthesis of aldosterone. Acta Endocrinol 1964;47:589.
29. Veldhius JD, Kulin HE, Santen RJ. Inborn error in the terminal step of aldosterone biosynthesis: Corticosterone methyl oxidase type II deficiency in a North American pedigree. New Engl J Med 1980;303:117.
30. Roy C. Familial pseudohypoaldosteronism. Arch Franc Pediatr 1977;34:37.
31. Kalia S, Tintinalli JE. Emergency evaluation of the cancer patient. Ann Emerg Med 1984;13:724.
32. Ginsberg LJ. A practical approach to tolerance testing in children. In Lifshitz F, ed. Pediatric Endocrinology. New York: Marcel Dekker.
33. Wilson RF. Science and shock: A clinical perspective. Ann Emerg Med 1985;14:714.

PART X

Hematology and Oncology

29

Sickle Cell Disease

Dilip L. Solanki

Sickle cell diseases (SCDs) are perhaps the most common human hereditary disorders worldwide and a common medical problem in most urban hospitals in the United States. These disorders are found in people of African, Mediterranean, Indian, and Middle Eastern heritage. In the United States, they are most commonly observed in Blacks and Hispanics from the Caribbean, Central America, and parts of South America. SCD is a generic term that encompasses a group of symptomatic disorders having in common the predominance of hemoglobin S. They are best classified by genotype. The type of hemoglobin produced is determined by the two beta globin genes located on chromosome 11 and the four alpha globin genes located on chromosome 16. Individuals who are homozygous for sickle beta globin gene have sickle cell anemia, the commonest SCD, occurring in 1 of every 500 births in the United States. The other relatively common SCDs are sickle cell hemoglobin C disease (Hb SC disease) resulting from inheritance of a sickle beta gene and a hemoglobin C beta gene, sickle cell beta thalassemia (Sβ thal) that results from inheritance of a sickle gene and a beta thalassemia gene. The latter disorder is further subdivided into sickle cell β+ thalassemia (Sβ+ thal) in which some normal beta globin is synthesized. If no beta globin is made, the disorder is called sickle cell β° thalassemia (Sβ° thal). Electrophoretically, Sβ° thal may be indistinguishable from sickle cell anemia. In Sβ+ thal, both hemoglobin S and hemoglobin A are present with a predominance of hemoglobin S. *This is to be distinguished from sickle cell trait in which both hemoglobins are also produced but with a predominance of hemoglobin A. Sickle cell trait is not a disease but rather a carrier state and should never be used to explain any illness of individuals carrying the trait.* Although there is tremendous variability and overlap between disease groups with respect to clinical severity and manifestation, the genotypic distinction between SS and other SCD is important for several reasons. Individuals with Hb SC disease and Sβ thal are less likely to be symptomatic early in life so that these disorders may remain undiagnosed until adolescence or adult life, have higher steady state hemoglobin levels that are important considerations in the detection of anemic crises, retain splenomegaly well into the late adolescence and adulthood and thus are at risk for splenic sequestration crises. They also are more prone to certain complications such as acute and chronic eye complications and sickling related hematuria, and rarely have sickled red cells on a routine blood smear.

Patients with SCD frequently suffer from acute painful vaso-occlusive crises and therefore become high consumers of emergency medical care. As a result, a complacency is developed that leads to a tendency to label *all* medical illnesses of these patients as sickle cell crisis. While crises tend to be self-limited and may require only conservative supportive treatment, SCD patients are at high risk for many serious and multisystem problems causing similar signs and symptoms that may require more aggressive, specific, and invasive care. These patients therefore present a complex challenge for the emergency physician who must be constantly vigilant to rule out potentially life-threatening disease.

The diagnosis of SCD is made by hemoglobin electrophoreses both on cellulose acetate at alkaline pH and citrate agar at acid pH combined with tests for sickling (solubility test or sickle cell preparation), clinical history, blood counts, peripheral blood smear, and measurement of minor hemoglobins A_2 and F. When available, parents and siblings should be studied by hemoglobin electrophoresis and measurement of HbA_2 and HbF. These serve to confirm the genotypic diagnosis and occasionally may be the only means of clarifying the genotype of the propositus. *The diagnosis cannot, and must not, be made from the sickling tests alone since neither available test will reliably distinguish sickle cell trait from SCD.* It cannot be too strongly emphasized that there are asymptomatic sickling syndromes (for example, SG Philadelphia) discovered on screening electrophoresis. Clinical and laboratory correlation is therefore of paramount importance in the diagnosis of SCD.

PATHOPHYSIOLOGY

There are two cardinal pathophysiologic features of SCD: (1) chronic hemolytic anemia and (2) vaso-occlusion resulting in ischemic tissue injury. The hemolytic anemia is caused primarily by the abnormal properties of Hb S, which causes the red cells to undergo repeated cycles of sickling and unsickling. This eventually leads to irreversibly sickled red cells, which, being rigid and fragile, undergo mechanical lysis in the circulation. The hemolysis is predominantly intravascular. Hemosiderinuria and depletion of serum haptoglobin therefore are consistent laboratory findings in addition to the elevated indirect bilirubin and lactate dehydrogenase. The severity of hemolysis and related abnormalities are directly proportional to the intensity of sickling. Since sickling in general is less intense in Hb SC disease and Sβ thal, the anemia and laboratory features of hemolysis are less prominent in these disorders than they are in Hb SS. Chronic hemolysis is responsible for the increased incidence of gallstones that rises with age and of hyperuricemia causing gout.

The mechanism of vaso-occlusion is less well understood. In the past, pathophysiology of vaso-occlusive tissue injury was dominated by an emphasis on the sickling phenomenon. It is now recognized widely that SCDs are exceedingly complex and that attempts to explain the vascular occlusion on the basis of a single feature are artificial. Available information supports an important contributory role for vascular endothelial cells, plasma proteins, granulocytes, lymphokines, and co-existing genetic factors in the genesis of vaso-occlusive episodes both acute and chronic. The organs at greatest risk are those with venous sinuses where the blood flow is slow and oxygen tension and pH are low (spleen, kidney, bone marrow) or those with a limited terminal arterial blood supply (eye, head of the femur, brain). Symptoms of vaso-occlusion may be acute (for example, pain crises, stroke, acute chest syndrome) or chronic (for example, aseptic necrosis of femoral head, splenic fibrosis, retinopathy).

CLINICAL PRESENTATION

Common acute illnesses of SCD children relevant to the emergency physician are infection, painful events, acute splenic sequestration, other anemic crises, acute chest syndrome, and stroke. Since management principles are distinct for each, these entities are discussed individually. However, it is important to keep in mind that more than one complication may occur concurrently in the same patient and that therefore all complications must be looked for. Clinical manifestations of Hb SS begin to appear by 6 months of age in about 6 percent of the children. By 8 years of age 96 percent of the children manifest sickle cell–specific symptoms.

Infection

Children with SCD are very susceptible to bacterial infections. This is a consequence of impaired splenic function, defective complement pathways, and serum opsonizing activities. Infections are a major cause of morbidity and mortality in the first few years of life. Indeed a life-threatening infection may be the first clinical manifestation of SCD in a child not detected during the newborn period. The organisms most frequently involved include *S. pneumoniae, H. influenzae, E. coli, S. aureus*, and *S. typhi*. Blood, lungs, bone, meninges, and urinary tract are the areas most often involved.

Pulmonary infections account for the majority of the cases. *S. pneumoniae* and *H. influenzae* are the organisms most often involved but *mycoplasma* and *chlamydia* infections also occur commonly and should be covered with erythromycin. Although prophylaxis with pneumococcal vaccine and oral penicillin have greatly reduced the frequency of pneumococcal infections, one must recognize that suboptimal antibody response against certain strains of *pneumococci* in some children and poor compliance to penicillin prophylaxis may leave such children at risk of pneumococcal sepsis. The long-term clinical efficacy of *H. influenzae* vaccine has not been well documented.

Osteomyelitis is to be considered in all patients with one or more localized areas of bone pain and high fever. It is most often caused by *Salmonella* infection although *staphylococcal* infection can also occur. Osteomyelitis is often multicentric and may lead to confusion with aseptic necrosis. The unique predisposition of SCD patients to salmonella osteomyelitis probably represents the ability of this organism to survive in the necrotic bone. The reservoir for salmonella is often the gallbladder. Urinary tract infections are most often caused by *E. coli* and are frequently complicated by septicemia.

The general guidelines for evaluation and treatment are given in Table 29.1. The emphasis should be on prompt and aggressive evaluation and institution of empiric antibiotic therapy. A few hours delay can make a significant difference for the patient

Table 29.1 Management of a febrile child with SCD

1. During physical examination, look for
   a. Respiratory distress and signs of pulmonary infection
   b. Meningeal signs
   c. Sepsis (rising fever, chills)
   d. Localized bone pain (osteomyelitis)
   e. Costovertebral angle (CVA) tenderness
   f. Right upper quadrant (RUQ) tenderness
   g. Degree of jaundice (biliary obstruction)
2. Laboratory studies
   a. CBC and reticulocyte count
   b. Blood cultures
   c. Chest X-ray
   d. Urinalysis, urine culture, and sensitivity
   e. Mycoplasma and chlamydia titer (pulmonary infection)
   f. Stool culture (if diarrhea is present)
   g. Lumbar puncture (all patients under 1 year of age and those with even minimal signs of meningitis)
   h. Bone films and scan, direct aspiration of involved area or joint by orthopedic surgeon for culture and gram stain
3. Hospitalize all patients, especially those under five years of age and with a documented temperature over 101° F
4. If meningitis is ruled out or not suspected, treat with cefuroxime or another appropriate antibiotic to cover *S. pneumoniae* and *H. influenzae*. The first dose of antibiotic must be given in the emergency department immediately after diagnostic studies are completed. *Treatment should be given even for minimal clinical indications.*

with pneumococcal sepsis. Initiation of antibiotic therapy in the emergency department is the method of choice. In some institutions, febrile children over the age of 5 years are not routinely hospitalized, but are often treated on an outpatient basis because these patients can be clinically evaluated much more easily than the younger ones. Such an approach would require close consultation with the hematologist and mechanism for a close follow up of such children.

Infections in SCD patients can be minimized by immunization and prophylactic penicillin and morbidity reduced by educating parents to seek prompt medical care for their febrile child.

Painful Events

These are believed to be caused by ischemic tissue injury resulting from the obstruction of blood flow produced by sickled erythrocytes. The frequency and severity of painful events are extremely varied. There is no clinical or laboratory finding that is pathognomonic of painful episodes, and the diagnosis is made solely on the basis of medical history. Musculoskeletal pain is the most common complaint.

Dactylitis, or hand-foot syndrome, is the first manifestation of vaso-occlusive crisis in many infants. The pain can be symmetrical, asymmetrical, or migratory, and it may or may not be associated with swelling, low grade fever, redness, or warmth. The abdomen is the second most common site of painful episodes.

The possibility that the pain is precipitated by a concurrent medical condition such as infection, should always be considered and searched for in every instance. It is extremely important to exclude nonsickle causes of pain such as cholecystitis, peptic ulcer, perforated viscous, urinary tract infection, intra-abdominal infection, osteomyelitis, or septic arthritis before labeling the patient as having a vaso-occlusive crisis. Pneumonia in children can present with abdominal pain. Table 29.2 lists clues to a nonsickle cause of pain.

Diagnostic evaluation of the painful events is dictated by site of pain and other associated manifestations and aimed primarily at ruling out nonsickle causes of pain. If fever higher than 101° F or if marked leukocytosis is present, an aggressive search for infection should be made. If chest symptoms are present, chest X-ray, arterial blood gases, and sputum studies are indicated to rule out pneumonia. Direct aspiration of a joint or bone lesion is indicated in cases of suspected arthritis or osteomyelitis; bone scans and X-rays are not always reliable in distinguishing infection from infarction. Electrolytes and blood pH should be obtained in all severely ill patients. Computed tomographic (CT) scan or an ultrasound of the abdomen is often helpful in detecting medical or surgical causes of abdominal pain.

Management of pain crisis has three essential elements: (1) identification and treatment of precipitating or associated events, (2) hydration, and (3) prompt relief of pain with analgesics. Dehydration that occurs frequently in these patients because of decreased fluid intake, increased insensible water loss, and hyposthenuria may promote sickling. Therefore intravenous (IV) hydration is indicated in most cases and is mandatory for clinically dehydrated patients. The choice of fluid is dictated by the patient's hydration status and electrolyte values. For uncomplicated pain crises, 5 percent dextrose with 0.45 percent normal saline is recommended as initial fluid. Children should receive 150 ml/kg/day with close monitoring to avoid iatrogenic congestive heart failure.

Analgesics are used with the goal of providing prompt pain relief. This is often not achieved because of inadequate understanding of the clinical pharmacology of analgesics, excessive concern about narcotic addiction, or misguided use of placebos. Despite the frequent need for analgesics, narcotic addiction is remarkably uncommon in this patient population. The choice of therapy is based on severity of pain and

Table 29.2 Clues to nonsickle causes of pain

Fever > 101° F, lethargy, dehydration	Localized bone pain with high fever
Severe abdominal pain	Headache, vomiting
Pain associated with extremity weakness or loss of function	Acute pulmonary symptoms
	Marked leukocytosis
Acute joint swelling	Pain unrelieved by conservative measures

potency, mode of action, and side effects of the drugs. Medication should be administered on a fixed schedule with dosing intervals not exceeding the duration of the desired effect. Potent narcotics should be used with the usual precautions and monitoring to avoid respiratory depression. A protocol for analgesic therapy is outlined in Table 29.3.

The goal of emergency department management is to assess the clinical problem, exclude nonsickle illnesses, to undertake a brief trial of therapy, and to decide whether to hospitalize the patient. Certain high-risk patients, such as those with abdominal pain, high fever, lethargy, and neurologic deficit, should be promptly

Table 29.3 Recommended initial dose and interval of analgesics necessary to obtain adequate pain control in SCD

	Max Dose (mg)	Route	Interval	Comments
Severe pain				
Morphine	0.15 mg/kg/dose (max 10 mg)	SC, IM	Q3h	Drug of choice
Meperidine	1.5 mg/kg/dose	IM	Q3h	Increased incidence of seizures; avoid in patients with renal or neurologic disease
Moderate pain				
Oxycodone (Percocet or Percodan)	1 to 2 tabs/dose (1 tab = 5 mg)	PO	Q4h	Patients over age five
Methadone	0.15 mg/kg/dose	PO	Q6h	Effective in patients usually requiring parenteral narcotics: **Not for routine use**
Meperidine	1.5 mg/kg/dose (max 100 mg/dose)	PO	Q3½h	
Mild pain				
Codeine	0.75 mg/kg/dose	PO	Q4h	May be effective up to six hours
Aspirin	1.5 gm/m^2/24 h	PO	Q4h	May be given with a narcotic for added analgesia
Acetaminophen	1.5 gm/m^2/24 h	PO	Q4h	May be given with a narcotic for added analgesia
Motrin (Ibuprofen)	300–600 mg/dose	PO	Q6h	

admitted. If the patient with severe pain remains comfortable for three to four hours after a parenteral narcotic, an oral narcotic may be administered and the child may be observed for another hour. If moderate or severe pain returns, the parenteral narcotic dose should be repeated. If significant pain persists, the patient should be hospitalized. If, on the other hand, pain is under control, the patient can be discharged on an adequate dose of an effective oral narcotic with a small discharge prescription. Many hospitals have guidelines for the duration of a patient's stay in the emergency department. These are usually difficult rules to follow, and each patient's care should be individualized. In general, patients who require continuing treatment with parenteral narcotics or who are unable to take adequate fluids by mouth warrant hospitalization.

Diazepam and chlorpromazine do not potentiate the analgesia of narcotics. Their use should be avoided except when a need for a potent tranquilizer clearly exists. Oxygen therapy most likely does not benefit vaso-occlusive crises and is indicated only if hypoxemia is present. When oxygen is used, the arterial O_2 tension must be monitored to document response and to avoid excessive levels that may induce anemic crises by suppression of erythropoiesis.

Sodium bicarbonate and vasodilators have no proven value in the management of vaso-occlusive crises.

Acute Splenic Sequestration Crises

This is a major cause of morbidity and mortality of SCD in the first two years of life and an absolute indication for hospitalization. Infant and young children whose spleens have not yet undergone multiple infarctions and fibrosis are at the greatest risk for this complication. In Hb SS, these begin to occur after five months of age and are unusual after two years of age. In those with other sickle cell diseases whose spleens remain enlarged, this complication can continue to occur later in life. Infection is often the precipitating cause.

These catastrophic events are characterized by sudden massive enlargement of the spleen filling the abdomen with resultant severe anemia and hypovolemia from pooling of a considerable portion of the blood volume. This is the most acutely dangerous crisis in the life of a young child with Hb SS. Infants can die within hours of the first sign of this disturbance. The usual clinical indications of this complication are weakness, dyspnea, pallor, abdominal pain, and signs of hypovolemia.

Laboratory studies show profound anemia with reticulocyte, lactate dehydrogenase (LDH) and indirect bilirubin levels above their usual values. Moderate to severe thrombocytopenia may be present.

Minor episodes characterized by modest increases in spleen size associated with a two to three gm decrease in hemoglobin level are very common. Although these resolve spontaneously, they predict for later severe episodes. Their recognition, therefore, is important in educating parents to look for pallor, to palpate for spleen size changes, and to seek prompt medical attention if either abnormality develops. Recognition of such episodes is facilitated by accurate documentation of steady state spleen size in every child with SCD.

Treatment is directed toward the prompt correction of hypovolemia with plasma expanders and red blood cells. If shock or hypotension can be reversed, there is rapid regression of splenomegaly and remobilization of trapped red cells. As a result, a rapid rise in hemoglobin can occur in a short time. Parents should be cautioned about the recurrent nature of this complication and educated in the recognition of the complication.

Aplastic and Megaloblastic Crises

Patients can present with increased dyspnea and fatigue and are found to be much more anemic than usual with very few or no reticulocytes. In the aplastic crises, the bone marrow shows a selective suppression of erythropoiesis and serum LDH and unconjugated bilirubin that are lower than is usual. Recent studies show that severe cases are frequently associated with human parvovirus infections. Some cases are caused by excessive oxygen therapy. Treatment is symptomatic with red cell transfusions if they are needed. These cases resolve spontaneously in 5 to 10 days.

Megaloblastic crises are rare and characterized by megaloblastic erythropoiesis and LDH and unconjugated bilirubin levels that are higher than usual. Folate deficiency is most often implicated. Treatment is symptomatic with red cell transfusions and folate replacement.

Acute Chest Syndrome

This acute illness is a common cause for hospital visits and is characterized by fever, chest pain, respiratory distress, and pulmonary infiltrates on a chest X-ray. In adults, the syndrome is often caused by pulmonary infarctions. In children, an infectious etiology is more likely. It can develop as an isolated event or occur in the course of a vaso-occlusive crisis. It often progresses rapidly from mild respiratory symptoms to respiratory failure. The resulting hypoxia can have profound systemic effects. Therefore, it is important to evaluate any child with SCD and respiratory symptoms carefully.

Laboratory studies should include complete blood count (CBC), retic count, arterial blood gases, chest X-ray, mycoplasma and chlamydia serology, and cultures of sputum, blood, and pleural fluid if present. Chest X-ray may be normal initially and for 2 to 3 days. Severe hypoxia with pO_2 below 60 indicates potentially life-threatening disease. Lung scans are generally not helpful in the etiologic diagnosis or in therapeutic decisions.

All patients with acute chest syndrome (ACS) should be hospitalized promptly. Oxygen adequate to raise the pO_2 over 70 mm Hg should be administered. Empiric therapy for infection should be started promptly as was outlined earlier. Exchange transfusion is indicated in those with hypoxemia unresponsive to oxygen administration and those with respiratory failure.

Neurologic Events

These occur in 10 to 20 percent of children with SCD, in almost all of those with Hb SS. Infarction, hemorrhage (both intracerebral and subarachnoid), and transient ischemic attacks (TIAs) are the most common presentations.

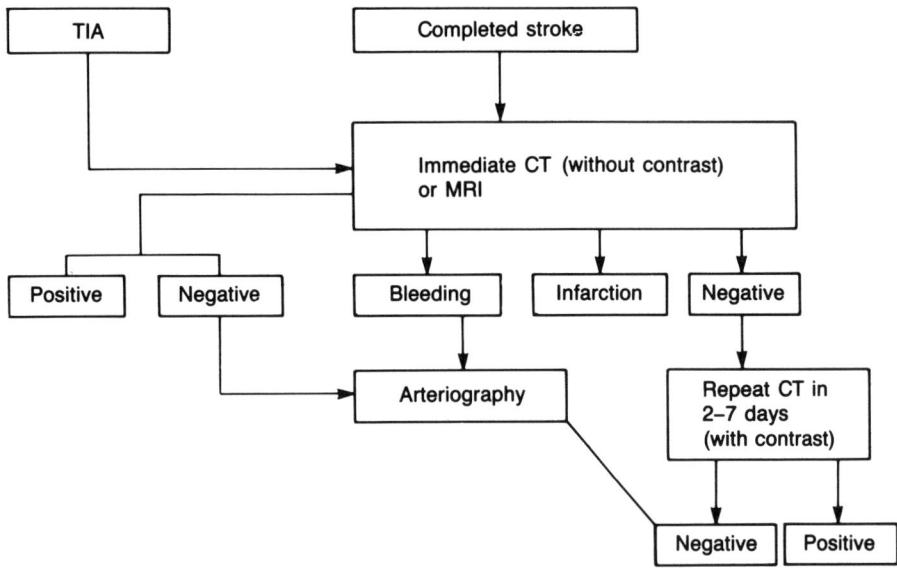

Figure 29.1 Suggested evaluation of neurologic events in SCD and TIA.

Clinical signs are usually obvious but may be difficult to distinguish from a limp caused by pain in young, nonverbal children. Hemiparesis is most common followed by aphasia, dysphasia, seizures, or monoparesis. Associated headache is common. Occasionally the patient may present in a complete or nearly comatose state. In about a quarter of the patients, the stroke may occur concurrently with other sickle cell complications such as pain crises, anemic crises, and acute chest syndrome.

Diagnosis is made on clinical grounds, but imaging procedures are generally necessary to distinguish between hemorrhage and infarction and to delineate the physical and functional location of the stroke. Most useful initial study is a CT without contrast or magnetic resonance imaging (MRI) (Figure 29.1). CT may be normal at the onset of infarction, but it is helpful in ruling out bleeding, abscess, tumor, or other abnormalities. MRI may be more sensitive but may not be as readily available. Lumbar puncture is indicated when infection or subarachnoid hemorrhage is suspected but must be undertaken only if CT or MRI shows no evidence of increased intracranial tension.

Arteriography may be helpful in patients with symptomatic TIA who have normal CT or MRI. This must not be done, however, without prior partial or total exchange transfusion to minimize hazards from sickling due to hyperosmolar dye.

For the patient with acute stroke, rapid evaluation and close monitoring for progression and development of increased intracranial tension are necessary. The involvement of a neurologist and/or a neurosurgeon is essential. Seizures, which are common, and increased intracranial tension should be treated by anticonvulsants and steroids respectively.

Partial exchange transfusion to reduce the Hb S level to less than 30 percent will help prevent progression of acute stroke and must be undertaken as soon as possible. Simple transfusion is not recommended. The outlook for hemorrhagic stroke and subarachnoid hemorrhage is less good, but they should be managed similarly.

SUGGESTED READING

1. Bainbridge R, Higgs DR, Maude GH, et al. Clinical presentation of homozygous sickle cell disease. J Pediatrics 1985;106:881–885.
2. Charache S, Lubin B, Reid C, eds. Management and therapy of sickle cell disease. NIH Publication NO. 89-2117, 1989.
3. Leikin S, Gallagher D, Kinney TR, et al. Mortality in children and adolescents with sickle cell disease. Pediatrics 1989;84:500–508.
4. Ohene-Frempong K. Stroke in sickle cell disease: Demographic, clinical and therapeutic considerations. Seminars in Hematology, 1991;28:213–219.
5. Poncz M, Kane E, Gill FM. Acute chest syndrome in sickle cell disease: Etiology and clinical correlates. J Pediatrics 1985;107:861–866.
6. Vichinsky E, Lubin B. Suggested guidelines for the treatment of children with sickle cell anemia. Hematology/Oncology Clinics of North America, 1987;1:483–501.

30

Oncologic Emergencies

Nirmal Bhaya

Cancer is the second leading cause of death in children between 1 and 15 years of age. Over the past four decades, there has been dramatic improvement in the prognosis of children with malignancies. The emergencies may arise because of the disease process itself or because of the chemotherapy and radiotherapy required to treat the malignancy. Hence it is important that emergency physicians be aware of the medical problems that immediately threaten the vital organ functions or that may compromise the long-term quality of life. All the conditions described are reversible if they are recognized and treated correctly in an appropriate and timely manner. The oncologist must be consulted to arrive at the best treatment plan for the individual child.

Emergencies in a child with neoplastic disease may result from

1. Bone marrow involvement caused by either the disease process or treatment resulting in various cytopenias
2. Metabolic abnormalities resulting from the rapid release of tumor metabolites
3. Mechanical emergencies resulting from space-occupying lesions causing extrinsic pressure or intrinsic obstruction.

The conditions are subdivided according to the emergencies involving each major system.

CARDIORESPIRATORY SYSTEM
Superior Vena Cava Syndrome and Superior Mediastinal Syndrome

Superior vena cava syndrome (SVCS) is a rare entity in pediatrics. In children with malignant anterior mediastinal tumors, the incidence appears to be about 12 percent at presentation. The most common causes of SVCS in children are Hodgkin's disease and non-Hodgkin's lymphoma. Benign tumors or inflammatory processes are rarely implicated. With the rising incidence of human immunodeficiency virus (HIV), tuberculous granuloma as a cause of SVCS should be strongly considered in the differential diagnosis.

The superior vena cava is a thin-walled structure with low intraluminal pressure, hence easily affected by extrinsic mechanical compression. The extrinsic obstruction is further aggravated by intravascular thrombosis in 50 percent of cases. The superior vena cava is surrounded by lymph nodes, thymus, and pericardium, and when these structures are involved with tumor or infection, they can compress the vena cava easily. In children compared to adults, the trachea is less rigid and has a relatively small intraluminal diameter; thus even a small degree of external compression or intrinsic edema causes airway obstruction. The end result of compression, clotting, and edema is that air flow as well as blood flow is reduced. Hence in a pediatric patient the terms *superior vena cava syndrome* and *superior mediastinal syndrome* have become almost synonymous.

The common symptoms of SVCS are brassy cough, dyspnea, orthopnea, stridor, and wheezing due to compression of tracheobronchial tree. Venous obstruction leads to plethora; edema and cyanosis of face, neck, and upper extremities; and suffusion of conjunctiva. Less frequently the child may present with symptoms of *wet-brain syndrome,* with anxiety, confusion, lethargy, headache, syncope, or seizures. These symptoms are aggravated by the supine position.

Complete history, physical examination, and chest X-ray should be sufficient to generate a differential diagnosis. Computerized tomography (CT) of the chest is helpful in delineating the location of mass and tracheal size. Venography is not usually needed to document caval obstruction.

It may be desirable to obtain tissue diagnosis prior to institution of therapy. This may not be feasible, however, in a child with significant airway compromise. Cardiovascular and respiratory changes associated with general anesthesia may be life threatening. In this situation, a bone marrow aspiration and the biopsy of the superficial lymph node under local anesthesia may suffice. One should avoid upper extremity and neck venipunctures.

The initial and primary mode of treatment is radiotherapy, 200–400 cGy/day. It is employed with steroids to reduce edema formation. Cytotoxic chemotherapy is a reasonable alternative. With treatment, most patients will achieve subjective improvement within three days and objective improvement within one week. Figure 30.1 outlines the approach to SVCS.

Effusions

Effusions may be caused by local invasion, metastatic spread of tumor or the sympathetic response to tumor in the chest or abdomen. Respiratory or cardiac compromise may occur if large amount of effusion develops rapidly. If patient presents with respiratory distress, emergency therapeutic and diagnostic thoracocentesis should be performed. Hypotension may develop following thoracocentesis, hence IV access should be established prior to thoracocentesis. Fluid should be sent for cell count, cytology, specific gravity, protein content and lactic dehydrogenase. Appropriate cultures (for example, TB) and assays of immunologic and biological markers should be obtained.

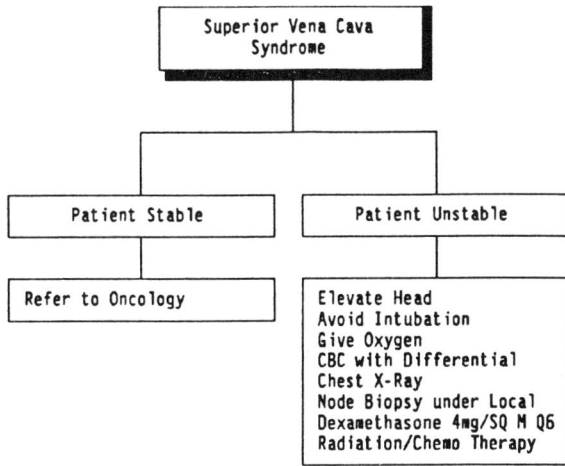

* Avoid Narcotic Sedation
* Avoid IV in Upper Extremities
* Radiation 50-100 Rads to midplane
* Hydrocortisone 2mg/kg Q6H

Figure 30.1 Emergency management of superior vena cava syndrome.

In a newly diagnosed patient with respiratory distress, it may be sufficient to remove fluid once followed by specific chemotherapy. Patients with recurring or resistant effusion may require sclerosing agents, for example, tetracycline.

Pericardial tamponade can be relieved by removing fluid under echocardiographic guidance. Definitive treatment includes chemotherapy, pericardial window, and sclerosing agents.

Diffuse Pulmonary Infiltrates

The appearance of diffuse pulmonary infiltrates and respiratory distress in an immunocompromised child is a medical emergency, requiring prompt diagnostic and therapeutic intervention. The diffuse pulmonary infiltrates may be infectious or noninfectious in origin. Infectious pneumonia may result from hematogenous spread or aspiration of upper airway pathogens. *Pneumocystis carinii* pneumonia is the most common cause of death in children with acute lymphoblastic leukemia in remission and are not neutropenic. Pneumocystis carinii is a protozoan that causes pneumonia by reactivation of latent infection.

Neutropenic patients can get pneumonia from a variety of gram-positive and gram-negative bacteria, which is discussed later in this chapter in the section entitled "Infectious Complications."

Drug reactions and radiation may induce pulmonary infiltrates. Chemotherapeutic agents like bleomycin, cyclophosphamide, methotrexate, busulfan, and chlorambucil are known to cause pulmonary infiltrates. Advanced leukemia, lymphoma, and metastatic lesions may involve pulmonary parenchyma.

Appropriate respiratory support should be started immediately. Oxygen should be administered and ventilation status monitored with pulse-oximeter and blood gases when appropriate.

After complete blood count (CBC), blood cultures, nasopharyngeal bacterial and fungal cultures, sputum and pleural fluid cultures when they are feasible, the patient should be started on an appropriate antibiotic. An approach to pulmonary infiltrates is outlined in Figure 30.2.

HEMATOPOIETIC SYSTEM

Hematologic complications result from replacement of the marrow with cancer cells or its suppression due to cytotoxic therapy. For treatment of various hematologic complications consult Figure 30.3.

Anemia

Most children with leukemia are anemic at the time of diagnosis. If the diagnosis is evident in the emergency department and the patient is stable, the oncologist should be consulted. If the patient has evidence of cardiovascular compromise (for example, extreme tachycardia and/or congestive failure) packed red blood cell (RBC) transfusion should be started in the emergency department.

If anemia is due to marrow suppression, transfusion is not usually required for asymptomatic patient. Causes like chronic blood loss, infection, hemolysis, or nutritional deficiencies should be ruled out.

Hemorrhage

Fatal hemorrhagic diathesis may develop in a cancer patient as a result of altered level or function of platelets and clotting factors, either by malignancy or by complications of therapy. If the patient presents to the emergency department with active bleeding, CBC, platelet count prothrombin time (PT), partial thromboplastin time (PTT), fibrinogen, and fibrin split products should be obtained. Once the etiology of hemorrhage is established, the treatment should be directed appropriately.

A platelet count of 20,000 to 30,000 is manifested by petechiae and mucocutaneous bleeding. At platelet counts below 10,000, the risk of severe spontaneous internal bleeding increases significantly. Management includes platelet transfusions. A dose of 6 units/m^2 or .2 units/kg raises the platelet count by 75,000/mm^3. Platelets are available as 30 to 60 ml/unit. The total volume infused should not exceed 10 ml/kg over two to four hours. Avoid giving deep intramuscular injections and deep venipunctures; drugs (such as aspirin, antihistamines), which alter platelet function, should be avoided.

Oncologic Emergencies | 341

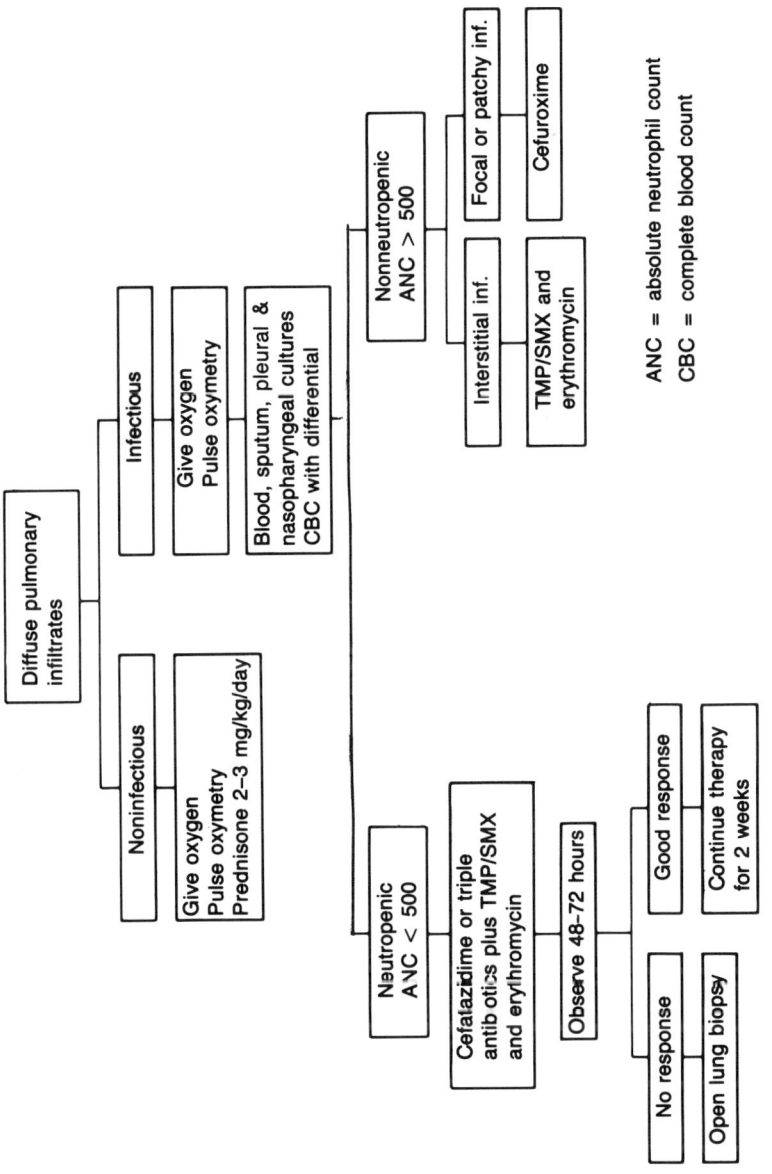

Figure 30.2 Approach to patient with pulmonary infiltrates.

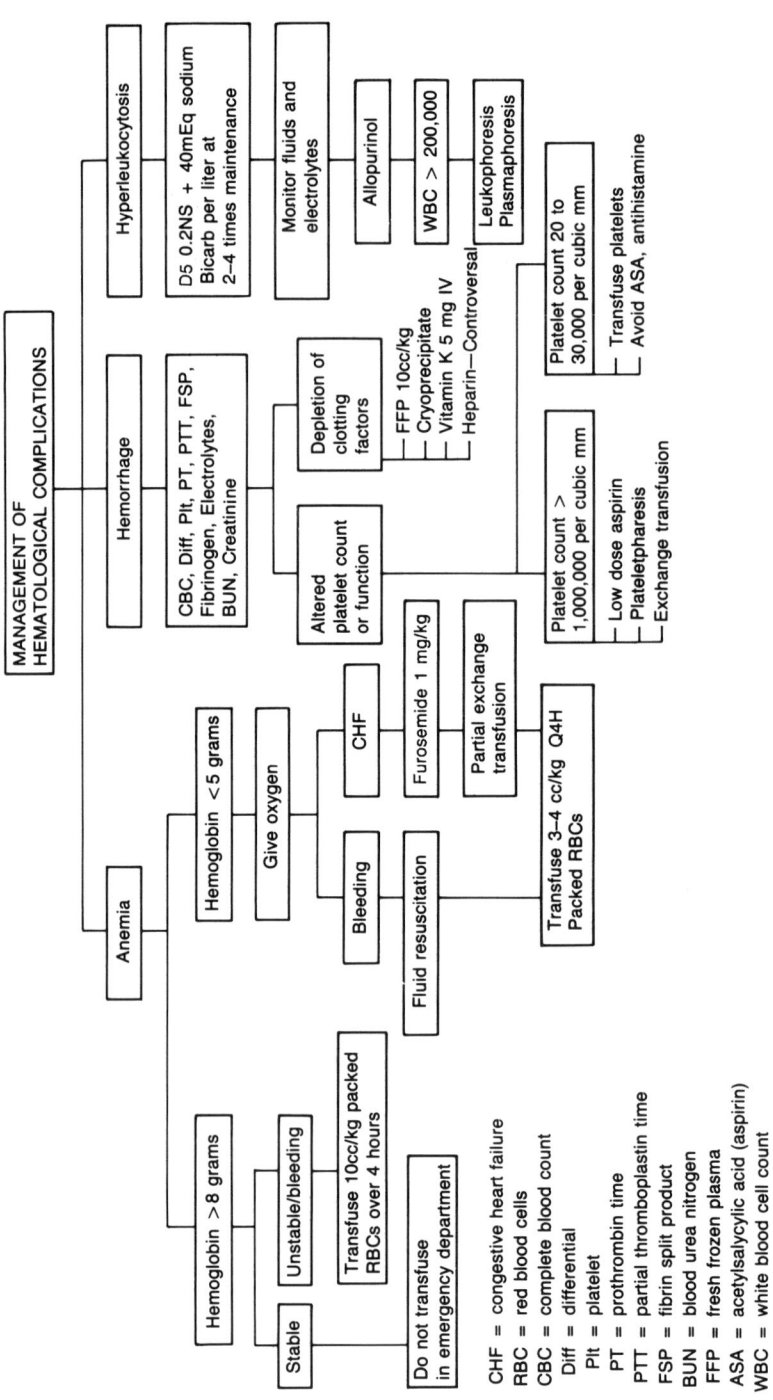

Figure 30.3 Management of hematologic complications in cancer patients.

Extreme thrombocytosis associated with Philadelphia chromosome positive acute myelogenous leukemia and following splenectomy, may cause severe hemorrhage or thrombosis. Treatment includes plateletpheresis or exchange transfusion.

Hemorrhage due to depletion of clotting factors may result from sepsis, acidosis, hypoxia, tissue factors released by tumor, or injury to normal tissue. In some patients with hypergranulocytic promyelocytic leukemia, a bleeding diathesis may occur at presentation or after initiation of therapy and may cause fatal central nervous system (CNS) bleeding in the first new days of illness. The laboratory studies of this condition show a picture of disseminated intravascular coagulation. The treatment includes fresh frozen plasma 10 ml/kg and cryoprecipitate to maintain the levels of clotting factors. The use of heparin in these situations is controversial. Vitamin K may also help by raising levels of factors II, VII, IX, and X. The dose of Vitamin K is 5 mg for infants and 10 mg for older children.

Hyperleukocytosis

Extreme leukocytosis occurs in about 5 percent of patients with acute leukemia at onset and during lymphoblastic crisis of chronic myelogenous leukemia. The lymphoblasts are exquisitely sensitive to chemotherapy, predisposing the patients to metabolic consequences of tumor lysis syndrome. The myeloblasts and monoblasts are rigid and sticky, which increase blood viscosity, leading to hemorrhage through weakened wall and thrombosis. Intracranial hemorrhage is the major cause of early death in patients with hyperleukocytosis. Pulmonary leukostasis may cause the symptoms of dyspnea, hypoxemia, right ventricular failure, and diffuse interstitial infiltrates on chest X-ray.

Immediate attention is recommended for patients with leukocyte count above 100,000/mm^3. Electrolyte and fluid status should be monitored closely. Dehydration must be corrected rapidly to decrease blood viscosity and to facilitate elimination of toxic metabolites. Red cell transfusions and diuretic therapy should be avoided as these measures increase the blood viscosity. In patients with white blood cell count (WBC) of more than 200,000/mm partial exchange or leukophoresis may lower the count, but does not alter the established areas of leukostasis (for treatment, see Figure 30.3).

INFECTIOUS COMPLICATIONS

Infectious complications have emerged as a major cause of morbidity and mortality in pediatric malignancies, and infection is the leading cause of death in leukemia. The following factors alter the defense mechanisms of cancer patients:

1. Alteration of mechanical barriers, (for example, mucosal ulcers due to methotrexate and insertion of Boviac-Hickman catheters for treatment)
2. Alteration of cell-mediated immunity
3. Alteration of humoral immunity due to splenectomy as in Hodgkin's disease
4. Alteration of neutrophil phagocytosis due to steroid use
5. Granulocytopenia, the single most important risk factor

Granulocytopenia is usually due to replacement of normal bone marrow by malignant cells or myelosuppression due to chemotherapy. Nearly all episodes of bacteremia and disseminated fungal infections occur in patients with absolute neutrophil count (ANC) of less than $500/mm^3$. The maximum risk of infection rises rapidly with an ANC of less than $100/mm^3$ and decreases sharply as the ANC reaches $1000/mm^3$.

Fever is defined as the occurrence of at least two temperature elevations over 38.4° C in 24 hours or a sustained temperature of more than 39° C for over 4 hours in the absence of an iatrogenic cause. The fever in granulocytopenic patient is usually from infectious causes, though it may be difficult to confirm. In about 20 percent of the patients, fever is due to noninfectious causes like the disease process itself or a blood transfusion.

Fever is difficult to evaluate in the neutropenic patient because of lack of an appropriate inflammatory response. The lungs, soft tissues (especially perirectal areas), and mucosal surfaces are the most frequent sites of serious infection. Careful head-to-toe examination including procedure sites (for example, bone marrow and venipuncture) is mandatory. For unknown reasons, meningitis is uncommon in granulocytopenic patients.

CBC, aerobic and anaerobic blood cultures, urine culture, chest X-ray, and renal and liver function tests should be obtained. Cultures from the infected site and cerebrospinal fluid (CSF) cultures should be obtained if indicated. Routine serial surveillance cultures should be obtained if indicated.

Fever in neutropenic patient is a life-threatening emergency. If proper antibiotic therapy is not instituted promptly, the infection disseminates very rapidly, leading to death in about 50 percent of patients in less than 24 hours. Empiric and broad-spectrum antibiotics should be started after expeditious and thorough evaluation in the emergency department. The choice of antibiotics varies from institution to institution, depending on local patterns of organism prevalence and resistance.

The most common infections in neutropenic patients arise from the patient's commensal flora, for example, *pseudomonas aeruginosa, E. coli, Enterobacteriaceae, Klebsiella, Staphylococcus aureus,* and *Staphylococcus epidermidis.* The antibiotic combination should be bactericidal and synergistic with gram-negative and gram-positive coverage. Most centers use the *triple drug regimen:*

1. Aminoglycoside-gentamicin or tobramycin 7.5 mg/kg/day IV (intravenous) every 8 hours
2. Oxacillin 200 mg/kg/day IV q 4 to 6 hours or Cephalothin 100 to 150 mg/kg/day IV every 6 hours
3. Antipseudomonal-carbenicillin or tricarcillin 300 to 400 mg/kg/day IV every 6 hours

If perirectal cellulitis is suspected, anaerobic coverage (for example, clindamycin 40 mg/kg/day) should be started. Antibiotic therapy with cefatazidime alone or in combination with amikacin has been shown to be comparable to triple drug regimen for microbiologically documented infection in neutropenic patients.

Septic shock is a major concern in a cancer patient. Bacteria, viruses, and fungi can all cause septic shock. Treatment consists of close monitoring of cardiovascular status, aggressive measures to maintain intravascular volume and blood pressure, and appropriate antibiotic therapy. Use of steroids in septic shock is controversial.

Viral Infections

Because of altered host defenses, the viral infections (for example, varicella and rubeola) can be disastrous in the cancer patient. The severity of illness is affected by the patient's age, immunity resulting from previous diseases or vaccine, and degree of immunosuppression. Pneumonia and encephalitis are major, life-threatening complications of measles and chicken pox.

A child exposed to varicella should receive varicella zoster immunoglobin (VZIG) within 72 hours of exposure. The dose is 0.1 ml/kg IM (intramuscular). The VZIG reduces the subsequent acquisition rate and decreases the severity of illness if varicella occurs.

If the patient develops varicella, the chemotherapy is withheld, and the patient is started on acyclovir 500 mg/m^2/dose IV every eight hours for seven days.

Exposure to rubeola should be treated with gamma globin 0.25 ml/kg IM. This provides some protection. Measles vaccine is contraindicated as is any other live virus vaccine.

METABOLIC EMERGENCIES
Tumor Lysis Syndrome

Tumor lysis syndrome is due to the rapid release of intracellular metabolites, resulting in hyperuricemia, hyperkalemia, hyperphosphatemia, and hypocalcemia. The quantities of these metabolites may exceed the excretory capacity of the kidneys, leading to renal failure. The syndrome is usually seen in patients who have large-cell burden of tumor or leukemia with hyperleukocytosis. Institution of chemotherapy or radiotherapy in these patients can precipitate fatal tumor lysis syndrome.

The rapid rise of potassium is the most dangerous abnormality and requires aggressive and prompt therapy. The patient should be put on a heart monitor and started on glucose, insulin, kayexalate, and renal dialysis if they are indicated.

Hyperuricemia should be treated with hydration at twice the maintenance rate and alkalinization of urine to pH above 6.5 to improve the dissolution for uric acid crystals.

Hyperphosphatemia requires hydration and diuretics. Calcium phosphate ($CaPO_4$) crystals become less soluble at a urine pH above six. Alkalinization should be discontinued in the face of severe hyperphosphatemia.

Symptomatic hypocalcemia may require calcium gluconate 100 to 200 mg/kg/dose IV. The patient should be put on a heart monitor to observe the effects of calcium administration closely.

Hypercalcemia

Hypercalcemia is a rare complication of childhood malignancy. This can be caused by an increased level of substances that cause increased bone turnover, osteolytic metastasis, or ectopic production of parahormone. The signs and symptoms include constipation, anorexia, nausea, vomiting, weakness, and, in severe cases, confusion and coma. An electrocardiogram (EKG) may show broad T-waves and a prolonged PR interval. Treatment consists of vigorous hydration followed by furosemide 1 mg/kg IV to maximize renal $Ca++$ excretion.

Syndrome of Inappropriate Secretion of Antidiuretic Hormone

The syndrome of inappropriate secretion of antidiuretic hormone SIADH is characterized by continuous release of antidiuretic hormone without any relation to plasma osmolality. It can occur because of CNS injury or disease, stress, and pain. The most common cause of SIADH in a cancer patient is either vincristine or cyclophosphamide. The vincristine is neurotoxic and has been shown to have a direct effect on supraoptic nuclei.

Treatment consists of fluid restriction if sodium is above 120 mEq/l and the patient is asymptomatic. If the patient is having seizures because of hyponatremia, combination furosemide and 3 percent sodium chloride should be administered.

GASTROINTESTINAL EMERGENCIES

Gastrointestinal emergencies in a cancer patient may arise from the esophagus to the perirectal area. The esophagus may be involved with candida or ulcers due to chemotherapy. The candida esophagitis may require administration of amphotericin B. The esophageal varices can present with severe life-threatening hemorrhage, which may be compounded by low levels of platelets and clotting factors. The esophageal varices usually result from hepatotoxic chemotherapy. Methotrexate may induce hepatic fibrosis.

The children with malignancy are prone to stress ulcers or Cushing's ulcers. These are commonly seen in children on corticosteroid therapy and in those with increased intracranial pressure. Treatment includes antacids, cimetidine, or newer H_2 blockers. If the child presents with hemorrhage, correct underlying abnormalities, and consider surgical management.

The small and large intestine may be affected by malignant process itself or by the effects of chemotherapy and radiotherapy.

Acute typhlitis caused by inflammation of ileocecal region presents with abdominal distention, right-sided abdominal pain, watery diarrhea, and fever. It is usually associated with neutropenia and thrombocytopenia. Most of these patients have recent histories of antibiotic use. The treatment includes bowel rest, nasogastric suction, broad spectrum antibiotics to cover against anaerobes, gram-negative organisms, and clostridium difficile. The surgical approach is indicated for perforation, severe bleeding, abscess formation and failure to improve with medical management.

The incidence of acute appendicitis in leukemia patients probably parallels the general population. In the past, cancer patients with appendicitis were treated with intensive medical therapy with disastrous results. The current approach is more optimistic and aggressive. Appropriate surgical management can be lifesaving. The steroids may mask the abdominal findings. Hence any degree of abdominal pain and tenderness in patients receiving steroids warrants that the diagnosis of acute peritonitis should be given serious consideration. The main differential diagnosis is acute typhlitis.

The perirectal abscess is usually seen in patients with neutropenia. Anorectal pain, tenderness, and discomfort with defecation indicate a perirectal abscess. The abscess may not be palpable, and only physical findings may be brawny, woody edema. It is usually caused by the mixtures of anaerobes or aerobes. Treatment includes sitz baths, broad spectrum antibiotics, and incision and drainage if there is abscess formation. Repeated rectal examinations should be avoided.

NEUROLOGIC EMERGENCIES

Encephalopathy in a cancer patient may be caused by disease itself, chemotherapy, or radiotherapy causing leukoencephalopathy and viral encephalitis. The child presents with altered mental status ranging from lethargy to coma usually six weeks after intrathecal methotrexate and craniospinal radiation. The diagnostic work-up includes CBC, serum glucose, electrolytes, hepatic and renal function tests, and coagulation profile. Emergency computerized axial tomography (CAT) may be required for definite diagnosis. If there are signs of increased intracranial pressure, IV dexamethasone 1 to 2 mg/kg and mannitol 1 to 2 gms/kg should be given. Seizures should be treated with appropriate anticonvulsants.

The spinal cord compression is due to the direct effect of tumor itself, either primary or metastatic. Other causes like radiation myelopathy, transverse myelitis, hematoma, and extradural abscess should be considered in differential diagnosis. Most patients present with back pain and tenderness to percussion. After complete neurologic evaluation, spinal radiographs, and CAT scan should be obtained. Recently magnetic resonance imaging (MRI) has proven useful in the evaluation of spinal cord diseases in children. Patients with severe progressive spinal cord dysfunction should be treated with dexamethasone 1 to 2 mg/kg IV. In patients with mild deficits, the dose of dexamethasone should be reduced to 0.25 to 1 mg/kg.

SUGGESTED READING

1. Albano EA, Pizzo PA. Infectious complications in childhood acute leukemias. Pediatric Clinics of North America 1988;35(4).
2. Allegretta GJ, Weisman SJ, Altman AJ. Oncologic emergencies I and II. Pediatric Clinics of North America 1985;32(3).
3. Azizkhan RG, Dudgeon OL, Buck JR, et al. Life threatening airway obstruction as a complication to the management of mediastinal masses in children. Pediatric Surgery 1985;20(6).
4. Barson WJ, Brady MT. Management of infections in children with cancer. Hematology/Oncology Clinics of North America 1987;1(4).
5. Jaffe D, Fleisher G, Grosflam J. Detection of cancer in the pediatric emergency department. Pediatric Emergency Care 1985;1(1).

6. Lange B, et al. Oncologic emergencies. In Pizzo PA, Poplack DG, eds. Principles and practice of pediatric oncology. Philadelpha: Lippincott, 1989.
7. Lange B, Halpern S. Oncologic emergencies. In Fleisher G, Ludwig S, eds. Pediatric emergency medicine. Baltimore: Williams & Wilkins, 1988.
8. Matthay KK. Oncologic disorders. Dieckman RA, ed. Pediatric emergency medicine. Moses and Grossman, 1991.
9. Maurer HS, Steinherz PG, Gaynon PS, et al. The effect of initial management of hyperleukocytosis on early complications and outcome of children with acute lymphoblastic leukemia. J Clinical Oncology 1988;6(9).
10. Schaller RT, Schaller JF. The acute abdomen in the immunologically compromised child. J Pediatric Surgery 1983;18(6).
11. Stellato TA, Shenk RR. Gastrointestinal emergencies in the oncology patient. Seminars in Oncology 1989;16(6).
12. Stokes DN. The tumor lysis syndrome—Intensive care aspects of pediatric oncology. Anaesthesia 1989;44.

PART XI

Miscellaneous

31

The Febrile Child under Two Years of Age

Roger Barkin

Infectious diseases represent a large number of encounters in the emergency department. Although many of these are self-limited and require support and recognition to institute appropriate therapy on an ambulatory basis, several of them do require immediate intervention to minimize morbidity and mortality. Children present unique challenges in that their clinical presentation varies by age as do the disease processes and the etiologic agents.

The febrile child, particularly the child under two years of age, presents unique challenges to the clinician. Over 10 percent of visits in this age group are for acute fevers. It is difficult to determine the etiology in the young child because of problems of obtaining a specific history and of defining physical findings.

Children are generally considered febrile when their rectal temperatures are 38.0° C (100.4° F) or higher. Oral temperatures greater than 37.6° C (99.7° F) are considered to be elevated. Although this figure is controversial, 37.3° C is defined as a febrile axillary value.

The *site* for temperature measurement must reflect proximity to major arteries, absence of inflammation, degree of precision required, safety, and insulation from external factors (drinking, and so forth). *Rectal* temperatures provide much more precision but obviously run the risk of rectal perforation and emotional trauma. Axillary temperatures are not practical in children under four years of age but are appropriate in thermostable environments or when absolute precision is not mandatory. Temperatures are not totally reliable in mildly febrile children (38–38.5° C). The oral, or sublingual, site is useful in cooperative older children who do not have rapid respiratory rates. The tympanic membrane has been used with great accuracy and reproducibility, using new technology that is increasingly available.

As temperatures rise above 40° C, the risk of meningitis increases. However, fevers higher than 42° C (107.6° F) usually are not infectious in origin (for example, central nervous system [CNS] involvement or heat stroke).

CLINICAL PRESENTATION

Historically parents usually report nonspecific observations related to behavior and associated signs and symptoms rather than those that permit an early focus on the involved system. It is particularly important, however, to define these alterations in behavior, activity, and eating habits and to determine if respiratory, gastrointestinal (GI), musculoskeletal, and dermatologic findings have developed. Urinary tract and CNS symptoms are reflected in changes in behavior, such as irritability and lethargy. Exposures to children with similar complaints are important to note as are recent events such as diphtheria and tetanus toxoids and pertussis vaccine (DTP) immunizations.

Early antipyretic therapy is imperative in facilitating observation. Many children who initially are irritable and disinterested in their environment will improve markedly with aggressive antipyretic management. Acetaminophen (15 mg/kg/dose *per os* [PO] or per rectum [PR]) should be administered to all children with temperatures higher than 38.5° C (101.3° F) on arrival in the clinic or emergency department to ensure optimal observation by reducing temperature and permitting a more accurate assessment of the child. Children with temperatures higher than 39.5° C (103° F) should also be sponged with tepid water. The response to antipyretics does not predict the prevalence of bacteremia.

The physical examination to assess responsiveness must be done systematically, focusing on careful observation of the child at play and encouraging the youngster to follow lights, bright objects, or a parent. Components of this overall assessment that are useful and reassuring include that the child

   Looks and focuses on the clinician and spontaneously explores the room
   Spontaneously makes sounds or talks in a playful manner
   Plays and reaches for objects
   Smiles and interacts with the parent or the practitioner
   Quiets easily when helped by parents

While the child is distracted with play objects, obvious physical abnormalities such as limitation of limb movement, rashes, and points of tenderness or pain should be defined. The chest, heart, and abdomen require a gentle hand and patience. Tachypnea disproportionate to fever must be carefully evaluated, usually by means of a

Table 31.1

Otitis media		36.9	Recognizable bacterial illness	9.4
Nonspecific illness		25.5	Bacteremia	6.1
Pneumonia		15.5	Cellulitis	0.9
			Meningitis	1.2
Recognizable viral syndrome		12.7	Urinary tract infection	0.6
Exanthem/enanthem	5.B		Other	0.6
Meningitis/encephalitis	3.6			
Gastroenteritis	1.8			
Croup	1.5			

Adapted from McCarthy PL. Controversies in pediatrics: What tests are indicated for the child under 2 with fever? Pediatr Rev 1979;1:51. Copyright American Academy of Pediatrics 1979. Reproduced with permission.

chest X-ray. Once these areas have been assessed, a full examination of the ears, throat, neck, and so forth is required.

In most children, the initial evaluation will define the cause of fever, and appropriate therapy can be initiated at the time of the assessment. With one group of children under 24 months of age who had acute onset of temperatures of 40° C (104° F) or over, the diagnostic categories and their relative percentages are presented in Table 31.1.

Routine laboratory considerations must include a complete blood count (CBC), urinalysis and urine culture, blood culture, lumbar puncture, and radiologic studies. These must obviously be individualized to reflect the findings of the physical examination and history.

SPECIFIC CLINICAL CIRCUMSTANCES
Infants under Two to Three Months of Age

A more extensive evaluation is required. The history is rarely more specific than the triad of fever, irritability, and poor feeding, and the physical examination may fail to reveal specific focal findings despite the presence of systemic infections, which may be enteric as well as the more common organisms infecting older children. Children under three months of age with a temperature higher than 38.5° C have a greater than 20-fold risk of having a serious infection than do older children with a similar temperature.

Prospective studies have demonstrated that clinical judgment is *not* useful in the assessment of the young febrile infant. There are no clear factors that are sensitive or specific to be relied on in decision making. Factors that have been most consistently associated with bacterial disease, however, include age under one month, history of lethargy, no contact with an ill person, breast feeding, polymorphonuclear neutrophil leukocyte (PMN) count greater than 10,000/mm^3, and band count over 500/mm^3. *No laboratory or historical factors should be used to exclude underlying bacterial infection.*

Children under two to three months of age with temperatures over 38° C (rectal) usually require blood cultures, urinalysis, and lumbar puncture unless they look remarkably well and close and frequent follow-up is absolute. Infants should generally be admitted and started on antibiotics (ampicillin 150 mg/kg/24-hr q 4 to 6 hr IV (intravenous) and gentamicin 5 mg/kg/24 hr q 8 hr IV or ampicillin, as above, and a third generation cephalosporin (cefotaxime: 150 mg/kg/24 hr q 6 hr IV, cefuroxime: 100–200 mg/kg/24 hr q 6 to 8 hr IV, *or* if the child is more than one month old, ceftriaxone: 50–100 mg/kg/24 hr q 12 hr IV). Treatment should be modified if a specific focus is detected or if cultures are positive.

Immunocompromised Children

Children with a history of recurrent serious bacterial infections should be evaluated for immunodeficiency. Children undergoing cancer chemotherapy or with a history of asplenia (congenital, traumatic, and so forth) are obviously at risk. Those with sickle cell disease have a 400-fold increased risk of pneumococcal septicemia if they are under five years of age and a 4-fold risk of *H. influenzae* septicemia if they are under nine years of age.

Such children require an aggressive and anticipatory approach to potential infections. A blood culture, ancillary tests, and early initiation of antibiotics is warranted.

Occult Bacteremia

Although bacteremia occurs in association with a host of clinical entities, including meningitis, arthritis, epiglottitis, cellulitis, pneumonia, and kidney infections, about six percent of febrile patients without a defined focus have positive blood cultures. Occult bacteremia is a significant problem in children, the high risk group being defined as

Age:	≤ 24 months
Fever:	≥ 39.4° C (102.9° F)
White blood cell count (WBC):	≥ 15,000 mm^3 (differential does not increase prognostic value)
Erythrocyte sedimentation dissociation (ESR):	≥ 30 mm/hr (difficult to use because of the length of time required to obtain a result)

It is essential to evaluate such children carefully to be certain that there is no underlying disease such a pneumonia or meningitis. There is no conclusive evidence that performing a lumbar puncture on a bacteremic child significantly increases the risk of subsequently developing meningitis.

Organisms that are frequently cultured include *Streptococcus pneumonia* and *Haemophilus influenza*. *Staphylococcus aureus* and *Neisseria meningitides* are less common pathogens. Children under two to three months of age may also have *Escherichia coli* and *Listeria monocytogenes*.

Children with occult bacteremia in whom a specific focus has been excluded are often started on antibiotics to produce an earlier clinical response and reduce potential complications.

MANAGEMENT

The management of the febrile child must reflect specific conditions that are diagnosed and those that must be considered in the differential diagnosis. Often the history and the physical examination may be useful. Laboratory studies may be confirmatory but often must await final culture results. In those patients in whom signs and symptoms are nonspecific, laboratory data is incomplete, and toxicity is present, anticipatory management is often warranted. An approach to such febrile children is outlined in Figure 31.1 and in the following guidelines.

1. Early antipyretic therapy will facilitate assessment. Previous antipyretic therapy requires a lower temperature threshold for imitating laboratory evaluation.

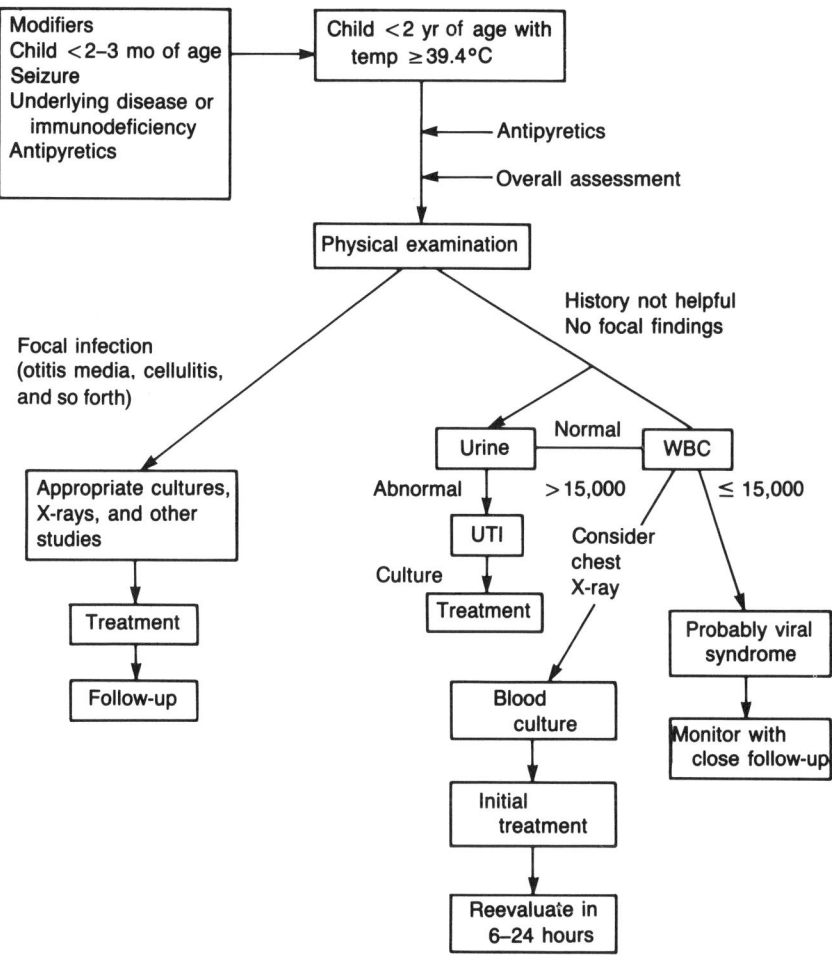

Figure 31.1 Evaluation of the febrile child under 2 years of age. Ceftriaxone 50 mg/kg/dose IM/IV; ampicillin 50–75 mg/kg/dose IM/IV; or amoxicillin 70–75 mg/kg/24 hr q 8 hr PO.

2. Underlying cardiac, pulmonary, neurologic, and immunodeficient (sickle cell, neoplasm, steroids, and so on) diseases require early evaluation and treatment, regardless of age and the height of fever.
3. Meningitis must be considered in any febrile child who has a seizure. Children 12 months of age and younger should have a spinal tap. A temperature of 41.1° C or higher is associated with a 10-percent incidence of meningitis in children under 2 years of age.
4. Children with fever and petechiae may have a viral illness, Rocky Mountain spotted fever, or invasive bacterial disease. Rapid intervention is required. Children with fever and petechiae who have a normal lumbar

puncture, WBC that is neither elevated nor decreased, normal absolute PMN and band count, and a temperature of less than 40° C have a reduced risk of bacterial infection.
5. If the temperature has been present for less than 24 hours, if the child looks well on the basis of overall assessment and is over six months old, and if no helpful history is detected, close follow-up for 6 to 12 hours may substitute for laboratory evaluation at the time of the first encounter. If the temperature remains elevated above 39.4° C at the follow-up appointment, evaluation should proceed.
6. Children with a WBC greater than 15,000 mm^3, from whom blood cultures have been obtained, may be treated with antibiotics with the potential of reducing complications. Alternative regimens include amoxicillin 50 to 100 mg/kg/24 hrs, ampicillin 50 mg/kg/dose IM (intramuscular), or ceftriaxone 150 mg/kg/24 hrs.
7. Follow-up is essential, usually in 6 to 12 hours, depending on clinical and logistic constraints.
   a. If the cultures remain negative, antibiotics may be stopped after 48 hours unless there was a specific focus initially or unless one develops. Follow-up until resolution of the illness is necessary.
   b. If the culture is positive, thereby documenting bacteremia, reexamination of the patient should determine treatment.
      (1) A patient who has a totally normal examination should continue taking high-dose antibiotics as an outpatient if daily contact can be maintained or as an inpatient if compliance is questionable. A total 10-day course is necessary. Most patients who have been treated initially will be improved on follow-up, but this does not preclude the importance of continuing antibiotics.
      (2) Febrile or toxic patients or those who develop a focus should be admitted for IV antibiotics and further evaluation. A total course of 10 days is necessary.

The febrile child under two years of age presents a unique challenge to the physician. The signs and symptoms are often nonspecific and the ancillary data is supportive of initial clinical impressions. Aggressive and anticipatory management is essential.

PARENTAL EDUCATION

Parental education is important in the management of the febrile infant. Obviously instructions are indicated in the management of the specific diagnosis entity, but additional information about fever control must be provided. This is of utmost importance in the initial assessment of the child and in addition may make the child more comfortable throughout the duration of the illness. Fever is a means of fighting infection, and the degree of fever does not always reflect the severity of illness.

1. Fever is a temperature over 100° F (37.8° C) orally or 100.4° F (38.0° C) rectally (Figure 31.1). If the fever is between 100° F and 101° F orally or rectally, the temperature should be taken again in one hour. Temperatures may be temporarily elevated from excess clothing or too much exercise. Oral temperatures can be raised by recently eaten warm food. Teething does not cause marked elevations of temperature.
2. Take the rectal temperature.
   a. Shake the thermometer down to below 97° F (36° C).
   b. Lubricate with Vaseline®, cold cream, or cold water.
   c. Gently insert the thermometer one-half inch into rectum. Often holding the child's stomach down on parent's lap is helpful.
   d. Leave in three minutes or until the silver line stops rising.
   e. Do not leave the child unattended. Hold the child still.
   f. Read by turning the sharp edge of the triangle toward you. Turn it slightly in each direction until you can see the end of the silver column.
   g. On the centigrade (Celsius) thermometer, each line is 0.1° C; on the Fahrenheit thermometer, each line 0.2° F. In unusual circumstances, auxiliary temperatures may be taken as a screen, holding the tip of thermometer under the dry armpit for four minutes. The elbow should be held against the chest. If the temperature is more than 99° F (37.2° C), recheck it by taking a rectal temperature.
3. Fever medication should be used if the temperature is above 101.5° F (38.6° C), if the child is very uncomfortable, or if any fever is present at bedtime. If the child is acting normally, fever medicines may be delayed until the temperature is 102.2° F (39.0° C).
   a. If the child is over three months of age, fever medicine should be given if the temperature is over 101.5° F (38.6° C). Acetaminophen (Tylenol or an equivalent) should be recommended every four to six hours.
   b. Do not recommend aspirin if the child has chickenpox or an influenza-like illness because of association between Reye's syndrome and aspirin.
4. Sponging is useful if the temperature remains over 104° F (40° C) after medicine. Recommend sponging or partially submerging your undressed child in lukewarm water (96–100° F). This can be done for 15 to 30 minutes as often as necessary. Some parents prefer laying the undressed child on a towel. If that is their preference another towel or washcloth soaked in lukewarm water should be placed on the child. The towel should be changed every 1 to 2 minutes for 15 to 30 minutes (1).
5. The child should be dressed lightly, and fluids should be pushed.
6. The physician should be called if
   a. The fever goes above 105° F (40.5° C)
   b. The fever lasts beyond 48 to 72 hours
   c. The child is under three months and has a rectal fever of over 104.4° F (38° C).

d. The child has a seizure (convulsion), abnormal movements of the face, arms, or legs; a stiff neck; purple spots; a fullness of the soft spot; looks sicker than expected; or develops difficulty breathing, burning on urination, decreased urination, abdominal pain; or marked change in behavior, consciousness, or activity.

SUGGESTED READING

1. Barkin RM, ed. Pediatric emergency medicine. Concepts and clinical practice. St. Louis: Mosby Yearbook, 1992.
2. Bell LM. Management of the febrile child under 2 years of age. In Barkin RM, ed. The emergently ill child. Rockville, Md.: Aspen Publishers, 1987.
3. Berkowitz CD. Assessment and management of the febrile infant under 2 months of age. In Barkin RM, ed. The emergently ill child. Rockville, Md.: Aspen Publishers, 1987.
4. Jaffe DM, Tanz RR, Davis AT, et al. Antibiotic administration to treat possible occult bacteremia in febrile children. New Eng J Med 1987;317:1175.
5. Lui CH, Lehan C, Speer ME, et al. Early detection of bacteremia in an outpatient clinic. Pediatrics 1985;75:827.
6. McCarthy PL. Controversies in pediatrics: What tests are indicated for the child under 2 with fever? Pediatr Rev 1979;1.
7. Powell KR, Mawhorter SD. Outpatient treatment of serious infections in infants and children with ceftriaxone. J Pediatr 1987;610:898.
8. Yamamoto LT, Wigder HN, Fligner DJ, et al. Relationship of bacteremia to antipyretic therapy in febrile children. Pediatr Emerg Care 1987;3:223.

32

Prehospital-Emergency Medical Services

George L. Foltin
Lou E. Romig

Physicians need to have an understanding of the structure and function of the emergency medical service (EMS) system that cares for their patients and to assure that the care delivered is appropriate for children. The elements essential for a well-functioning EMS system are contained within the components listed in Table 32.1. These include medical direction, prehospital transport agencies, interfacility transport agencies, dispatch, communications, protocols (for triage, treatment, transport, and transfer), receiving facilities, specialty care units, quality assurance, public education, and disaster management. The development of these essentials was a major goal of the Emergency Medical Services Act of 1973 (PL 93-154), which encouraged the growth of EMS systems nationally in the 1970s. Assuring that existing EMS systems have adequate resources to provide appropriate care to children has been the purpose of the emergency medical services for children (EMS-C) initiative which has existed since 1985.

THE PREHOSPITAL SETTING
Epidemiology

Children comprise approximately 30 percent of all patients who use emergency department facilities. In the prehospital setting, EMS systems report that from 3 percent to 5 percent of ambulance runs are for children under 12 years of age. In systems that consider patients to be pediatric up to 18 years of age, the number jumps to as high as 10 percent (1,2,3,4).

Problems that result in requests for ambulance usage are approximately 50–50 between medical and trauma in most systems that have reported pediatric epidemiology. When the figures are broken down by age, children over two years of age use ambulances predominantly for trauma-related problems. Vehicular injuries (including passenger and pedestrian- and bicycle-struck incidents) are the most common followed by falls and burns (5). The medical problems encountered by prehospital care providers in their pediatric patients are different than those encountered in adults. Cardiac-related problems are quite rare in children. Seizures, respiratory distress, near

Table 32.1 EMS systems components

Access and system entry   Patient and citizen education including prevention, bystander cardiopulmonary resuscitation (CPR) training, and how to gain access into the 911 system.

Prehospital care   Telephone triage, first response by bystanders, police, and fire. Treatment and transport by EMTs and paramedics. Triage decisions for specialty referrals such as trauma centers.

In-hospital emergency care   Resuscitation, stabilization, and admission or transfer to a higher level of care.

Definitive care   Pediatric intensive care unit, operating room.

Rehabilitation   Begins at the moment the patient enters the system. A crucial component to ensure a favorable outcome.

---

drowning, and poisonings are conditions the prehospital care providers will encounter (2,4) (Table 32.2).

Motor vehicle trauma is the number one killer of children. Several studies have suggested that a significant percentage of these deaths are preventable, pointing out the importance of organized pediatric trauma systems in which prehospital providers play a crucial role.

The Need for Pediatric Focus

The number of pediatric patients a given prehospital provider encounters yearly is dependent on the call volume of the EMS system and the demographics of the population served. Even prehospital providers who work in an urban setting may not handle more than two pediatric patients a week. The rural provider may receive a pediatric call as seldom as once a month. Overall, less than five percent of children transported by ambulance will have a life-threatening problem and less than one percent will be in full cardiopulmonary arrest (5,8).

Table 32.2 Common pediatric prehospital emergencies

Respiratory distress	*Status epilepticus*
Trauma to the airway	
Head injury with apnea	*Near drowning*
Upper airway obstruction	
Lower airway disease	*Poisoning*
Unconscious	Sudden infant death syndrome
Shock states	*Child abuse*
Dehydration	
Sepsis	
Hemorrhage	

On the other hand, a significant proportion of children transported by ambulance have potentially serious illnesses or injuries. A study at a Midwestern pediatric tertiary center demonstrated an eight-fold higher admission rate for children brought by ambulance as opposed to those arriving by other means. Of these 1 percent died in the emergency department and 14.4 percent required immediate operative or intensive care (3). Another study performed at a tertiary referral center in New York City demonstrated a five-fold admission rate for children who arrived by ambulance as opposed to those arriving by other means, and 36 percent of these patients required an advanced life support (ALS) decision in the prehospital setting (6).

The low encounter rate by prehospital providers to sick children results in problems for both emergency medical technicians (EMTs) and paramedics: (1) Hands on experience may be difficult to obtain; (2) skills that have been acquired for handling pediatric patients might deteriorate; and (3) there may be lack of confidence in ability to assess and treat a sick child (Table 32.3).

Training

Historically training for prehospital personnel has been deficient in pediatric emphasis with limited training on recognition, management, and equipment for use with children. The nature of field personnel's task requires that they make rapid, prioritized decisions based on protocols. The development of protocols designed especially for pediatrics is essential to enable prehospital personnel to provide appropriate care to children. Training and equipment needs will be defined by the scope of the protocols for both basic and advanced life-support providers.

Prehospital providers should be made aware that a large portion of their training about adults also applies to children. They merely need to be taught the unique pediatric knowledge base along with focus on the key differences in applying their

Table 32.3 Scope of practice for prehospital providers

EMT	Paramedic
100 hours of training	Minimum 600 hours of training
Deliver BLS	All EMT skills and can deliver ALS
BVM (bag-valve-mask) ventilation	Intubation
Airway adjuncts, oropharyngeal and nasopharyngeal airways	Establish vascular access
Suction devices	Deliver medications
Esophageal obturator airway (EOA)	Perform defibrillation
Deliver supplemental oxygen	Perform cricothyroidotomy
Immobilize the c-spine	Perform needle thoracostomy
Apply PASG (pneumatic antishock garment)	
Deliver first aid	
Defibrillate using an automatic defibrillator	

skills to children. Prehospital providers need to realize that they are expanding on previously learned material rather than learning a whole new field.

Many courses have been developed nationwide for both initial training and continuing medical education (CME) for prehospital providers at all levels. Many of these courses are valuable, and information about them can be obtained through publications such as the *Pediatric Resources For Prehospital Care* (7). The American Heart Association/American Academy of Pediatrics Pediatric Advanced Life Support (PALS) course has been successfully adapted for EMS providers in a number of centers (8). The national Department of Transportation (DOT) guidelines for initial EMT and paramedic training, which include a greater emphasis on caring for children, are currently under revision.

Some special considerations are airway/breathing, spinal immobilization, and circulatory and neurological compromise as is discussed in the next four sections.

Airway/Breathing

As formal pediatric EMS education becomes more available, prehospital personnel (both BLS and ALS) are being made aware of the vital role of adequate airway and ventilatory management in the child. One of the old myths, however, is that the pediatric airway is difficult to manage beyond bag-valve-mask and that paramedics should not perform advanced techniques such as intubation and needle thoracostomy. Some EMS systems in the United States allow paramedic intubation of adults but not of children. That attitude is slowly changing. ALS personnel are now learning these advanced techniques as they apply to children. Many students' experiences are limited to classroom sessions with mannequins. Some are learning on cadavers and anesthetized surgical patients. An increasing number are learning by intubating live animals in controlled laboratory settings or under the supervision of veterinary personnel in animal clinics and hospitals (9). As important as learning the skill, is the change in attitude that the training provides. The paramedic realizes that skills learned on adults can be applied to children with key differences. This may, very well, allow the field personnel to perform successfully on the relatively rare occasions when those skills are needed.

Although training in advanced airway and ventilatory skills is now available and emphasized, current educational programs are also emphasizing the basics. Paramedics are being taught to be aggressive but also to recognize when aggressive invasive techniques are not indicated. Children will often respond well to meticulous noninvasive intervention such as airway positioning, suctioning, and high-flow oxygen. Paramedics are learning that they may best serve the patient by settling for an adequate airway, rather than the definitive one. They are extending their understanding to encompass optimal airway management instead of merely immediate management. The well-trained medic recognizes that the rapid transport of a head-injured child undergoing good bag-valve-mask hyperventilation may represent better overall care than transport delayed for a potentially traumatic field intubation of the same trismic, combative patient. This approach serves as an example that prehospital personnel are capable of learning to recognize the fine lines between conservative management, aggressive intervention, and overtreatment in the pediatric EMS patient.

Spinal Immobilization

Spinal immobilization is a skill that all prehospital providers routinely provide to the adult patient but that they sometimes find difficult for the child. Faced with a multivictim auto crash, limited equipment, and a combative child with an obvious head injury, it may be difficult to immobilize a squirming child with only a Kendricks extrication device (KED) board, towel rolls, and tape and with no cervical collar. The indications to initiate spinal precautions for both children and adults are intuitively clear although they are little substantiated by research. Along with kinematic, physiological indications and medicolegal considerations, judgment must often be incorporated into the decision-making process. Medics should be allowed the opportunity to practice immobilizing infant mannequins to a back board, and key scenarios should be discussed. For example when faced with a scared, combative 18-month-old with no obvious injuries who just fell off a bed onto a hardwood floor and when knowing that the fight to immobilize the child may worsen any injuries, the paramedic's judgement may lead to transporting the child lying quietly on the stretcher in the parent's arms. On the other hand, severely injured small children should not be hand-carried but rather should be afforded the same rigorous immobilization as the adult passengers in the same vehicle crash would probably receive.

Circulatory Compromise

The clinical assessment of circulatory adequacy in the child is an art that can be taught. Those expert in pediatric assessment can teach prehospital personnel to assess mental status changes, heart rate, capillary refill, and pulse character rather than to rely solely on blood pressure measurements. After determining the patient's status, they must decide if and how they should intervene in the short time they have.

Rapid vascular access for severely ill and injured children has long been a point of frustration for prehospital personnel. Paramedics often are reluctant even to attempt intravenous (IV) access in a sick pediatric patient.

A recent development in pediatric EMS has been the general acceptance of intraosseous access. Studies have demonstrated paramedic intraosseous success rates of 80 percent, 85 percent, and 94 percent, respectively (10,11,12).

For many medics the mere availability of the technique has made them more comfortable and confident in dealing with the critically ill or injured child. As with respiratory management, emphasis on the relatively invasive intraosseous procedure is currently balanced by a move away from mandatory vascular access. The concept of *prophylactic IVs* is being discouraged for nontraumatized children, recognizing that the stress of IV insertion may compromise the patient's condition. Field personnel rarely need IV lines strictly for administration of medications. Most of the pediatric medications available to EMTs can be given by inhalant, subcutaneous, rectal, or endotracheal routes.

Since poor circulatory status is rarely of primary cardiac origin in children as opposed to that in adults, a paramedic should consider and address the possibilities of hypoxia, hypothermia, and increased intracranial pressure when managing a child with symptomatic bradycardia prior to using atropine therapy.

Rural versus urban considerations play an important role in deciding the need for vascular access. This translates into probable expected long transport times for the rural patient versus known short transport times in an urban setting. The difficulty in resource allocation occurs in that the pediatric patient, who is least likely to require vascular access due to a short transport (urban), is most likely to be transported by an ALS-capable medic since that is where the majority of them practice.

Neurological Compromise

Prehospital personnel often have difficulty evaluating the mental status of a child. The subtle early changes in mental status exhibited by children are often difficult to pick up, especially in situations where the child has valid psychological reasons to be scared, agitated, or irritable. Furthermore, the preverbal child cannot be examined using the customary adult mental status examination. As they are in regard to adults, the use of nonprecise terms such as *obtunded, comatose*, and *unresponsive* are open to interpretation and should not be used when communicating with medical control. Glasgow Coma Scale (GCS) scores cannot be applied to young children and the pediatric adaptations of the scores have not been validated.

Some EMS systems are now using the AVPU (alert, responsive to voice, responsive to pain, or unresponsive) system for radio or phone reports, which can easily be applied to children. The advantages of this system are that it is quick, easy to assess in all age groups, and involves no math. It can be used for serial evaluations since each category represents a theoretical increment in cortical function. The GCS score, however, still has its place and may be required on EMS report forms.

Seizures are a very common chief complaint among pediatric EMS patients and are frightening to both parents and field personnel. Paramedics are restricted in their choices of therapy; most services carry only diazepam or lorazepam. Until recently, they were also restricted to IV drug administration. Protocols for rectal drug administration are slowly being adopted and have been enthusiastically received by field and emergency department personnel alike. Since the pediatric patient is most likely to have had a febrile seizure, very commonly the patient will no longer be actively seizing. Paramedics must be taught that under no circumstances should they deliver an anticonvulsant to a patient who is not actively seizing. In addition, since the most common reason for respiratory depression in a child with status epilepticus is secondary to administration of a benzodiazipine, prehospital personnel must be trained and ready to manage the airway. Both paramedics and EMTs need to be taught that maintenance of a patent airway with sound BLS technique alone will result in a good outcome for the seizing pediatric patient. Furthermore the most harmful etiologies for reversible seizures are hypoglycemia, hypoxia and poisonings.

Access to Care

As was outlined in Table 32.1, education of parents and other caretakers of children in accessing EMS assistance is a critical part of a fully functioning EMS system. This includes prevention, which is far more effective and efficacious than care rendered after sudden injury. Important areas for lay public education are outlined in Table 32.4.

Table 32.4 Patient education for appropriate use of emergency medical services for children (EMSC)

Prevention (TIPP [the injury prevention program])
Post important phone numbers, 911, local emergency number, regional poison information center, physician's phone number
Teach children to dial 911 in an emergency
Encourage parents to take a first aid and a CPR course
Define when to access EMS versus when to contact the physician
Define when to contact the poison information center

The ideal setup for EMS-system access is through the use of *enhanced 911 (911e)*, which automatically supplies the address of the caller, improving the effectiveness of system response. Unfortunately many communities do not yet even have a 911 program in place. Calls to 911 are answered by a dispatcher who must trigger an EMS response and provide prearrival instructions to the caller. Only recently has attention been focused on the dispatcher's need for education in pediatrics (6).

THE HOSPITAL SETTING
Triage

The movement toward organized trauma systems has been accompanied by efforts to make transport decisions for all ages based on objective physiological and kinematic criteria either alone or in conjunction with on-line medical control. While efforts have focused mainly on adults, criteria (both research- and practice-based) have been developed for the field triage of pediatric trauma patients to pediatric trauma centers. The pediatric trauma score (13) is the most widely accepted single criterion but is not in widespread use.

All pediatric care is not equal. A facility that provides excellent care for adults may not be able to provide the same level of care for children. Most parts of the country do not have criteria for triage of sick, nontraumatized children. Facilities that excel in pediatric care are in place, but prehospital personnel may have to transport medical patients to the nearest facility. Systems loosely based on the trauma system concept are slowly being developed for pediatric medical patients. The prototype is a system developed in California (14). In this voluntary system, emergency departments criteria for staffing, educational, and equipment guidelines are outlined in order to be designated as *emergency department approved for pediatrics* (EDAP). These facilities act as primary receiving centers for pediatric patients. Patients may be transported directly or by transfer to a higher level of care, a pediatric critical care center (PCCC). These centers are also designated according to guidelines.

Medical Control/Protocol Development

Paramedics and EMTs are able to provide medical care in the field as "physician extenders." They act under the license and legal liability of a physician medical director or directors. Agencies and their medical directors develop written protocols—usually in cooperation with a voluntary advisory committee reflecting the medical opinion of local experts in EMS and emergency medicine—specifying actions that can and should be taken under clearly defined circumstances. These protocols act as standing orders and procedures legally authorized by the medical director. These constitute a form of indirect (off-line) medical control that in many systems is augmented by direct (on-line) medical direction by a physician or nurse. Most EMS services have adult-oriented protocols for both traumatic and medical incidents. Relatively few have specific pediatric protocols although this is rapidly changing.

Those with expertise in pediatric emergency care must be involved in EMS systems in both off-line and on-line medical control. This should include participation in supervisory and administrative aspects of protocol development and education.

REFERENCES

1. Tsai A, Kallsen G. Epidemiology of pediatric prehospital care. Ann Emerg Med 1987;16:284–292.
2. Johnston C, King W. Pediatric prehospital care in a southern regional emergency medical service system. Southern Medical Journal 1988;81(12):1473–1476.
3. Romig L. EMS utilization by the pediatric patient population of a midwestern metropolitan area. Ped Emerg Care (abs) 1988;4(4):297.
4. Seidel J, Hornbein M, Yoshiyama K, et al. Emergency medical services and the pediatric patient: Are the needs being met? Pediatrics 1984;73:769–772.
5. Seidel JS. EMS-C in urban and rural areas: The California experience. In Haller JA Jr, ed. Emergency medical services for children, Report of the ninety-seventh Ross conference on pediatric research, Columbia, Ohio, Ross Laboratories 1989;22–30.
6. Pon S, Foltin G, Tunik M, et al. Utilization of prehospital care by pediatric patients in New York City. Ped Emerg Care (abs) 1989;5(4):286.
7. Luten R, Foltin G, eds. Pediatric resources for prehospital care. Elks Grove, Ill.: Prehospital Care Committee, Section of Emergency Medicine, American Academy of Pediatrics, 1990.
8. Romig L. A pre-hospital modification of the AHA Pediatric Advanced Life Support course. Ped Emerg Care (abs) 1989;5(4):286.
9. Tunik M, Foltin G, Robinson G, et al. Teaching paramedics to intubate infants. Ped Emerg Care (abs) 1988;4(4):298.
10. Smith R, Keseg D, Manley L, et al. Intraosseous infusions by prehospital personnel in critically ill pediatric patients. Ann Emerg Med 1988;17(5):491–494.
11. Miner W, Corneli H, Bolte R, et al. Prehospital use of intraosseous infusion by paramedics. Pediatric Emergency Care 1989;5(1):5–7.
12. Seigler R, Tecklenburg F, Shealy R. Prehospital intraosseous infusion by emergency medical services personnel: A prospective study. Pediatrics 1989;84(1):173–177.
13. Tepas J, Mollitt D, Talbert J, et al. The pediatric trauma score as a predictor of injury severity in the injured child. J Ped Surg 1987;22:14–18.
14. Los Angeles Pediatric Society. The emergency department approved for pediatrics (EDAP), pediatric critical care center (PCCC) information manual. Los Angeles: Los Angeles Pediatric Society, American Academy of Pediatrics, and Los Angeles County Department of Health Services, 1984.

33

Child Abuse

Gwendolyn Gibson
Robert Block

Child abuse has been variably defined and classified. This chapter will focus on physical injuries to children that are likely to present to an emergency department. Physical abuse is any nonaccidental injury to a child caused by a parent or a caretaker. It includes beating, shaking, burning, poisoning, scalding, or other traumas. Children may also present with signs or symptoms of neglect. These may include failure to thrive (FTT), dehydration, starvation, and severe illness for which proper medical care has been ignored. Physicians must be constantly aware of abuse as a potential diagnosis and maintain a high index of suspicion especially when history given by a caretaker is inconsistent with physical findings. Unexplained or multiple trauma; trauma inconsistent with various age-related, alleged self- or sibling-inflicted, injuries; or excessive delay in seeking medical treatment should raise suspicions about abuse.

All states have mandatory reporting statutes requiring physicians and nurses to report all cases where abuse is suspected. It is not the physician's job to diagnose abuse independently but rather to report suspected abuse to the proper authorities (child welfare and in some states law enforcement) and to participate in a multidisciplinary investigation. It is critically important to recognize and report suspected abuse because children whose injuries are not recognized as abuse and who are inappropriately released to parents or caretakers may be abused again and again. Sometimes these children will reappear in the emergency department with severe, irreparable damage or death. Conversely physicians must not overzealously label all trauma to children as abuse. Parents should not be confronted in a hostile manner even if abuse is highly likely. Rather explain that state law mandates the reporting of certain medical findings, and the investigation usually can corroborate a history of accident if that is the true cause of the injury or condition. Because it is quite likely that medical records will be subpoenaed for juvenile, civil or criminal court action, documentation should be thorough, detailed, explicit, and legible. Photographs and drawings are often helpful.

Physical abuse is sometimes a single attack, more often it is a pattern of repeated behavior. Bruises and welts are the most frequent evidence of physical abuse. They can reflect the shape of the object used to hit a child and may be in various stages of healing. Typical sites for inflicted bruises are the buttocks and lower back (paddling), genital area and inner thighs, cheeks (slap marks), earlobe (pinch marks), upper lip and frenulum (forceful feeding), and the neck (choke marks).

Human bite marks leave distinctive, paired, crescentic bruises that contain individual teeth marks. The point-to-point distance between the center of the canines should be measured. A distance greater than three cm indicates the injury was inflicted by someone with permanent teeth.

Dating bruises can be an important part of the physical abuse evaluation (Table 33.1). Evaluation of bruises should include laboratory studies such as the PT (prothrombin time)/PTT (partial thromboplastin time), a bleeding time, and a platelet count.

Accidental bruises, certain skin disorders, and cultural practices may be mistaken for abuse. Accidental bruises usually occur over boney prominences. The most common sites in children are on the knees and shins. Bruises on the forehead of two-year-olds are not uncommon. Most falls produce a bruise on a single surface. Bruises over the soft parts of the body should raise suspicion. Common cultural beliefs such as *cao gio* (coining), an Asian practice of rubbing a coin on the back and chest to relieve fever, chills, and headaches, can be confused with abuse. A common skin condition often mistaken for bruising is Mongolian spots which occur in 95 percent of Black babies, 81 percent of Oriental and American Indian babies, 70 percent of Hispanic babies, and 10 percent of white babies. Other conditions mistaken for abuse are allergic shiners and *Haemophilus influenzae* periorbital cellulitis.

Child abuse is frequently the cause of *burns*, the fourth most frequent cause of death from all causes in children under 1 year of age and the third most frequent in children from 1 to 14 years of age. Scald or immersion burns are the most common cause of thermal injury to children who have been abused. They leave the characteristic stocking or glove pattern that is observed on the physical examination. A child can receive a full thickness burn in less than two seconds in water at 150° C. Contact burns are the second most frequent cause of abusive burns. Usually they result from contact with a hot metal object and can reflect the shape of the object. Cigarette burns are another type of contact burn and are round, isolated lesions with deep dermal injury.

A child who presents with multiple fractures at multiple sites and in various stages of healing should be presumed to be abused until it is proven otherwise (Figure 33.1). Osteogenesis imperfecta is, after all, a rare condition. Epiphyseal-metaphyseal injury is virtually diagnostic of physical abuse in an infant. An infant cannot generate enough force to fracture a bone at the epiphysis. To evaluate a child of any age for old

Table 33.1 Dating bruises

Age of Bruise	Appearance
0–2 days	Swollen, tender, bright red to blue
1–5 days	Red, blue, or purple
5–7 days	Green
7–10 days	Yellow
10–14 days	Yellow to brown
2–4 weeks	Clearing

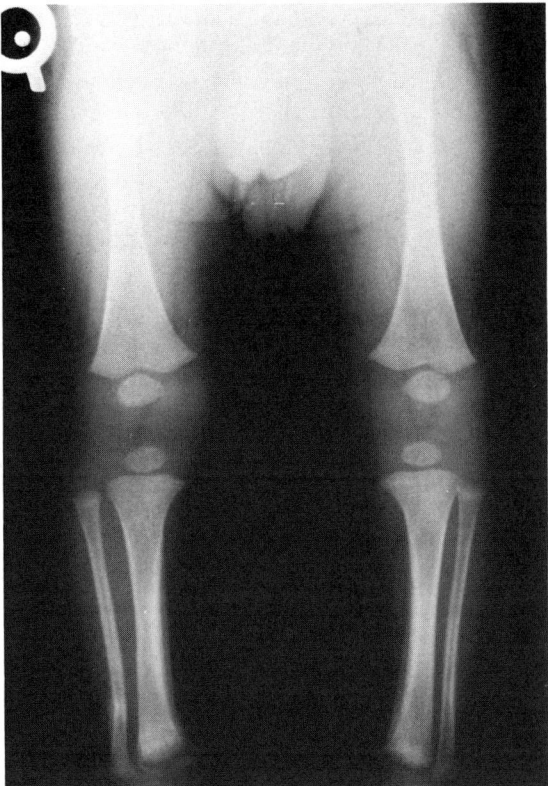

Figure 33.1 Child abuse showing old and new fractures. "Bucket handle" of distal tibia.

injuries, a skeletal survey is required. The study includes X-rays of the ribs, shoulder girdle, hips, spine, long bones, bones of the hands and feet, and skull. A complete skeletal survey should be done on all children less than two years of age who are possible abuse victims. Children older than two years generally don't need a skeletal survey unless there is localized tenderness on examination.

Abdominal injury is the second most common cause of death among battered children. A ruptured liver or spleen and intestinal perforation are the most common injuries. Most injuries are caused by a punch or kick that compresses the organ against the anterior spinal column. Unfortunately there are no visible bruises or marks on the abdomen in over half such cases. Therefore, a high index of suspicion is required in any abdominal crisis of undetermined etiology in a child.

Head injury is the most common cause of death from child abuse. Head injuries caused by abuse are the most common cause of cerebral palsy outside the neonatal period and a significant cause of mental retardation. Skull fractures should arouse suspicion of abuse when found in a child less than one year of age and probably less than two years of age.

In 1974, Caffey described a syndrome of severe central nervous system (CNS) injury and mental retardation in infants called the *shaken infant syndrome*. Shaking an infant or young child produces a whiplash injury to the brain. As the infant is shaken, the brain moves to and fro causing injury to the bridging vessels that leads to subdural hematoma or subarachnoid hemorrhage. Retinal hemorrhages and changes in sensorium are characteristic findings. There may be no bruises or signs of skull fracture to warn of CNS damage. Rib fractures where the child was squeezed during shaking may be present. These children may present with a clinical picture of sepsis, seizures, or nonspecific neurologic signs that, in infants less than six months of age, may only occur after considerable time has passed.

Other types of abuse that may present in an emergency department and that require a high index of suspicion are passive crack cocaine or marijuana inhalation and intentional poisoning. Munchausen syndrome by proxy describes the condition of a child whose illness is simulated and/or produced by a parent or caretaker who repeatedly presents a child for medical evaluation. Denial by the perpetrator of any

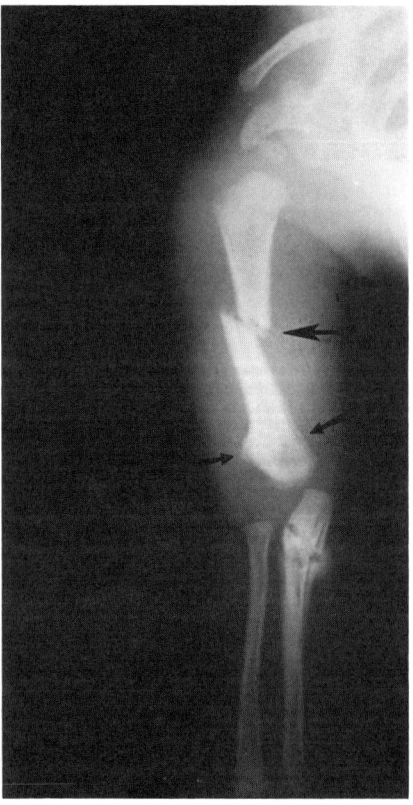

Figure 33.2 Child abuse showing periosteal elevation and spiral fracture.

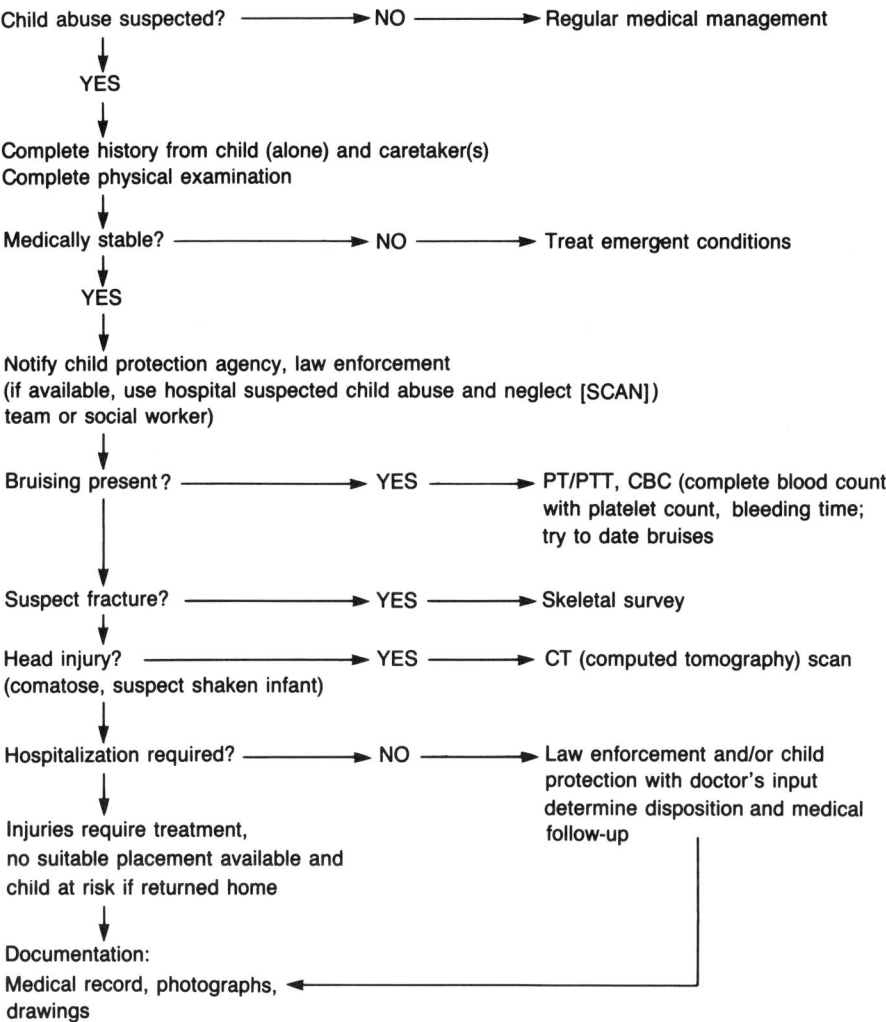

Figure 33.3 Physical child abuse decision tree.

knowledge of the etiology and quick resolution of symptoms when the child and perpetrator are separated are indicators of possible Munchausen by proxy.

CONCLUSION

The physical and psychological trauma to a child who has been abused or neglected can be severe. Children who survive may have long-term consequences of critical importance. Competence on the part of the physician who must suspect and recognize child abuse and participate with others to investigate and manage the case is vital. Correct action in a case of child abuse is every bit as important as it is in any significant childhood injury (Figures 33.2 and 33.3).

SUGGESTED READING

1. Caffey J. The Whiplash-shaken infant syndrome: Manual shaking by the extremities with whiplash-induced intracranial and intraocular bleedings, linked with residual permanent brain damage and mental retardation. Pediatrics 1974;54:396.
2. Helfer RE, Kempe R. The battered child, 4th ed, Chicago: University of Chicago Press, 1987.
3. Ludwig S, Kornberg A. Child abuse—a medical reference, 2d ed. New York: Churchill Livingstone, 1992.

34

Sexual Abuse

Gwendolyn Gibson
Robert Block

Child sexual abuse includes behaviors such as intercourse, sodomy, oral-genital stimulation, fondling, exhibitionism, and involving a child in prostitution or pornography. It may be a one time occurrence but often represents an abusive relationship spanning several years. Sex abuse has been defined as the engaging of a child in sexual activities that the child cannot comprehend for which the child is developmentally unprepared and cannot give informed consent and/or that violates the social and legal taboos of society.

The time of the last incident is important information that should be obtained on initial presentation of a child to an emergency facility for alleged sexual abuse. If the abuse occurred within 12 hours, the patient needs to be seen immediately because forensic evidence including sperm and acid phosphatase may still be present. If the incident is 12 to 48 hours old, some forensic evidence may still be present, and the child needs to be examined as soon as possible. If the incident occurred more than 72 hours prior to presentation, an appointment for evaluation can be scheduled in a more appropriate setting. An examination occurring within 72 hours of sexual assault should include forensic studies. Most centers have rape kits available, complete with instructions on how to collect specimens legally and medically correctly. A pediatric kit is recommended for children, but an adult kit can be modified for pediatric use.

Prior to the physical examination, time should be taken to obtain a history from the child, preferably interviewing the child away from the parents. An extensive history is not required from a child who has previously disclosed, but enough information should be obtained to aid the physician in medical assessment and treatment. Commonly a child will initially give a history of minimal sexual contact. In subsequent interviews, however, the child will disclose more detailed information regarding the abuse. Consequently thorough examinations need to be performed with any history of sexual abuse. The information should be carefully recorded, using the child's own words in quotation marks as often as possible. Care should be taken to avoid leading questions. It is not unusual after an initial disclosure for a child to recant the history. This may be due to several reasons. The child may have received pressure from others to recant, may have become fearful from being removed from home and family, or may be overwhelmed by the consequences of the disclosure. In any case, the child's initial history should not be discounted.

The primary goal of the genital examination is to identify and treat trauma and other sequela of abuse and to provide physical evidence of sexual abuse. Prior to the examination, it is important to establish rapport and to comfort the child with a thorough explanation of what is about to happen in order to minimize the perceived unpleasantness of the situation and to alleviate fear. Children are examined in the frog-leg position on the examination table. Young children can be examined lying in their mother's or in a trusted caretaker's lap while the adult sits or lies on the examination table. A prepubertal girl's genital anatomy is diagramed in Figure 34.1. It is essential to have an adequate strong light source and magnification for a proper examination. A colposcope is ideal but not necessary. A speculum is rarely necessary in evaluating a young child.

An acutely assaulted child or adolescent may demonstrate perineal swelling, lacerations or bruising and hymenal tears with bleeding and discharge. Physical signs of chronic abuse include a thickened, rolled hymenal border; attenuation of hymenal tissue; scarring; and discharge. Care must be taken in evaluating the size of the hymenal opening. It varies with age and the degree of relaxation of the child, the amount of labial traction used, and the shape of the hymen itself. Most often the physical examination will be normal, even with a history of penetration given by the child. Consequently a normal physical examination does not negate a history of sexual abuse.

The presence of sexually transmitted diseases beyond the neonatal period is uncommon in normal prepubescent children. Among sexually abused children

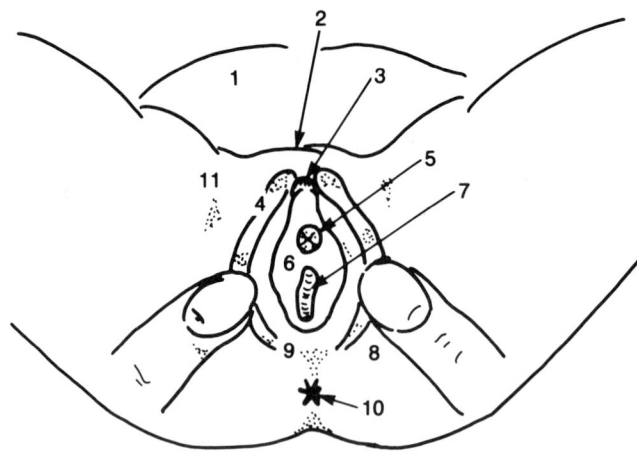

1. mons pubis
2. clitoral hood
3. clitoris (glans)
4. labia minora
5. urethral meatus
6. hymen
7. vagina
8. fossa navicularis
9. posterior fourchette
10. anus
11. labia majora (retracted)

Figure 34.1 Female child genital anatomy.

chlamydia is the most frequently isolated organism. In the evaluation of a child for sexual abuse, the incubation periods of organisms and the child's history must be taken into consideration. The American Academy of Pediatrics' Committee on Child Abuse and Neglect does not recommend routine cultures and screening of all sexually abused children. The positive yield of cultures is very low in asymptomatic prepubertal children, especially in those whose history indicates fondling only. The Centers for Disease Control (CDC) has slightly different guidelines, recommending cultures of all victims for Neisseria gonorrhea and chlamydia and a serologic test for syphilis. If cultures are obtained, they should include throat, vagina, and rectal sites. A chlamydia culture is required because nonculture or raped tests are inconclusive in children. The use of Dacron or Calgi swabs moistened with sterile nonbacteriostatic saline to obtain cultures or secretions is recommended. Calgi swabs may be toxic to herpes and chlamydia, and wood swabs are toxic to gonococcus.

Neisseria gonorrhea has an incubation period of 3 to 10 days. Vaginal infections due to gonorrhea may be asymptomatic in 44 percent of children, and pharyngeal infections are symptomatic in only 25 percent. Gram stain alone should not be used for diagnosis. Positive culture results should be confirmed by two methods, either biochemical, enzyme substrate, or serology. The presence of gonorrhea is indicative of sexual abuse.

Condyloma acuminata (venereal warts) has an incubation period of 1 to 20 months. The prolonged latency period makes identification of the source of infection difficult. There are over 50 known types of human papilloma virus responsible for condylomata. Genital types are 6, 11, 16, 18, 31, and 35. It is important that a biopsy and subtyping be performed prior to treatment to aid in identifying a source. The presence of condyloma in a child over two years of age should be considered sexual abuse until it is proven otherwise.

Trichomonas vaginalis is unusual in prepubertal children. Its incubation period may be as little as five days or as long as four weeks. A wet prep is only 50 percent sensitive. Most trichomonas infections in prepubertal children are a result of sexual abuse.

Herpes simplex virus Type 1 (HSV-1) may be spread nonsexually, but HSV-2 infection strongly suggests sexual transmission. The incubation period is 2 to 16 days with an average of 6 days. Lesions should be cultured and typed. A detailed history of HSV infection among parents and other contacts is very important. HSV in infants may be congenital or spread through nonsexual contact from an infected adult, but abuse should always be suspected.

Syphilis has an incubation period of approximately 3 weeks with a range of 10 to 90 days. In 1990, the consensus was for routine testing of abuse victims. Syphilis is a definite sign of sexual abuse if there are no indicators for perinatal infection.

Human immunodeficiency virus (HIV) infection presents a new challenge although the risk of transmission of HIV by abuse is small at present. If possible, serologic testing of the abuser should be performed. The CDC recommends screening children at the time of abuse with repeat testing 12 weeks later based on prevalence of infection or suspected risk (alleged perpetrator with a clinical profile of acquired immunodeficiency syndome/AIDS-related complex [AIDS/ARC] or behaviorally at risk) or at patient or parent insistence.

Certain conditions may be mistaken for sexual abuse. Lichen sclerosis et atrophicus and labial adhesions are two. Nonabusive causes of vulvovaginitis may be a foreign body, a chemical irritation, or infections such as β hemolytic streptococci, salmonella, shigella, yersinia, and candida. Gardnerella vaginalis is more common among children who have been sexually abused but is seen in nonabused children also.

When the clinician is examining boys for possible sexual abuse, the oropharynx should be carefully examined for signs of trauma and/or infection. The penis should be inspected for signs of trauma, and the urethra carefully inspected for inflammation, bleeding, or discharge. To examine the anus, the child is best placed in the lateral decubitus position. This is less threatening than knee-chest positioning and allows adequate visualization of the anus with gentle separation of the buttocks.

Evidence of abuse includes tears, abrasions, or scars of the anus; swelling; bleeding; discharge; or semen. In chronic anal penetration, anal sphincter tone may be relaxed and the skin and mucous membranes hypertrophied. Anal findings are very difficult to interpret, however, unless there is acute trauma, significant anal dilatation, or complete loss of anal tone. Circumferential bruising without trauma elsewhere on the buttocks (except for bruises from fingers) is often suggestive of anal assault.

Physicians who see children who have been abused may be called as expert witnesses in court. Although court appearances are often seen by some doctors as time-consuming, frustrating experiences, failure to perform this role with the same professional abilities as are used in the medical environment can result in an unjust outcome for the patient. Physicians asked in court for opinions, explanations, and conclusions, rather than merely a recitation of findings, will be qualified as experts. As such, they are entitled to fair reimbursement that should be discussed before the court appearance. A pretrial conference with the appropriate attorney is helpful to both the doctor and the lawyer. Most courts will respect a cooperating physician's busy schedule and will place doctors on call for a targeted time.

SUGGESTED READING

1. American Academy of Pediatrics, Committee on Child Abuse and Neglect. Guidelines for the evaluation of sexual abuse of children. Pediatrics, 1991;87;254.
2. Gellert GA, Durphee MJ, Berkowitz CD. Developing guidelines for HIV antibody testing among victims of pediatric sexual abuse. Child Abuse and Neglect 1990;14:9.
3. Herman-Giddens ME, Grothingham TE. Prepubertal female genitalia: Examination for evidence of sexual abuse. Pediatrics 1987;80:203.

PART XII

Environmental

35

Snakebite Poisoning

James S. Walker

Children are commonly bitten by animals. Very few animal bites sustained by children elicit more emotional response and parenteral concern, however, than do snakebites. Man's fear of, and adversarial relationship with, snakes have been propagated since Adam's and Eve's reptilian encounter in the Garden of Eden. Accordingly from many parents' standpoint, it seems that almost every snake is poisonous and that therefore every snakebite is life threatening. In reality, true life-threatening conditions as a result of venomous snakebites are quite rare. Nonetheless poisonous snakebites represent a true emergency to the physician from the vantage point that critical decisions must be made in a timely manner.

EPIDEMIOLOGY

From 1985 to 1990, the incidence of snakebites (both poisonous and nonpoisonous) reported by the American Association of Poison Control Centers (AAPCC) National Data Collection System has ranged from 2000 to 3000 bites per year (1–6). The reported incidence of indigenous poisonous snakebites for 1990 was 904 crotalid and 18 coral (1–6). Recognizing that all snake bites are not reported to the AAPCC, one can only speculate the true incidence of venomous and nonvenomous snakebites per year in the United States. One source estimates that at least 1000 additional venomous snakebites go unreported (7). Historically an estimate of 8000 venomous snakebites per year is quoted frequently in the literature (8). The number of mortalities from venomous snakebites is very low—ranging from 10 to 15 per year (7,9). According to the AAPCC statistics, however, there have been only 2 deaths reported in the United States from 1985 to 1990 as a result of indiginous poisonous snakebites (1–6). The few fatalities that are a result of poisonous snakebites are usually associated with a delay in treatment, direct intravenous (IV) injection of the venom or underlying disease (10,12). Pediatric patients do not have a higher case fatality or mortality rate than do adults (11,13).

The poisonous snakes indigenous to the United States are members of the family Crotalidae (pit viper) or the family Elapidae. The rattlesnake (*crotalus* species), water moccasin (*Agkistrodon piscivorus*), and copperhead (*Agkistrodon contoris*) are pit vipers and are responsible for 95 percent to 99 percent of venomous snake bites (1–6). These snakes have developed an infrared or head sensing structure (pit) located between the eye and nostril on either side of the head that facilitates tracking prey. The eastern and western diamondback rattlesnakes are the most dangerous species of the pit vipers. Rattlesnakes account for 65 percent of venomous snakebites (11). The coral snake is the only member of the Elapidae family in this country and along with imported exotic snakes, accounts for the remaining 1 percent to 5 percent of poisonous snakebites (1–6).

The states with highest bite rates are in the Southeastern and Southwestern United States. Specifically these top ten states include North Carolina, Texas, Arkansas, Mississippi, Louisiana, Arizona, New Mexico, Oklahoma, Florida, and Alabama (14). Furthermore, California and Georgia should not be completely forgotten (14). With respect to the delineation of the most frequently offending snake, one can generalize that the eastern diamondback rattler (*Crotalus adamanteus*) is the most dangerous species in the Southeast and that the western diamondback rattlesnake (*Crotalus atrox*) is the most dangerous species in the Southwest (14,20).

If a stereotypical illustration of a poisonous snakebite could be made, it would best depict the following scenario: The typical victim of a pit viper bite is a young male (age 11 to 19) who is bitten on the hand while trying to handle the snake (14,16). The incidence of pit viper bites is much higher in males than it is in females (4:1) (16). When females are bitten, they tend to sustain the bite to a lower extremity as compared to a male who has a propensity to be bitten on an upper extremity (16). Generally 67 percent of all pit viper bites tend to involve the hand and upper extremity and 33 percent the lower extremity (14,16). Furthermore one-half of all bites occur between 2 and 9 PM (14). Not surprisingly, many bites are associated with alcohol ingestion by the victim (14). The peak snakebite season is from April through October since snakes are poikilothermic and hibernate or are relatively inactive during the winter (14,16).

SNAKE IDENTIFICATION
Pit Vipers

The ability to identify whether the offending snake is venomous or nonvenomous is of paramount importance. This identification process, however, does not have to be made in great detail. Use the following adage in snake identification, "I don't know what it is, but I know what it is not." A review of simple taxonomy enabling the clinician to recognize pit vipers will be provided. One should never attempt to identify a pit viper by skin color or pattern. Furthermore, clinicians should be careful when handling these snakes, even when the snake is dead or appears dead, as a dead snake can cause a significant envenomation by means of postmortem reflexes (16). The care and caution to be used in handling a live snake are obvious. It is wise to have only experts handle live snakes.

There are six characteristics that are helpful in identifying a pit viper: (1) triangular-shaped head, (2) vertical elliptical pupils, (3) "pits" between the eyes and nostrils, (4) fangs, (5) rattles on the tail, and (6) a single row of subcaudal plates (10,17). From this list, it may appear that identifying a pit viper should be simple. This is not the case. There are many pitfalls in the identification process, especially if the clinician is unfamiliar with snakes. In some instances, the head will be mutilated beyond recognition or the snake will be decapitated. The single most diagnostic characteristic is the presence of a single row of subcaudal plates just distal to the anus (Figure 35.1). If the snake still cannot be identified, seek the assistance of a herpetologist. If the snake is not available, rely on the victim's companions or observers to describe the snake. This means of identification, however, can be misleading.

Coral

Two genera of poisonous coral snakes are found in the United States. They have round pupils, no facial pits, fixed fangs, and small heads. A distinguishing characteristic is the skin color and pattern. The coral snake has contiguous red and yellow rings with black rings. This unique color pattern gave rise to the mnemonic: "Red on yellow, kill a fellow; red on black, venom lack." The eastern corral snake (*Micrurus fulvius*) inhabits the southern United States from Florida to Texas. The Sonoran or Arizona coral snake (*Micrurioides euryxanthus*) is found in New Mexico and Arizona. Generally coral snakes are docile. They chew rather than bite because of their small mouths and fixed fangs (10,14).

PATHOPHYSIOLOGY OF ENVENOMATION
Location of the Bite

The location of the bite is of extreme clinical importance (18). Incidental injection of venom into an artery or vein greatly enhances the potential for systemic dissemination and subsequent systemic manifestations of envenomation (17). Commonly this may result in the victim's death. Bites to the head and faces are much more serious than bites sustained on an extremity. The localized edema associated with a head or facial bite often results in airway compromise (16,17,19). The need for a

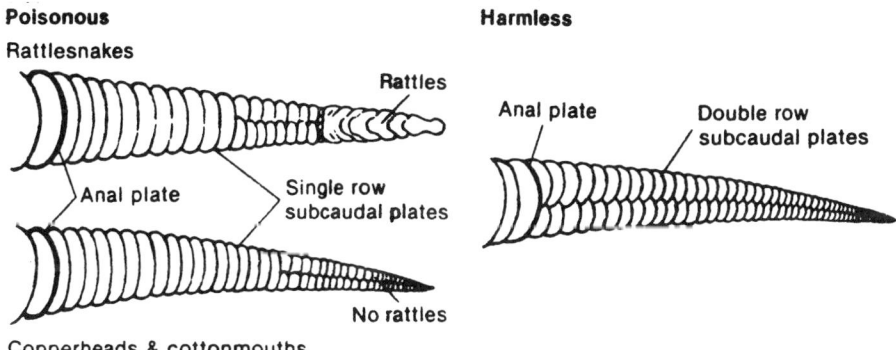

Figure 35.1 Helpful differentiating anatomical characteristic of pit viper. (Adapted from Wingert WA. A quick handbook on snakebites. Res Staff Physician 1977;5:59. Used with permission.)

surgical airway in the setting of a venom-induced coagulopathy is not without hazards. Bites on an upper extremity tend to have a worse prognosis than bites sustained to a lower extremity (17).

Venom

Snake venom represents a complex mixture of enzymes, large and small proteins, polypeptides, free amino acids, biogenic amines, lipids, metal ions, and other components yet to be identified. The function of this venom is to immobilize, kill, and digest prey (8,11). The potency of the venom and the amount of venom injected varies among species of snakes as well as among individual snakes. Individual variation occurs within the same species as a result of age, size, and time lapse from the last feeding. The venom of older snakes is thought to be less toxic than is that of younger snakes. The capacity or ability to deposit venom in the victim increases exponentially with the length of the snake. Furthermore venom composition may vary seasonally because of changes in feeding patterns or physiological changes such as hibernation (16,20).

Venom Composition

With respect to pit vipers, rattlesnake venom ($LD_{50} = 2.20$) is much more potent than the venom found in copperheads ($LD_{50} = 10.92$) and cottonmouths ($LD_{50} = 4.17$) (10). This difference in toxicity and potential for lethality can be attributed to the increased amounts of hyaluronidase; phospholipase; A,B,C,D proteases; L-amino acid oxidase; amino acid esters; thrombin-like enzymes; AT Pase; DNase; RNase; phosphodiesterase; and a host of other enzymes (10,16). It is apparent that the end result of a significant Crotalus envenomation is extensive local tissue destruction, intravascular coagulation fibrinolysis, hypovolemic shock, and death. Generally an envenomation by a cottonmouth or copperhead does not result in systemic manifestations and the localized reaction is much less than that of a rattlesnake (15).

Envenomation by a coral snake causes minimal localized tissue reaction, and the predominant systemic effect is a blockade of the neuromuscular transmission resulting in respiratory arrest. The venom of the Mojave rattlesnake (*Crotalus scutulatus*) is unique in that it, also, causes neuromuscular paralysis and has very little hemolytic activity (15,16).

Organ System Involvement

The primary target organs of a Crotalid envenomation are the blood, cardiovascular, musculoskeletal, respiratory, and central nervous systems. The treating physician must bear in mind that several organ systems may be affected from a single envenomation.

1. *Blood.* The previously mentioned small peptides, phospholipase, and thrombinlike enzymes interact to produce a consumptive coagulopathy or disseminated intravascular coagulation (DIC) syndrome as a result of intimal damage. Hemolysis and thrombocytopenia are also present. Spontaneous bleeding may occur in the lungs, kidneys, peritoneum, vagina, rectum, and other areas of the gastrointestinal (GI) tract. In general, the vascular endothelium and the clotting system are the two clinical aspects of envenomation (8,16,22).
2. *Cardiovascular.* The early cardiovascular collapse seen in a patient bitten by a rattlesnake is usually attributed to their hemolysis and vascular intimal damage. Serotonin and bradykinin release may contribute to the hypotension. Also some venoms have a direct cardiotoxic effect (8,16).
3. *Pulmonary.* Pulmonary edema may result from extravasation of proteins through damaged alveolar membranes (8,16).
4. *Renal.* Renal dysfunction can result from rhabdomyolysis, hypotension, and consumptive coagulopathy (8,16).
5. *Musculoskeletal.* Localized myonecrosis as well as subcutaneous hemorrhage and skin necrosis are commonly present. The myonecrosis may cause significant rhabdomyolysis and even development of a compartment syndrome in a extremity (8,16).
6. *Nervous.* Most rattlesnake envenomations have little effect on the nervous system. The venom of the Mojave rattlesnake, however, is neurotoxic by producing neuromuscular weakness and paralysis.

CLINICAL PRESENTATION OF ENVENOMATION

The signs and symptoms found after a crotalid envenomation are quite variable and nonspecific. It is important to remember that pit vipers rarely discharge the full content of their venom glands at a single bite. They may release a quantity of venom varying from none to almost the entire content of the gland. Many explanations for the amount of venom delivered are teleologic. The pertinent point is that 20 percent to 30 percent of all poisonous snakebites will have no envenomation (10). For the remaining 70 percent to 80 percent of the victims, the clinical effects are categorized into local and/or systemic.

The primary local manifestations of crotalid envenomation are edema and pain. The most consistent symptom associated with pit viper bites is an immediate burning pain in the area of the bite. The pain is out of proportion to that produced by a simple traumatic puncture wound. This is especially true for a bite made by the eastern and western diamondback rattlesnake. The next most common finding is the swelling or edema associated with and surrounding the bite. This edema initially is subcutaneous and may progress to involve the entire extremity. Petechiae, ecchymosis, and hemorrhagic bullae are other early local signs. The development of a compartment syndrome in an extremity is the most significant complication of a localized envenomation.

Many systemic symptoms, including weakness, nausea, fever, vomiting, sweating, perioral anesthesia, metallic taste in the mouth, muscle fasciculations, and hypotension, commonly occur after pit viper envenomation. Anaphylaxis and other types of allergic reactions to the snake venom have also been reported in individuals bitten on more than one occasion (23). Death from pit viper bites is usually a result of DIC, hypotension, or pulmonary edema. It is felt that cardiovascular and renal toxicity are secondary to the hypotension.

To facilitate the objective evaluation of pit viper envenomation, a graduation scale of envenomation was derived. The method of grading rattlesnake bites by numbers (grade 1, 2, 3, 4, or 5) on the basis of selected signs and symptoms is inadequate and confusing. Every finding should be taken into consideration when determining the severity of the envenomation. It is less perplexing to describe the envenomation in functional and physiologic terms like trivial, minimal, moderate, and severe (11).

Trivial envenomation. Manifestations remain confined to bite area. Puncture(s) are present. No localized edema or pain. No systemic signs or symptoms. No laboratory changes.

Minimal envenomation. Manifestations confined to area of bite with minimal edema, erythema, and pain immediately beyond that area. Perioral paresthesia may be present but no other systemic signs or symptoms. No laboratory changes.

Moderate envenomation. Manifestations extend beyond immediate bite area. Significant systemic signs and symptoms. Moderate laboratory changes.

Severe envenomation. Manifestations involve entire extremity or part. Serious systemic signs and symptoms. Very significant laboratory changes.

MANAGEMENT

Emergency department management of poisonous snakebites is filled with controversy and debate. There is no standard of care. Depending on the regional location, one can find camps of management that range from electric shock, cryotherapy, steroids, surgical excision, debridement, routine fasciotomy, antihistamines, cholinergics, or antivenin to just plain supportive care. Many alleged successful treatments are anecdotal or teleogical. Unfortunately very few of these treatment modalities are adequately supported by research. Consequently for valid recommendations for treatment, one should rely on the management strategies used by institutions that evaluate poisonous snakebites frequently. Such an institution is the University of Arizona. The following treatment protocol was derived by Doctors Richard Dart and John Sullivan at the University of Arizona (22,24). An algorithm illustrating emergency department management is shown in Figure 35.2.

Prehospital

I. The principle of management is rapid, safe transport to medical care.
   A. Rest

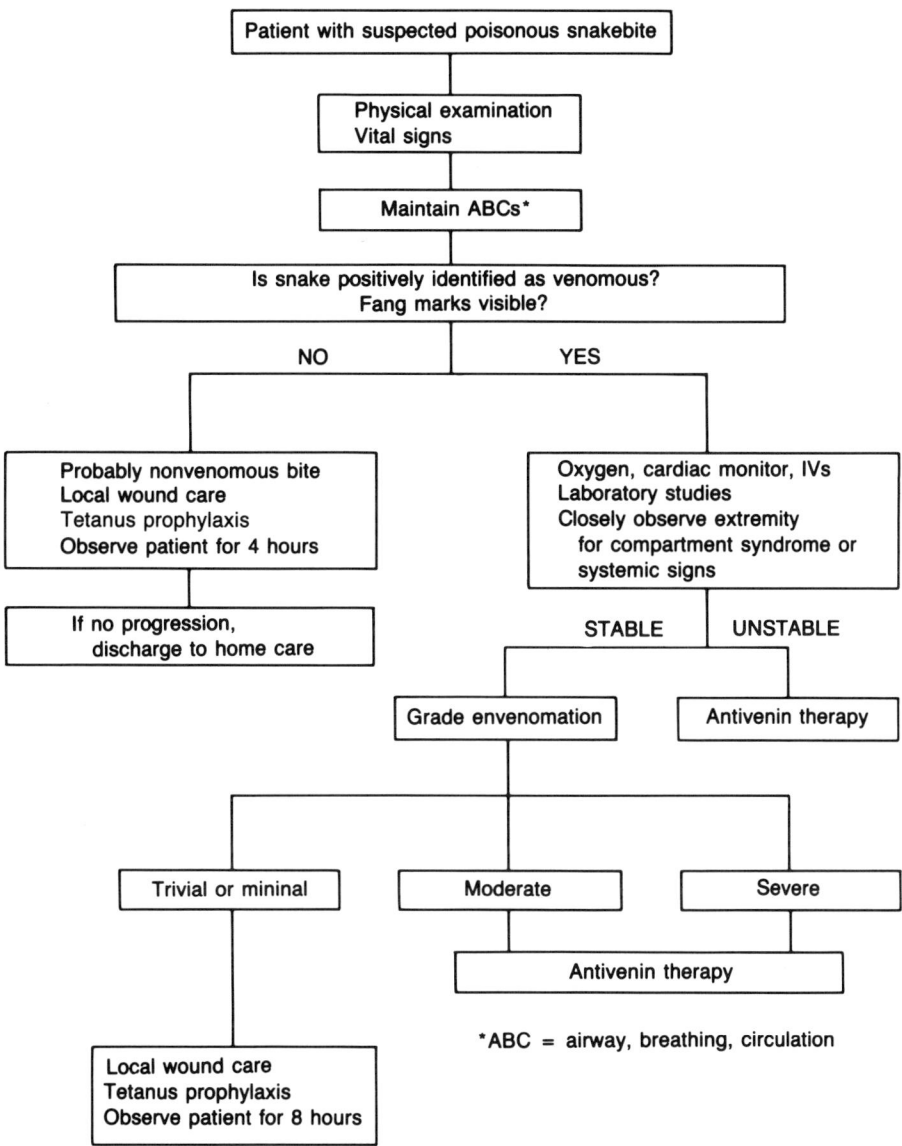

Figure 35.2 Management algorithm: Suspected poisonous snakebite. Adapted from Nelson BK (Medical Toxicol 1989;4:17–31) and Burgess JL, Dart RC (Ann Emerg Med 1991;20:795–801).

B. Immobilization
C. Constriction band (long transports)
D. Wound suction may be effective using new technology. A device called Extractor™ has been developed that can remove venom from the bite site. The complications and impact on envenomation have not been ascertained.
E. If a prehospital system is involved, place the patient on a cardiac monitor, administer oxygen, and start an IV line of normal saline. Maintain the bitten part at heart level.

Emergency Department

I. Distinguish among venomous, nonvenomous, or other animal bites, or plant-thorn injury.
II. Briefly determine where and when the injury occurred and under what conditions.
III. Establish a time and sequence of manifestations.
   A. Rattlesnakes, cottonmouth, and copperhead snakes
      1. Local
         a. May include punctures, pain, edema, erythema, bleeding, ecchymosis, and lymphangitis
         b. Any or all of these may be unapparent.
      2. Systemic: May include hypotension, weakness, sweating or chills, perioral and/or peripheral paresthesia, task changes, nausea and vomiting, and fasciculations. Coagulopathies and shock may occur in some envenomations
   B. Coral snakes
      1. Local: Minimal reaction, punctures may be obscure
      2. Systemic: May include drowsiness, weakness, dysphagia, dysphonia, diplopia, ptosis, headache, weakness, and respiratory distress
IV. Establish control of airway and breathing, and establish IV access.
V. Same as prehospital management for determining characteristics of bite and first aid measures. First aid measures rarely of use in emergency department setting.
VI. Grade of envenomation in pit viper bites: Varies with amount and kind of venom, when injected, and health of patient; in 10 percent to 25 percent of bites, no venom may be delivered. Grading of the bite is determined by the most severe symptom or sign (for example, a patient with no swelling but having a systolic blood pressure of 70 mm/Hg should be considered severely envenomated). Severity of envenomation may worsen with time.
   A. Trivial or minimal envenomation
      1. Manifestations remain confined to or around the bite area.
      2. No systemic symptoms and signs
      3. No laboratory changes

B. Moderate envenomation: Any one or combination of
   1. Manifestations extend beyond the immediate bite area but generally are less than the entire extremity.
   2. Significant systemic symptoms and signs
   3. Moderate laboratory changes; that is, decreased fibrinogen and platelets and hemoconcentration; mild coagulopathy.
C. Severe envenomation: Any one or combination of
   1. Manifestations involve the entire extremity or part.
   2. Serious systemic symptoms and signs
   3. Marked laboratory changes

Laboratory Tests

These tests should be repeated daily or as indicated for patient management. For moderate and severe envenomations, this usually means every 3 to 4 hours for at least 12 hours (Table 35.1).

I. Complete blood count (CBC)
II. Coagulation profile (prothrombin time [PT], partial thromboplastin time [PTT], fibrinogen, fibrin split products, platelet count)
III. Electrolytes, blood urea nitrogen [BUN], creatinine, glucose
IV. Creatinine phosphokinase (CPK)
V. Urinalysis
VI. Type, screen, and hold blood at time of admission if there is moderate or severe envenomation

Medical Treatment

I. Rattlesnakes, cottonmouth, and copperhead snakes
   A. Evaluate status of preadmission treatment
      1. If a tourniquet or a tight band has been placed, apply a less constricting band proximal to the tourniquet, start IV infusion of an isotonic crystalloid solution, and remove the tourniquet slowly.
      2. Determine drug and alcohol status.
   B. Start IV infusion of crystalloid solution (for example, lactated Ringers or sodium chloride). If shock or severe bleeding is present, consider albumin solutions or whole blood.

Table 35.1 Essential laboratory data in evaluating and managing poisonous snakebites.

CBC to include platelet count	PT, PTT
Urine Analysis (UA)	Serum fibrinogen, fibrin split products
Chemistry panel (to include BUN, creatinine, electrolytes, CPK)	Type, screen, and hold blood (packed red blood cells)

1. Consider use of antivenin.
2. Cleanse the wound.
3. Loosely immobilize and slightly elevate the affected part in a functional position.
4. Give tetanus prophylaxis if it is needed.
5. When the patient is stable, give appropriate analgesic if it is indicated.
6. Place the patient on a cardiac monitor.

C. Antivenin
1. Read the package insert.
2. Check allergy history, especially allergies to horse serum products.
3. Administer a skin test *if antivenin is indicated*, and keep epinephrine at the bedside.
   a. Never do the skin test unless it is certain that antivenin will be administered.
   b. A skin test consists of the intradermal injection of 0.02 ml of skin test solution provided with the antivenin by the manufacturer.
   c. If the skin test is positive (wheal or flare within 20 to 30 minutes), and antivenin is deemed necessary, request a consultation through the regional poison center. Antivenin may be administered in many cases despite a positive skin test.
4. Administer antivenin (crotalid) polyvalent IV initially at a slow rate and then at a faster rate (approximately 10 minutes per vial) if no reaction occurs.
   a. Minimal or trivial envenomation—no antivenin; moderate—5 to 10 vials; severe 10 to 30 vials.
   b. To administer, add 10 cc of normal saline to each vial. Mix by rolling between the hands, then dilute by injecting into normal saline IV bag (for example, 5 to 10 vials in 250 cc). Give it intravenously by continuous infusion. Reduce the volume of diluent in small children.
   c. Attempt to give the total dose during the first one to two hours.
   d. Use after 24 hours is currently limited to reversal of coagulopathy.
   e. In allergic patients, put five vials of antivenin in 500–1000 ml saline. Infuse solution very slowly in a patient pretreated with diphenhydramine 50 mg IV just before infusion. Have epinephrine at the bedside. Suggest poison center consultation before treatment.
   f. Guide to dosage of antivenin should include symptoms, signs, and laboratory tests. Measure the circumference of the involved part just proximal to the bite and 10 to 20 cm

above this point. Record vital signs every 15 minutes during antivenin administration and every 4 hours thereafter to document the progression of the edema. Also mark the border of edema progression.
   D. General recommendations
      1. Observe the snakebite patient for a minimum of 8 hours.
      2. Do not leave the patient unattended.
      3. Do not delay immediate or vigorous treatment, if the patient has a moderate or severe envenomation.
      4. The use of ice or other cold applications is discouraged.
      5. Do not apply a tourniquet.
      6. Do not use steroids as a primary treatment except in severe hypersensitivity reactions.
      7. Vasopressors should be used only to treat hypotension as short-term agents in severe hypersensitivity reactions.
      8. Heparin is generally not recommended for coagulopathies.
      9. Do not make incisions.
      10. Do not surgically explore for assessment of severity.
      11. Do not consider fasciotomy unless objective evidence of true compartment syndrome exists. Despite the usual presence of edema in crotalid bites, vascular compromise is rarely expected. Consider a trial of mannitol before fasciotomy.
      12. Consult a poison center for all bites (for informational purposes). In moderate to severe bites, allergic patients, or cases with complicating factors, ask to speak directly to toxicologist on call. The phone number for the Arizona Poison Control Center is (602) 626-6016.

COMMENTS ON ANTIVENIN

Antivenin has been reported to reduce the morbidity and mortality associated with pit viper envenomations despite the lack of randomized human trials (8). Uncontrolled series and case reports have supported the ideation that antivenin is effective in reversing coagulation defects (8). Furthermore similar evidence suggests that antivenin not only neutralizes but also reverses the localized manifestations of envenomation.

The administration of antivenin, however, is not without criticism or complication. The primary enigma of antivenin use is the development of a hypersensitivity reaction. In several studies, the incidence of an immediate hypersensitivity reaction (anaphylaxis) was 5 percent to 33 percent. The incidence of a delayed hypersensitivity reaction (serum sickness) was 36 percent to 75 percent. The Western Envenomation Database, a collaborative effort between the Section of Emergency Medicine of the University of Arizona and Arizona Poison and Drug Information Center, reports a 23.2 percent incidence of acute and a 62.0 percent incidence of delayed allergic reaction to antivenin (22).

It should be noted that the antivenin dosages should not be reduced in children as the amount of venom requiring neutralization is the same as it is in adults (8). As a consequence, the risks of hypersensitivity reactions are probably higher in children (8). Furthermore there does not appear to be a linear relationship between the dose of antivenin and the severity of serum sickness. It appears, however, that the potential for hypersensitivity is related to the methods of preparation, purification, and concentration of the antivenin (8). It should be recognized that the Wyeth antivenin (Crotalidae) is polyvalent as well as being extracted from horse serum. Accordingly one can discern such a high incidence of hypersensitivity reaction.

A better antivenin is badly needed. New antivenins are currently under investigation (25). Researchers at the University of Wisconsin are evaluating an antivenin extracted from egg yolk. Scientists at the University of Arizona are searching for a highly purified polyvalent antivenin (25). None of these preparations are universally available or clinically proven to be efficacious at this time.

CONCLUSION

The management of snakebites is quite controversial, even among experts. Many recommended procedures or measures have not been adequately supported by research. If treating physicians do not have much experience in the management of poisonous snakebites, they may rely on the advice and protocols of physicians who commonly treat snakebites. The preceding recommendations are listed in a succinct manner to facilitate execution. The important point is to individualize each victim's treatment strategy and not to approach it in a cookbook fashion.

REFERENCES

1. Litovitz TL, Norman SA, Veltri JC. 1985 Annual Report of the American Association of Poison Control Centers National Data Collection System. Am J Emerg Med 1986;4:427–458.
2. Litovitz TL, Martin TG, Schmitz BF. 1986 Annual Report of the American Association of Poison Control Centers National Data Collection System. Am J Emerg Med 1987;5:405–445.
3. Litovitz TL, Schmitz BF, Matyunas N, et al. 1987 Annual Report of the American Association of Poison Control Centers National Data Collection System. Am J Emerg Med 1988;6:479–515.
4. Litovitz TL, Schmitz BF, Holm KC. 1988 Annual Report of the American Association of Poison Control Centers National Data Collection System. Am J Emerg Med 1989;7:495–545.
5. Litovitz TL, Schmitz BF, Bailey KM. 1989 Annual Report of the American Association of Poison Control Centers National Data Collection System. Am J Emerg Med 1990;8:394–442.
6. Litovitz TL, Bailey KM, Schmitz BF, et al. 1990 Annual Report of the American Association of Poison Control Centers National Data Collection System. Am J Emerg Med 1991;9:461–509.
7. Russell FE. Snakebite. In Conn HF, ed. Current therapy 1968. Philadelphia: Saunders, 1968; 830–832.
8. Nelson BK. Snake envenomation: Incidence, clinical presentation and management. Med Toxicol 1989;4:17–31.
9. Russell FE. Snakebite venom poisoning in the United States. Annu Rev Med 1980;31:247–259.
10. Russell FE. Snake Venom Poisoning. Port Washington, N.Y.: Scholium International, 1983.

11. Russell FE. Snake venom poisoning. Vet Hum Toxicol 1991;33:584–586.
12. Parrish HM. Mortality from snakebites, United States 1950–1954. Public Health Rep 1966;72:1027–1030.
13. Parrish HM, Goldner JG, Silberg SL. Comparison between snakebites in children and adults. Pediatrics 1965;36:251–256.
14. Wingert WA. Poisoning by animal venoms. Top Emerg Med 1980;2:89–118.
15. Lindsey D. Pit viper envenomation: Controversy, change and current practice. Unpublished manuscript. 1989 and 1990 ACEP Wound Care Course.
16. Ellenhorn MF, Barceloux DG. Envenomations from bites and stings. In *Medical Toxicology; Diagnosis and Treatment of Human Poisoning*. New York: Elsevier, 1988; 1112–1132.
17. Podgorny G: Venomous reptiles and arthropods of the United States and Canada. In Haddad LM, Winchester JF, eds. *Clinical Management of Poisoning and Drug Overdose*. Philadelphia: Saunders, 1983; 275–301.
18. Wingert WA. A quick handbook on snakebites. Res Staff Physician 1977;5:59–62.
19. Gerkin R, Curry S, Vance M, et al. Life-threatening airway obstruction from rattlesnake bite to the tongue. Vet Hum Toxicol (Abs) 1986:28:487.
20. Gregory UM, Russell FE, Brewer JR, et al. Seasonal variation in rattlesnake venom proteins. Proc West Pharmacol Soc. 1984;27:233–236.
21. Clement JE, Pietrusko RG: Pit viper snake bite envenomation in the United States. Clin Toxicol 1979;14:515–538.
22. Burgess JL, Dart RC: Snake venom coagulopathy: Use and abuse of blood products in the treatment of pit viper envenomation. Ann Emerg Med 1991;20:795–801.
23. Hogan DE, Dire DJ. Anaphylactic shock secondary to rattlesnake bite. Ann Emerg Med 1990;19:814–816.
24. Dart RC, Sullivan JB: Management of poisonous snakebite. Unpublished manuscript. 1989 and 1990 ACEP Wound Care Course.
25. Sullivan JB. Past, present, and future immunotherapy of snake venom poisoning. Ann Emerg Med 1987;16:938–944.

36

Mammalian Bites

Steven C. Jackson

Over two million mammalian bites are reported annually in this country (1,2). One percent of all emergency department visits are for treatment of mammalian bite wounds. Annual health care cost for treatment of bites is over 30 million dollars (1,3,4). Children, because of their size, lack of caution, and aggressive play are more prone to bites than are adults. Bite wounds have a high incidence of disability, disfigurement, and infection. Deaths, though low in incidence, do occur directly or indirectly from mammalian bites. Education of children, parents, and pet owners can prevent many bites from occurring.

EPIDEMIOLOGY

It is estimated that there are 52 million dogs and 56 million cats kept as pets in this country. There are 2 million human and animal bites reported annually. Since many bites go unreported, the incidence is far greater. Over 50 percent of all mammalian bite wounds occur in children (2,3,4). Thirty percent of patients hospitalized for bites are children under 10 years old. Fifty percent of bites leave permanent disfiguring scars, and 30 percent of bites cause time lost from school (5,6). Children are most often bitten on the extremities. They have a higher percentage of bites to the face and head than do adults.

Most (75 percent to 80 percent) of all mammalian bites are from dogs and most commonly occur in boys during the summer months (2). The majority of dog bites occur near the dog's home. The dogs are usually known by the victim (2,5,6). Over 30 percent of dog bites are provoked, either intentionally or accidently.

Cats are the most popular pets in American households. Cats are the second most common cause of bite wounds, implicated in 20 percent to 25 percent of bites (7).

Human bite frequency is estimated at 3.6 percent of all bites. Human bites to children are common, making up 1 per 600 to 615 pediatric emergency department visits. The upper extremities in children are bitten 42 percent of the time and the head and neck 32 percent (8). Biting activity is highest in institutionalized children (9,10). Human bites to a child may be an indication of child abuse. Baker reported that 9 percent of human bites to children were the results of abuse (8,10).

PATHOPHYSIOLOGY

While the majority of mammalian bites are minor, serious injury can occur. The jaws of large dogs can exert pressure of between 200 and 400 pounds per square inch. These powerful jaws can crush and tear, creating extensive but rarely life-threatening injuries. An average of 10 deaths per year occur directly from dog attacks. Over 30 percent of all deaths occur in infants less than one year of age. Most of the remaining deaths are in children one to eight years old (5). These deaths result secondarily from hemorrhage and shock. Central nervous system (CNS) injury may occur when the infant's head is grabbed by the dog's powerful jaws. Extensive soft tissue injury often results in cosmetically disfiguring wounds. Injury to underlying bones, nerves, tendons, and blood vessels is frequent.

The most common and significant complication of animal and human bites is infection. All bite wounds are heavily contaminated with the oral bacteria flora of the animal or human biter. Crushed, devitalized tissue and anaerobic conditions create an ideal culture media for bacterial growth. Most wound infections consist of localized cellulitis or abscess. More serious infections include lymphangitis, tenosynovitis, osteomyelitis, septic arthritis, meningitis, brain abscess, endocarditis, fulminant sepsis with multiple organ failure, and death (11). The incidence of infection and the severity of infection depend on a number of factors. These include species of animal, location of bite, severity of injury, promptness of rendered effective treatment, and underlying medical condition of the victim.

Infection rates of mammalian bites vary among studies. The average reported infection rate is 11 percent to 12.5 percent (12,13). Puncture wounds and bites to the hand have the greatest risk of becoming infected (11,13,14). Bites to the face and scalp have a relatively low risk of infection. Dog bites become infected 4 percent to 18 percent of the time (12). Cat and human bites become infected more frequently than do dog bites (7,15). Cat bite infection ranges from 29 percent to 50 percent of the time (4,13). This higher infection rate for cat bites is secondary to the cat's long slender teeth causing deep punctures that close over and are difficult to clean. Estimates of infection rates for human bites are 9.3 percent to 50 percent (8,9). Human hand bites frequently become infected (25 percent to 58 percent) (8,9).

There have been a total of 208 organisms, 147 aerobes, and 61 anaerobes isolated from mammalian bite wounds (16). Common pathogens isolated from dog bite wounds are *Streptococci spp, Pasteurella multocida, Staphylococci aureus*, enterobacteria, and multiple anaerobes including *Bacteroides spp* (14,17,18). The oral flora of cats is similar to dogs with a higher percentage of *Pasteurella multocida* isolated (1). Common pathogens found in human bite wounds include *Staphylococci spp, streptococci spp, Eikenella corrodens, Hemophilus spp*, and anaerobes (1,3,17,19). The majority of bite wounds contain a mixture of numerous bacteria (3,14,17,19,20). There is an average of 2.8 bacterial species isolated from each animal bite and 5.8 bacterial species per human bite. There are a greater number of anaerobes in the human bite wound than there are in the animal. In over 50 percent of human bites, anaerobes can be isolated while the percentage drops to only 30 in animal bites (2,20,21). Most bites contain a high percentage of penicillin-resistant organisms (16,17,20).

Pasteurella multocida is a gram-negative coccobacillus found in the oral flora of many domestic and wild animals. This organism can be isolated from 20 percent to 50 percent of dog bites and 50 percent to 80 percent of cat bites (22). It is rarely transmitted to humans by cat scratches or by licking from a dog. *Pasteurella multocida* infection is characterized by a rapidly developing cellulitis (within 24 to 48 hours). A wide spectrum of serious infections can occur including osteomyelitis, septic arthritis, pneumonia, endocarditis, meningitis, and septicemia (21,22,23,24). Life-threatening infections occur primarily in young or immunocompromised individuals.

Capnocytophaga canimorsus (formerly Centers for Disease Control [CDC] Group DF-2) is a gram-negative bacteria found in the oral flora of dogs (25). Transmitted primarily from dog bites and rarely from cat bites, it is associated with a fulminant sepsis with a mortality of 27 percent. Serious disease occurs in immunocompromised individuals. Common risk factors are splenectomy, leukemia, steroid therapy, and chronic lung disease (25,26,27,28).

Other diseases transmitted from dog bites include rabies, tetanus, brucellosis, blastomycosis, leptospirosis, and mycobacteriosis (11). Cat bites can transmit rabies, tetanus, cat scratch fever, sporotrichosis, and tularemia (11,15,24). Diseases potentially transmitted by human bites include hepatitis B, syphilis, tuberculosis, actinomycosis, and human immunodeficiency virus (HIV) infection (1,4,29,30).

Since the 1950s, there has been a dramatic decline in the number of humans and domestic animals with rabies. The decrease is thought to be secondary to animal vaccinations and stray animal control (31). In the 1950's, eleven people per year died of rabies in the United States. Currently an average of 1 case of rabies per year is diagnosed. Most of these cases are contracted outside the United States. Cats are now the most common domestic animal to acquire rabies. In 1988, there were 192 rabid cats, 171 rabid cattle, and 128 rabid dogs. Wild animals account for 88 percent of rabies in this country. The most common rabid wild animals are skunks, raccoons, bats, and foxes (31).

DIAGNOSIS

A thorough history should be obtained on any child with a mammalian bite. Determine whether the child was bitten by an animal, another child, or an adult. For animal bites, information about the species and about whether the attack was provoked are essential. Determine the rabies vaccination status of the animal. It is important to determine the age of the bite wound and whether prehospital treatment was rendered. The child's underlying medical conditions and current medications, allergies, and immunization status must also be noted.

Perform a thorough physical exam. Examine each wound carefully. Bites often appear innocuous but prove to be more extensive on careful examination. Describe and diagram each wound, noting its location and type (that is, puncture, abrasion, laceration, or avulsion). A neurovascular examination, noting functional integrity, should be performed. All joints should be placed through passive and active ranges of motion. Look for signs of infections such as erythema, edema, tenderness, or presence of purulent drainage. Each wound should be explored, noting any foreign material and amount of crushed tissue. All lacerated tendons, nerves, and blood vessels should be identified. Fractures and joint violations must be noted. X-rays should be obtained on most bites to identify fractures, foreign bodies, or osteomyelitis. Bites to the hands should be X-rayed. Gram stain and culture all infected bite wounds.

Two areas to be especially careful in examining are bites to the hands and scalp. Bites to these areas have a high incidence of complications (1,3,30). A *clenched-fist* injury occurs during a fight when the fist strikes another person's mouth. The child may present with a small laceration or puncture wound over the fourth or fifth metacarpal phalangeal joint. The child may not admit to being involved in a fight. The tooth often lacerates the extensor tendon, fractures the bone, or enters the joint. This type of injury has the highest rate of complication of any bite with an infection rate of 50 percent (1,30).

Dog bite to the scalp should be examined carefully. The dog may grab the infant or small child's head and crush it between its powerful jaws. The dog's teeth may crush bone and even pierce the calvarium thus entering the brain (32,33). Often there is a depressed skull fracture underlying what at first looks like only a small scalp puncture. Skull X-rays and/or computed tomography (CT) of the head should be liberally ordered to detect any skull or CNS injury.

MANAGEMENT

All life-threatening bite wounds are treated by following the ABCs (airway, breathing, circulation) of trauma management. Fortunately most bite wounds are not life threatening and the child can be managed as an outpatient. Obtain early consultation with the appropriate specialist for extensive lacerations or bites to the hands. The goals in management of most bite wounds are to prevent infections, treat existing infection, prevent disfiguring scars, and avoid prolonged disability. Early appropriate treatment of bites reduces the infection rate. A number of studies have shown that those treated within eight hours have lower infection rates than do those who delay treatment (1,11,30,34).

The most important aspect of bite-wound treatment is meticulous wound cleansing and careful debridement. Copious wound irrigation markedly reduces wound infection rates. Wounds should be irrigated with one to two liters of sterile normal saline using a 20 to 35 ml syringe and a 19 to 20 gauge needle or intravenous (IV) catheter (1,11,12,13,35,36). Pressure (five to eight psi) created by this sized syringe and catheter is optimal for mechanical cleansing of bacteria and debris. Low pressure irrigation, that is, bulb syringe or soaking the wound, does not exert enough mechanical force to dislodge bacteria. Pressure greater than eight psi can damage tissues and spread bacteria deeper into tissues (37,38). The jet of saline should be directed at various angles to best loosen the bacteria and debris. Any devitalized tissue should be carefully debrided, and any adherent foreign material should be picked out. Puncture wounds are usually difficult to irrigate. If necessary, a thin rim of epidermis and dermis is trimmed (35).

The decision to close the wound depends on the age and the anatomical location of the wound, the type of bite (human or animal), and the type of wound, that is, puncture versus laceration.

In general, any extensively crushed, contaminated wound that cannot be adequately irrigated and debrided should be left open. Most wounds older than eight hours are left open, except dog bites to the face, which can be closed if they are less than 12 hours old (35). Most human and cat wounds should be left open (8,35,36). The exception may be a laceration to the face that is less than eight hours old. Bites to the hands should not be sutured (30,34,35). Puncture wounds should not be sutured. Most dog bites can be closed.

Wounds left open can be repaired by delayed closure in three to five days or left to heal by secondary intention. This method of repair is indicated for wounds with a high potential for infection. An indication for delayed primary closure would be a severe human bite laceration in a cosmetically important area. After irrigation, the wound is loosely packed with saline soaked gauze. In three to five days if the tissues appear healthy without signs of infection, the wound can be sutured and closed.

All bite wounds should be rechecked in 48 hours. Extremities with bite wounds should be splinted and kept elevated. Consider admitting to the hospital those patients who have open fractures or violation of a joint from the bite.

The use of prophylactic antibiotics is controversial. Most authorities recommend antibiotics for three to five days on all cat and human bites. All children with bites to the hands and feet should receive prophylactic antibiotics (12,39). Antibiotics should be prescribed if any underlying structures are injured. All immunocompromised children who are bitten should be started on antibiotics.

No single antibiotic covers all the pathogens found in mammalian bites. Amoxicillin/clavulanic acid covers most of the pathogens in human and animal bites and is recommended by most authorities (1,3,16,17,19,39). Erythromycin, sulfamethoxazole-trimethoprim, cephalexin, cefaclor, tetracycline, and dicloxacillin show poor activity against many of the common pathogens of mammalian bites (16,17,24). Tetracycline can be used for penicillin-allergic patients. Tetracycline is contraindicated, however, in children under eight years old. Erythromycin may be used in those cases.

Amoxicillin/clavulanic acid is recommended for empiric therapy of established infections. The dosage is 20 to 40 mg/kg/day; the higher dosage is used for the more extensive infections. Ticarcillin/clavulanic acid is a good choice for empiric therapy if IV therapy is required (3,6,35). Further antibiotic therapy should be guided by the wound culture results. The child should be immunized against tetanus and rabies as indicated (Tables 36.1, 36.2, and 36.3).

Most states require that dog bites be reported to the local health department. Suspected child abuse should be reported to the appropriate child protection agency.

PREVENTION

Preventive measures can reduce the number of children bitten each year. Children should be taught to respect animals. They should avoid situations where an animal may act aggressively and never approach a stray or unknown animal. They should avoid contact with a sleeping or eating dog. Children should avoid entering private property unless they are accompanied by the owner of that property. They should be taught not to run when they are approached by a potentially aggressive dog. Parents should never leave an infant or small child alone with a dog. Pet owners must

Table 36.1 Guide to tetanus prophylaxis in wound management

History of Tetanus Immunization (Doses)[a]	Clean Minor Wounds		All other	
	Td[b]	TIG	Td[b]	TIG[c]
Unknown	Yes	No	Yes	Yes
0–1	Yes	No	Yes	Yes
2	Yes	No	Yes	No
3 or more	No[d]	No	No[e]	No

[a]Including bite wounds
[b]For children less than 7 years of age, DTP (DT if pertussis vaccine is contraindicated). For persons 7 years or more of age, Td is preferred to tetanus toxoid alone.
[c]Tetanus immune globulin. The current recommended dose is 250 units intramuscular (IM). Td should be given at the same time but at a separate site.
[d]Yes, if more than 10 years since last dose.
[e]Yes, if more than 5 years since last dose.
Adapted from Immunization Practices Advisory Committee, MMWR 1990;39:39.

Table 36.2 Rabies postexposure treatment guide

Species of Animal	Condition of Animal	Treatment of exposed person
Dogs and cats	Healthy and available for 10 days of observation	No prophylaxis unless animal develops symptoms of rabies[a]
	Rabid or suspected rabid	RIG and HDCV[b]
	Unknown	Consult public health officials
Wild (skunks, racoons, bats, foxes, and other carnivores)	Regard as rabid unless geographic area is free of rabies or animal proven negative by laboratory tests[c]	RIG and HDCV
Other (livestock, rodents and lagomorphs)	Consider individually	Consult public health officials: bites of squirrels, rats, mice, other rodents, rabbits, hares almost never require antirabies prophylaxis

[a]Begin immunization at the first sign of rabies of dog or cat
[b]RIG = rabies immune globulin
  HDCV = human diploid cell rabies vaccine
[c]The animal should be killed and tested as soon as possible. Discontinue vaccine if immunofluorescence test results of the animal are negative
Adapted from Recommendations of the Immunization Practices Advisory Committee, MMWR 1991;40:4.

Table 36.3 Rabies postexposure prophylaxis schedule

Vaccination Status	Treatment Regimen[a]
Persons not previously vaccinated	Local wound cleaning
	RIG, 20 IU/Kg; one-half the dose infiltrated around the wound and the remainder IM
	HDCV 1.0 ml IM; one each on days 0, 3, 7, 14, 28
Previously vaccinated[b]	Local wound cleaning
	HDCV 1.0 ml IM on days 0 and 3; RIG should not be administered

[a] Applicable for all age groups, including children
[b] Prior postexposure vaccinations with HDCV or previous vaccinations with another type of rabies vaccine and documented positive antibody response to prior vaccination
Adapted from Recommendation of the Immunization Practices Advisory Committee, MMWR 1991;40:7.

take the responsibility of supervising, leashing, or confining their pets. Each community should have an effective animal control and rabies vaccination program. All animal bites should be investigated by the health department. Children should be taught never to bite. Children who are bitten should be treated early at an appropriate facility.

CONCLUSION

Mammalian bites are frequent and underemphasized, causing considerable disability and suffering in children. Bites often look deceptively innocuous but on close examination have extensive tissue destruction and injury to underlying anatomical structures. Infection is a common complication of mammalian bites.

The cornerstone of bite-wound management is early, meticulous wound care with gentle debridement and extensive saline irrigation. Prophylactic antibiotics should be prescribed for all human and cat bites, all bites involving the hands or feet, and those involving underlying anatomical structures. A full 10-day course of antibiotics should be prescribed for an established infection. Education of parents, children, and pet owners as well as effective animal control will prevent many bites from occurring.

REFERENCES

1. Goldstein EJ, Richwald GA. Human and animal bite wounds. Am Fam Physician 1987;36:101–109.
2. Harris D, Imperato PJ, Oken B. Dog bites—An unrecognized epidemic. Bull NY Acad Med 1974;50:981–1000.
3. Brook I. Human and animal bite infections. J Fam Practice 1989;28:713–718.

4. Rest JG, Goldstein EJ. Management of human and animal bite wounds. Emerg Med Clin North Am 1985;3:117–126.
5. Pinckney LE, Kennedy LA. Traumatic deaths from dog attacks in the United States. Pediatrics 1982;69:193–196.
6. Feder HM, Shanley JD, Barbera JA. Review of 59 patients hospitalized with animal bites. Pediatr Infect Dis J 1987;6:24–28.
7. Wright JC. Reported cat bites in Dallas: Characteristics of the cats, the victims and the attack events. Pub Health Rep 1990;105:420–424.
8. Baker MD, Moore SE. Human bites in children, a six-year experience. AJDC 1987;141:1285–1290.
9. Lindsey D, Christopher M, Hollenbach J, et al. Natural course of the human bite wound: Incidence of infection and complications in 434 bites and 803 lacerations in the same group of patients. J Trauma 1987;27:45–48.
10. Gold MH, Roenigk HH, Smith ES, et al. Human bite marks. Clin Pediatr 1989;28:329–331.
11. Goldstein EJ. Infectious complications and therapy of bite wounds. JAPMA 1989;79:486–491.
12. Callaham M. Prophylactic antibiotics in common dog bite wounds: A controlled study. Ann Emerg Med 1980;9:410–414.
13. Aghababian RV, Conte JE. Mammalian bite wounds. Ann Emerg Med 1980;9:79–83.
14. Ordog GJ. The bacteriology of dog bite wounds on initial presentation. Ann Emerg Med 1986;15:1324–1329.
15. Chretien JH, Garagus VF. Infections associated with pets. Am Fam Physician 1990;41:831–845.
16. Goldstein EJ, Citron DM. Comparative activities of cefuroxime, amoxicillin-clavulanic acid, ciprofloxacin, enoxacin, and ofloxacin against aerobic and anaerobic bacteria isolated from bite wounds. Antimicrob Agents Chemother 1988;32:1143–1148.
17. Brook I. Microbiology of human and animal bite wounds in children. Pediatr Infect Dis J 1987;6:29–32.
18. Goldstein EF, Citron DM, Vaguolgyi AE, et al. Susceptibility of bite wound bacteria to seven oral antimicrobial agents, including RN-985, a new erythromycin: Considerations in choosing empiric therapy. Antimicrob Agents Chemother 1986;29:556–559.
19. Goldstein EJ, Reinhardt JF, Murray PM, et al. Outpatient therapy of bite wounds—Demographic data, bacteriology, and a prospective, randomized trial of amoxicillin/clavulanic acid versus penicillin ± dicloxacillin. Int J Dermatol 1987;26:123–127.
20. Goldstein EF, Citron DM, Finegold SM. Role of anaerobic bacteria in bite-wound infections. Rev Infect Dis 1984;6:S177–S183.
21. Chapple CR, Fraser AN. *Pasteurella multocida* wound infections—A commonly unrecognized problem in the casualty department. Injury 1986;17:410–411.
22. Weber DJ, Wolfson JS, Swartz MN, et al. *Pasteurella multocida* infections—Report of 34 cases and review of the literature. Medicine 1984;63:133–154.
23. Kumar A, Devlin HR, Vellend H. *Pasteurella multocida* meningitis in an adult: Case report and review. Rev Infect Dis 1990;12:440–448.
24. Levin JM, Talan DA. Erythromycin failure with subsequent *Pasteurella multocida* meningitis and septic arthritis in a cat-bite victim. Ann Emerg Med 1990;19:1458–1461.
25. Brenner DJ, Hollis DG, Fanning GR, et al. *Capnocytophaga canimorsus sp.* nov. (Formerly CDC Group DF-2), a cause of septicemia following dog bite, and *C. Cynodegmi sp.* nov., a cause of localized wound infection following dog bite. J Clin Microbiol 1989;27:231–235.
26. Job L, Horman JT, Grigor JK, et al. Dysgonic Fermenter-2: A clinico-epidemiologic review. J Emerg Med 1989;7:185–192.
27. Hantson P, Gautier PE, Vekemans MC, et al. Fatal *Capnocytophaga canimorsus* septicemia in an previously healthy woman. Ann Emerg Med 1991;20:93–94.
28. Carpenter PD, Heppner BT, Grann JW. DF-2 bacteremia following cat bites—Report of two cases. Am J Med 1987;82:621–623.

29. Shirley LR, Ross SA. Risk of transmission of human immunodeficiency virus by bite of an infected toddler. J Pediatr 1989;114:425–427.
30. Mann RJ, Hoffeld TA, Farmer CB. Human bites of the hand: Twenty years of experience. J Hand Surg 1977;2:97–104.
31. Eng TR, Hamaker TA, Dobbins JG, et al. Rabies surveillance, United States, 1988. MMWR 1988;38:1–18.
32. Steinbok P, Flodmark O, Scheifele DW. Animal bites causing central nervous system injury in children—A report of three cases. Pediat Neurosci 1986;12:96–100.
33. Watson DW. Severe head injury from dog bites. Ann Emerg Med 1980;9:28–30.
34. Dreyfuss UY, Singer M. Human bites of the hand: A study of one hundred six patients. J Hand Surg 1985;10A:884–889.
35. Trott A. Care of mammalian bites. Pediatr Infect Dis J 1987;6:8–10.
36. Stucker FJ, Shaw GY, Boyd S, et al. Management of animal and human bites in the head and neck. Arch Otolaryngol Head Neck Surg 1990;116:789–793.
37. Stevenson TR, Thacker JG, Rodeheaver GT, et al. Cleansing the traumatic wound by high pressure syringe irrigation. JACEP 1976;5:17.
38. Wheeler CB, Rodeheaver GT, Thacker JG, et al. Side-effects of high pressure irrigation. Surg Gynecol Obstet 1976;243:775.
39. Brakenbury PH, Muwanga C. A comparative double blind study of amoxicillin/clavulanate vs placebo in the prevention of infection after animal bites. Arch Emerg Med 1989;6:251–256.

37

Hypothermia

Steven C. Jackson

Hypothermia is defined as a core temperature of 35° C and below. Accidental hypothermia is an important and underdiagnosed cause of morbidity and mortality in children. The incidence of hypothermia is increasing (1). It occurs from exposure of healthy children to a cold environment or can complicate various disease states. Infants are especially vulnerable to hypothermia because of a relatively large surface area, low subcutaneous fat, and immature thermal regulation. The increase in outdoor activities during cold winter months has increased the incidence in older children. Children's inexperience and general lack of caution make them frequent victims of exposure.

PHYSIOLOGY

The body's temperature is maintained at 37° C by a balance of heat production and heat loss. Body heat is preserved by heat conservation and heat generated by cell metabolism. When the body's core temperature falls below 37° C, compensating physiologic mechanisms are activated. The hypothalamus is the primary thermoregulating structure in our body. The anterior hypothalamus detects changes in body temperature and the posterior hypothalamus directs physiologic responses to these changes (2). Stimulation of the sympathetic nervous system causes vasoconstriction limiting heat loss. It also causes an increase in muscle tone thereby doubling heat production. If the body continues to cool, muscles will shiver, increasing thermogenesis 5 times. The hypothalamus also stimulates the endocrine system, increasing the metabolic rate and heat production. One of the body's most important adaptations to cold is behavior modification. That is, steps are taken to get out of the cold and to put on warm clothes. The increase in voluntary muscular activity can increase heat production 25 times. Neonates cannot shiver. They conserve heat by vasoconstriction and generate heat by lipolysis of specialized tissue called brown fat (3).

The body loses heat by four mechanisms: radiation, conduction, convection, and evaporation (2). The amount of heat loss from each is dependent on weather conditions, body size, and protective insulation (subcutaneous fat, clothes). Radiation is the transfer of heat from the body to the environment by electromagnetic waves (infrared heat rays). The amount of heat lost by radiation depends on the amount of exposed body surface as well as on the ambient temperature. At an ambient temperature of 20° C (68° F) up to 60 percent to 70 percent of body heat is lost by radiation.

The percentage in an infant may even be larger. An infant's exposed head loses up to 50 percent of body heat at an ambient temperature of 9° C (39° F). Conduction is the transfer of heat from direct contact of the body with other objects. It normally accounts for 2 percent to 3 percent of body heat loss but will increase 20 to 30 times when the body is submerged in cold water. Convection is heat lost into moving air. Heat lost by convection increases on cold, windy days and decreases with insulating clothes. Heat lost by convection is usually 10 percent to 12 percent. Evaporation accounts for 20 percent to 25 percent of the body's total heat loss on a cold day. Five hundred and eighty calories are lost for each gram of water that evaporates from the skin or respiratory tract (2). On cold days most evaporatory heat loss occurs from respiration and insensible water loss from the skin. Wet newborns in the delivery room rapidly lose heat by evaporation.

PATHOPHYSIOLOGY

The pathophysiology of hypothermia is related to the degree of core temperature lowering (4). Hypothermia can be divided into three stages: mild (35° to 33° C), moderate (32° to 29° C), and severe (less than 29° C). As was previously noted, the initial stage of hypothermia is excitatory. The basal metabolic rate increases along with heart rate, respiratory rate, and blood pressure. At 32° C bodily functions begin to slow. Basal metabolic rate begins to drop 10 percent for each degree centigrade core temperature lowering. Oxygen consumption also declines, becoming 50 percent at 30° C and 20 percent of normal at 20° C (Table 37.1).

As the body cools below 32° C there is a depressant effect on cardiovascular function. The conductive system of the heart is effected to a greater degree than is the myocardium. Hypothermia causes widening of the QRS and prolongs the PR and QT

Table 37.1 Temperature and pathophysiology correlation in hypothermia

| Core Temperature | | Pathophysiologic Changes |
°C	°F	
37.6	99.6	Normal rectal temperature
35	95	Metabolic rate increases, vasoconstriction, shivering maximal
34	93.2	Blood pressure, heart rate, respiratory rate increased
33	91.4	Confusion, ataxia, slurred speech
32	89.6	Stupor, decreasing oxygen consumption
31	87.6	Heart rate, blood pressure, respiratory rate decreases
30	86	Shivering stops
29	85.2	Atrial fibrillation
28	82.4	Increased risk of ventricular fibrillation, basal metabolic rate 50 percent
27	80.6	Unconscious
26	78.8	Deep tendon reflexes (DTRs) absent
23	73.4	Pupils fixed and dilated
20	68	Asystole, flat EEG

interval. Bradycardia and atrial arrhythmias are commonly seen. Ventricular fibrillation can be precipitated at core temperatures below 29° C (4).

There is a progressive slowing of nerve conduction (5,6). This initially appears as confusion, ataxia, clumsiness, and slurred speech and progresses to deep coma. Shivering, prominent in mild hypothermia ceases at lower core temperatures. Depressed brain-stem function further decreases heart rate, blood pressure, and respiratory rate. Most neurologic reflexes are absent below 27° C, and the victim is usually unconscious at 26° C. Pupils are fixed and dilated at 23° C. The person appears dead. The electroencephalogram (EEG) becomes flat at 20° C (4).

Hypothermia causes a cold diuresis by the kidneys. This diuresis of dilute urine can increase urine output three times. The concentrating ability of the kidneys is diminished from a decreased responsiveness to antidiuretic hormone (ADH) and a loss of distal tubular absorptive function (5). Nitrogenous waste, endogenous acids as well as exogenous drugs, will accumulate as kidney function decreases.

The respiratory system also slows after the core temperature falls below 32° C. The respiratory rate and minute volume declines. The cough reflex is lost and noncardiogenic pulmonary edema may develop. Respiration ceases at 24° C.

Cooling causes gastric dilatation and a paralytic ileus. Hepatic metabolism gradually declines, including detoxification of drugs. Pancreatitis is not uncommon in hypothermia.

The combination of a cold diuresis and interstitial edema causes a decrease in intravascular plasma volume. The resulting hemoconcentration increases blood viscosity. Decreased temperature shifts the oxyhemoglobin dissociation curve to the left, releasing less oxygen to the tissues. Severe hypothermia may cause prolonged bleeding and coagulation times as well as disseminated intravascular coagulation. The leukocyte and platelet count may be low from hepatic and spleen sequestration (7).

Pituitary, adrenal and thyroid function is well preserved until very cold core temperatures. Insulin becomes nonfunctional at 31° C(6).

PREDISPOSING CONDITIONS

Accidental hypothermia is an environmental disease. Healthy children exposed to severe cold weather conditions will become hypothermic. Outdoor winter activities and cold water immersion are commonly associated with hypothermia. Inadequate household heating during cold winter months is a common urban cause for it.

There are a number of conditions that predispose a child to hypothermia. Neonates, and especially premature infants, have special problems in temperature regulation. The ratio of their large-surface area to mass, their thin subcutaneous fat layer, and their inability to shiver make them vulnerable to cold stress. Premature infants lack adequate brown fat stores and conserve heat by vasoconstriction. Intense vasoconstriction leads to anaerobic metabolism and acidosis that further reduces their resistance to cold (3).

Conditions predisposing a child to hypothermia can be divided into defects of temperature regulation, thermogenesis, and heat conservation. Dysfunction of the heat-regulating hypothalamus can occur from central nervous system (CNS) hemorrhage, meningitis, encephalitis, neoplasm, kernicterus, or severe congenital CNS anomalies (6). Drugs such as phenothiazines, tricyclic antidepressants, barbiturates, and narcotics can also impair thermoregulation. Other drugs associated with hypothermia include carbon monoxide, organophosphates, and glutethimide. Hypothermia in adolescents is commonly associated with ethanol use. Impaired thermogenesis in children can occur from malnutrition, hypoglycemia, hypothyroidism, hypopituitarism, and hypoadrenalism. Increased heat loss can occur from large burns and exfoliative dermatoses. Spinal cord injuries and many neuromuscular diseases impair cold perception, vasoconstriction, and shivering. Sepsis in infants is associated with hypothermia (8). Other conditions predisposing to hypothermia include trauma, diabetic ketoacidosis, chronic renal failure, and congenital heart disease.

HISTORY, PHYSICAL EXAMINATION

A complete history should be obtained. It may be necessary to question the child's parents or friends or the paramedics. Attempt to determine how, when, and where the child became hypothermic. When and where was the child found? What was the duration of cold exposure? Was there any history of trauma or water submersion? Has the child's condition improved or deteriorated? What treatment has been given? Inquire about any underlying medical conditions.

A thorough physical examination must be performed. The diagnosis and treatment are based on an accurate core temperature. The thermometer must be capable of reading low temperatures. In the field, a low-reading glass thermometer is adequate. In the emergency department, a low-reading electronic probe or thermocouple is quick and accurate. Obtaining an accurate core temperature is vital. In hypothermia, a temperature gradient often exists between the core and surface (shell) (9). Oral and axillary temperatures are inconsistent and do not accurately assess core temperature. Rectal, esophageal, bladder, and tympanic membrane temperatures closely correlate with the core temperature. In severe hypothermia, two separate core temperatures should be monitored. The airway and all ventilations must be assessed. The pulse may be difficult to detect because of bradycardia and intense vasoconstriction. A full minute should be taken to assess the pulse before concluding that none is present. In the emergency department, a doppler may assist in finding a pulse and recording a blood pressure. A thorough head-to-toe examination must be performed, searching for signs of trauma, complications of hypothermia, and/or any underlying medical condition. A neurologic examination must be complete. The neurologic impairment is correlated with the degree of core temperature depression. For example, if the patient has a core temperature of 34° C and is comatose, another reason for the coma besides hypothermia should be sought.

LABORATORY

Laboratory tests are used to detect complications of hypothermia and any underlying medical condition. Laboratory tests to be obtained include complete blood count (CBC), glucose, electrolytes, prothrombin time (PT), partial thromboplastin time (PTT), liver function tests, arterial blood gases, urinalysis, and toxicologic screen. Bacterial cultures should be obtained for suspected infection. A septic work-up is routinely performed on hypothermic infants (8). A chest X-ray and electrocardiogram (EKG) are obtained. Further tests are ordered based on the history and physical examination.

The hematocrit is often elevated from plasma volume depletion. Leukocytes are elevated in infection and depressed with hepatic and splenic sequestration. Glucose may be high or low. Hypoglycemia can occur from malnutrition and depletion of glycogen stores. Hyperglycemia occurs from impaired insulin function, decreased renal clearance, and reduced hepatic metabolism. Elevated blood urea nitrogen (BUN) and creatinine may reflect impaired renal function as well as dehydration. Serum potassium concentration depends on serum pH, duration of cold diuresis, and renal function. Extremely elevated potassium levels occur from extensive cellular destruction. Liver function tests are often elevated, and an elevated amylase may occur with pancreatitis.

Hypothermia may affect the arterial blood gases in several ways. Metabolic acidosis is usually present. This occurs from lactic acidosis because of shivering and poor tissue perfusion, impaired hepatic metabolism, impaired buffering capacity of the cold blood, and reduced renal clearance of acids (10). The levels of PO_2 and PCO_2 will depend on the balance of the metabolic supply and demand and on whether the reduced cardiopulmonary function is adequate for the metabolic demand. Arterial blood gases (ABG) should not be corrected for temperature (11).

The chest X-ray must be examined for signs of trauma, infection, and noncardiogenic pulmonary edema. The EKG may show widened QRS, prolonged QT and PR intervals, and J waves. J or Osborn waves are terminal (usually upright) deflections at the junction of the QRS and ST segment. They are frequently seen at core temperatures below 32° C. Osborn waves may also be present in nonhypothermic patients such as cardiac ischemia, CNS lesions, and a normal variant in children (4). Bradycardia is the most common arrhythmia. Atrial fibrillation with a slow ventricular response is frequently present. Ventricular fibrillation can occur at temperatures below 29° C. Hypothermia will cause an irritable myocardium and a number of disturbances such as hypoxia, acid base and electrolyte abnormalities, and rough handling of the patient will precipitate ventricular fibrillation (6).

MANAGEMENT

Hypothermia, within limits, protects the body's cells against hypoxia. Hypothermia lowers the metabolic rate and cellular oxygen requirements. This affords some protection against the reduced cardiac output. Numerous cases in the medical literature have reported good neurologic outcomes after prolonged hypothermia induced cardiac arrests (12). Death may be difficult to determine in the severely hypothermic patient. Vigorous resuscitation should continue until the body is rewarmed to above 32° C (Figure 37.1).

The goal of management in hypothermia is to support the cardiopulmonary system, prevent further heat loss, rewarm the body's core, and correct any complications. Management may vary depending on the location and sophistication of available resuscitation equipment.

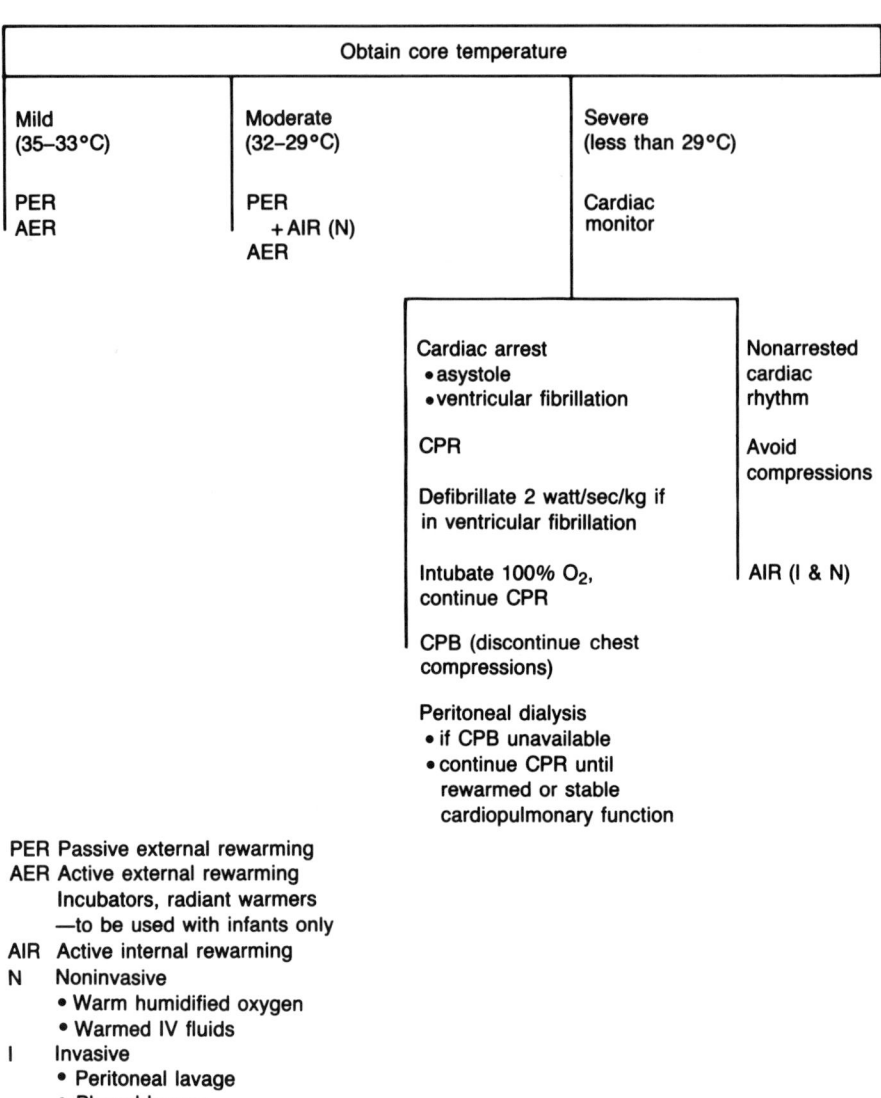

Figure 37.1 Hypothermia management

First aid management in hiking or camping situations should consist of removing victims from the cold and placing them in tents and wrapping them in sleeping bags. Victims should not be allowed to hike further but rather should be made to rest and given warm food and drink. Other members of the camping party should go for help.

Prehospital therapy by paramedics should consist of cardiopulmonary support, gentle handling, and rapid transport to the hospital. An accurate core temperature is important. The airway and all ventilations should be assessed, and oxygen should be started. The pulse should be palpated for a full minute before the decision is made that it is absent. If a cardiac monitor is available, check for cardiac activity. If the child is in cardiac arrest, begin cardiopulmonary resuscitation. If no monitor is available, start cardiopulmonary resuscitation (CPR) if the patient is severely hypothermic, no pulse is felt, and no other signs of life are present. If a weak pulse or any organized cardiac rhythm is present, do not begin CPR. If ventricular fibrillation is present on the monitor, attempt a single defibrillation using 2 joules/kg (13). An intravenous (IV) line should be established. No cardiac drugs should be given. The only rewarming techniques should be covering the patient with blankets and using warm humidified oxygen.

In the emergency department, reassess the airway, breathing, and circulation (ABCs), and obtain an accurate core temperature. Place the patient on a cardiac monitor. If the patient remains in cardiac arrest, continue CPR. If the cardiac arrhythmia is ventricular fibrillation, attempt defibrillation using 2 joules/kg. Further countershocks should not be performed until the victim is rewarmed to above 28° C. Often ventricular fibrillation will spontaneously convert to a more stable rhythm at above 28° C. Intubate severely hypothermic children even if they are not in cardiac arrest as the airway is usually severely compromised and aspiration is common. Ventilations with 100 percent oxygen and chest compressions should be continued while the patient is rewarmed. The optimal rate of cardiopulmonary resuscitation in hypothermia has not been established (10). The rate should be guided by the arterial blood gases. The cold myocardium is relatively unresponsive to cardiac drugs and pacing as well as to countershocks (13). Pharmacotherapy should be avoided in severe hypothermia, as not only are drugs ineffective but they may also accumulate to toxic levels when the patient is rewarmed. IV fluids should consist of D_5NS. Lactated Ringers solution should be avoided because the liver cannot metabolize lactate. A central venous catheter should be used to monitor fluid status. A Foley catheter should be placed. Urine output inaccurately reflects the victim's fluid status because of the renal concentrating defect (2).

It is vitally important to maintain optimal cardiopulmonary function prior to and during rewarming, and the rewarming should never precede stabilization of cardiopulmonary function. Rewarming the hypothermic victim without optimizing oxygenation and cardiac output will tax the already compromised patient, increasing metabolic requirements and thus hypoxic injury (14,15).

REWARMING TECHNIQUES

There are two methods of rewarming: passive and active. Passive rewarming decreases further heat loss and allows endogenously produced heat to rewarm the body. Passive rewarming is simple and noninvasive and is the method used to treat mild hypothermia. It consists of removing affected children from the cold and covering them with blankets. Active rewarming is employed when endogenous thermogenesis is inadequate. This occurs in such groups as premature infants, neonates, children with underlying illnesses disturbing heat production, and severely hypothermic children. Active rewarming can be divided into external and internal rewarming. Active external (surface) rewarming is the application of heat to the skin (shell). Examples of active external rewarming include use of hot packs, radiant warmers, heated blankets, incubators, and hot water baths. The use of active external rewarming should be discouraged. An exception is the use of radiant warmers and incubators in mildly or moderately hypothermic infants. Most methods of external active rewarming in hypothermia is either not necessary, inconvenient, or, in cases of severe hypothermia, harmful. In severe hypothermia, surface rewarming causes vasodilation. This may result in hypovolemic shock, metabolic acidosis, pulmonary edema, or core temperature afterdrop (a decrease in core temperature after rewarming has started). The flow of cold acidotic blood back to the core can precipitate ventricular fibrillation in the already compromised myocardium. Hot water baths are impractical, and hot packs can cause severe thermal burns.

Active internal rewarming is the application of heat directly to the body's core and is recommended for severe hypothermia. Examples of active internal (core) rewarming are use of warm IV fluids, warm humidified oxygen, gastric lavage, peritoneal dialysis, pleural lavage, mediastinal irrigation, hemodialysis, and cardiopulmonary bypass. The first two methods are simple and noninvasive. IV fluids are warmed to 40 to 45° C and infused. Rewarming by IV fluids is slow and limited by the amount of fluids required. Use of humidified heated oxygen is an effective and simple method of core rewarming (16). Oxygen is heated to 40 to 45° C and administered by mask or endotracheal tube. The rate of rewarming varies from 0.5 to 2.5° C/hr depending on the temperature of oxygen and the respiratory minute volume. Warm gastric lavage slowly warms the core, limited by gastric surface area. Gastric distension and aspiration are hazards with gastric lavage. A more invasive core rewarming technique is peritoneal dialysis (lavage). Two catheters are placed in the peritoneal cavity and a continuous flow of warm (40° to 45° C) fluid is maintained. Rewarming rates range from 4° to 6° C/hr and no special fluids are required (9). The heat from the fluid is transferred directly to the intraperitoneal organs and indirectly to the heart and kidneys. Its advantage is rapid rewarming rates, simplicity, and availability in most emergency departments. Contraindications are previous abdominal surgery and intra-abdominal trauma. Pleural lavage involves placement of two thoracotomy tubes and continuous irrigation of the pleural cavity with warmed saline (17). Mediastinal lavage and hemodialysis are infrequently used, being reserved for special circumstances. Cardiopulmonary bypass (extracorporeal) rewarming rapidly rewarms the core at 10° to 12° C/hr while supporting the cardiovascular system. Unlike other active internal rewarming techniques external chest compressions can be stopped with cardiopulmonary bypass. Disadvantages include its unavailability at many hospitals and the risk of heparinization in trauma patients.

Most mildly hypothermic children have stable hemodynamics and can be safely warmed passively. Infants with mild to moderate hypothermia are rewarmed in an incubator and with radiant warmers. Severely hypothermic children in cardiac arrest require core rewarming by cardiopulmonary bypass (12,15). If using this technique is not possible, rewarm by peritoneal dialysis and warm humidified oxygen. These techniques should also be used for severely hypothermic children with more stable cardiovascular function. For moderate hypothermia, the combination of core rewarming with heated O_2 and IV fluids as well as covering with blankets is usually adequate.

A special category of near-drowning children is that of ice water submersion. There have been a number of remarkably good recoveries in children after prolonged ice-water submersion. Bolte and colleagues report on a 2½-year-old girl submerged for 66 minutes in cold water who survived with good neurologic recovery (18). All the cases are children who were severely hypothermic on removal from the water. Children submerged in ice water cool rapidly because of their relatively large surface area and low subcutaneous fat insulation. The rapid cooling is thought to protect cellular function from hypoxic damage. The diving reflex is a series of physiologic responses to cold water immersion. The diving reflex was once thought pivotal in good neurologic recovery in children. Recent data has shown it not to be important in cold water survival (19).

PREVENTION

Hypothermia prevention should focus on children vulnerable to hypothermia as well as on those with increased cold stress. Infants are especially vulnerable to the cold. Newborns should be dried and wrapped in blankets immediately after delivery. Their heads should be covered, and examination should be performed under a radiant warmer. Adequately heated homes and good nutrition must be insured for all young children. Underlying medical conditions predisposing a child to hypothermia should be recognized, and special precautions should be taken to prevent hypothermia in these children. Children involved in winter outdoor activities should be taught to dress adequately and to change clothes immediately if they become wet. They should be taught how to recognize hypothermia, and how to administer basic first aid to a victim.

CONCLUSION

Hypothermia is an important cause of mortality and morbidity in children. Although it is most common in cold winter months, it can occur in temperate climates and at warmer times as well. Hypothermia is an environmental illness. There are a number of conditions that predispose to this condition. Infants are especially vulnerable to hypothermia because of their large surface area and immature thermoregulation. An accurate core temperature is important in the diagnosis and treatment of hypothermia. Mild hypothermia can be treated conservatively. Severely hypothermic children should be aggressively treated. Cardiopulmonary support is essential for a good neurologic recovery. Core rewarming techniques should be used for severe hypothermia.

REFERENCES

1. Health Studies Branch, Division of Environmental Hazards and Health Effects. Hypothermia prevention. MMWR 1988;37:780–782.
2. Edlich RF, Chang DE, Birk KA, et al. Cold injuries. Compr Ther 1989;15:13–21.
3. Fant M, Cloherty IP. Temperature control. In Cloherty JP, Stark AR, eds. Manual of neonatal care. Boston: Little, Brown, 1985.
4. Danzl DF. Accidental hypothermia. In Rosen P, ed. Emergency medicine, concepts and clinical practice. St. Louis: Mosby, 1988.
5. Moss J. Accidental severe hypothermia. Surg Gynecol Obstet 1986;162:501–513.
6. Paton BC. Accidental hypothermia. Pharmacol Ther 1983;22:331–377.
7. Wong KC. Physiology and pharmacology of hypothermia. West J Med 1983;138:227–232.
8. Daga R, Gorodischer R. Infections in hypothermic infants younger than 3 months old. Am J Dis Child 1984;138:483–485.
9. Lonning PE, Skulberg A, Abyhom F. Accidental hypothermia review of the literature. Acta Anaesthesiol Scand 1986;30:601–613.
10. Danzl DF, Pozos RD, Auebach PS, et al. Multicenter hypothermia survey. Ann Emerg Med 1987;16:1042–1055.
11. Delaney KA, Howland MA, Vasallo S, et al. Assessment of acid-base disturbances in hypothermia and their physiologic consequences. Ann Emerg Med 1989;18:72–82.
12. Kelly KJ, Glaeser P, Rice TB, et al. Profound accidental hypothermia and freeze injury of the extremities in a child. Crit Care Med 1990;18:679–680.
13. Orlowske JP. Drowning, near-drowning, and ice-water submersions. Pediatr Clin North Am 1987;34:75–92.
14. Moss JF. The management of accidental severe hypothermia. State J Med 1988;88:411–413.
15. Cohen DJ, Cline JR, Lepinski SM, et al. Resuscitation of the hypothermic patient. Am J Emerg Med 1988;6:475–478.
16. Shields CP, Sixsmith DM. Treatment of moderate-to-severe hypothermia in an urban setting. Ann Emerg Med 1990;19:1093–1097.
17. Iversen RJ, Atkin SH, Jaker MA. Successful CPR in a severely hypothermic patient using continuous thoracostomy lavage. Ann Emerg Med 1990;19:1335–1337.
18. Bolte RG, Block PG, Bowers RS, et al. The use of extracorporeal rewarming in a child submerged for 66 minutes. JAMA 1988;260:377–379.
19. Ramey CA, Ramey DN, Hayward JS. Dive response in children in relation to cold-water near-drowning. J Appl Physiol 1987;63:665–668.

38

Heat Injuries

James S. Walker

Children frequently present to the emergency department because of an abnormally elevated body temperature or hyperthermia. Fever (rectal temperature greater than or equal to 38° C) has long been recognized by physicians, parents, and even patients themselves as an indication of illness. Fever is not synonymous with hyperthermia, however. Rather fever is a type or subset of hyperthermia (1,2). There are many different etiologies for hyperthermia (Tables 38.1, 38.2, and 38.3). Fever represents the resetting of the thermoregulatory control center in the hypothalamus to a new level by endogenous and exogenous pyrogens (1,2,3). This pyrogen-induced febrile response has many homeostatic mechanisms and does not always warrant treatment (1,2,3). Nonpyrogen-mediated mechanisms of hyperthermia represent an imbalance in heat production or heat loss and usually do not involve resetting of the thermoregulatory control center of the brain. This helps explain why nonpyrogen-induced hyperthermia does not respond to antipyretic medications such as aspirin or acetaminophen. Furthermore this offers an explanation of why nonpyrogen-mediated hyperthermia tends to be higher than pyrogen-mediated hyperthermia and of why the frequency of hyperpyrexia is greater (1,2,3).

Hyperpyrexia is defined as a rectal temperature greater than or equal to 41.1° C (3). Body temperatures above this level disrupt enzymatic processes at the cellular level and cannot be tolerated for long periods of time without developing significant sequela. Only rarely will a patient with an infection present with hyperpyrexia (3). More commonly hyperpyrexia in the pediatric population will be associated with environmental heat-related injuries. Although less common in incidence, neuroleptic malignant syndrome is another etiology for hyperpyrexia that is clinically important and that is becoming more frequent among adolescents and teenagers who tend to experiment with drugs.

ENVIRONMENTAL HEAT-RELATED INJURIES

First it should be recognized that heat-related injuries span a wide range of pathological adversities from benign heat cramps to lethal heat stroke. Heat stroke represents a true medical emergency caused by excessive heat storage when high ambient temperatures prevent heat dissipation by radiation or convection and when sweat evaporation is limited by ambient humidity. A multitude of other factors may

Table 38.1 Mechanisms of hyperthermia

Hyperthermia	
"Resetting" of the thermoregulatory center located in the hypothalamus	No effect on thermoregulatory center located in the hypothalamus
Pyrogens (endogenous and exogenous)	Nonpyrogenous agents

Table 38.2 Pyrogen-induced etiologies for hyperthermia

1. Infections (exogenous pyrogens)
    a. Bacterial
    b. Viral
    c. Parasitic (to include ticks)
    d. Fungal
2. Rheumatic diseases (exogenous pyrogens)
    a. Rheumatoid arthritis
    b. Juvenile rheumatoid arthritis
    c. Kawasaki's disease
    d. Henoch-Schonlein purpura
    e. Polymyositis
    f. Dermatomyositis
    g. Juvenile ankylosing spondylitis
    h. Systemic lupus erythematosus (SLE)
    i. Scleroderma
    j. Polyarteritis nodosa/cutaneous polyarteritis
    k. Takayasu's arteritis
3. Hypersensitivity reactions (exogenous pyrogens)
    a. Serum-sickness
    b. Stevens-Johnson syndrome
    c. Drug reactions
    d. Immunization reactions

Table 38.3 Nonpyrogenous etiologies for hyperthermia

1. Drugs/toxicology
    a. Anticholinergics
    b. Sympathomimetics
    c. Salicylates
    d. Phenothiazines
    e. Cocaine
    f. Lithium
2. Metabolic diseases
    a. Hyperthyroidism
    b. Cystic fibrosis
3. Central nervous system (CNS) disorders
    a. CNS lesions in hypothalamus/brain stem
    b. Head injuries
    c. Status epilepticus
4. Miscellaneous
    a. Alcohol withdrawal
    b. Environmental heat injuries
    c. Neuroleptic malignant syndrome
    d. Malignant hyperthermia

also predispose to heat stroke. It is estimated that up to 4000 deaths per year are attributed to heat injuries (4,5). More pertinent to this text are the estimated 5 to 10 adolescent and teenage football players who die each year from heat injuries.

Pathophysiology of Thermoregulation

A brief review of physiology is necessary to understand the factors that surround heat injuries properly. Heat is generated by all living organisms as a result of metabolism. More specifically this arises from exothermic intracellular metabolic reactions. This basal metabolic activity may produce 60 to 70 kcal/hr in the adult (6). Heat production mechanisms, however, include exercise or active energy metabolism in addition to basal metabolism. In fact, moderate exercise generates about 300 kcal/hr of heat and strenuous exercise can generate up to 900 kcal/hr of heat (6). Furthermore one must take into consideration the potential addition of further heat from ambient environmental sources by means of conduction, convection, and radiation. It becomes readily apparent that, if there were no heat-loss mechanisms, heat injuries would be universal. Accordingly the body temperature represents a balance between heat-production and heat-loss mechanisms (6,7).

Heat can be diffused or disseminated from the body by means of evaporation, conduction, convection, radiation, and transpiration. Evaporation is accomplished by sweating and represents a major source of heat loss in humans; conduction is loss or gain of heat through direct contact of the body with a cooler surface or medium such as water; convection is loss or gain of heat through contact with moving air surrounding the body. Radiation is gain or loss of heat through energy emission from the skin surface, and transpiration is the loss of heat through exhaled water vapor. Subsequently for conduction, convection, and radiation to be effective as a means of heat loss, there must be a significant thermal gradient between the body and the ambient environment. When the ambient temperature is close to the body temperature, evaporation becomes the only effective means of heat loss. Moreover when the relative humidity of the ambient environment is high, evaporation is negated. Hence a high ambient temperature and a high relative humidity significantly impair heat loss. As a direct consequence, there is increase in heat storage and thus an increase in the core temperature.

Acclimatization to heat characterizes a physiological change or adjustment in which a person becomes more tolerant to the effects of heat. Generally these adaptations are manifested predominantly in terms of metabolic and circulatory efficiency. Metabolic adaptations include: (1) increased myoglobin content in skeletal muscle, (2) increased mitochondrial density in skeletal muscle, (3) increased levels of renin-angiotensin, and (4) increased secretion of aldosterone (1,7). Circulatory adjustments to heat include: (1) increased stroke volume, (2) increased maximal cardiac output, (3) decreased peak heart rate, and (4) increased glomerular filtration rate (1,7). The cumulative effect of these metabolic and circulatory transformations facilitate the delivery of heated blood from the muscle and viscera to the skin for cooling. There is also less heat production by the skeletal muscle by increased aerobic metabolism and increased volumes of sweat with a lower sodium concentration. This acclimatization process may take from 10 to 60 days to accomplish depending on the degree of exposure to the heat stress.

The spectrum of heat injuries depicts an inability to physiologically react to environmental conditions, insufficient correction of fluid and electrolyte losses, and the result of coming into contact with a host of various heat sources. A vivid example of such an exogenous heat source is the child left unattended in a locked car in a parking lot in summer. The ambient temperature in this scenario can reach to 60° C. Another predisposing situation is the high school football player who is attending two football practice/drills a day in August. An additional clinical scenario includes a febrile, dehydrated infant who is bundled up in heavy clothes and blankets by well-meaning parents. The rampant use of cocaine and other drugs by many adolescents and teenagers also predisposes them to heat stroke.

Heat Cramps

Heat cramps are severe, painful involuntary contractions of large skeletal muscle groups of the abdomen and extremities (more commonly of the lower extremities) that occur during or following vigorous physical exercise. They tend to appear in fit and relatively acclimatized children. These cramps are associated with profuse sweating. Although the true etiology is not known, it is speculated that the large amounts of sweat accompanied by inadequate sodium replacement (drinking tap water) induces a localized hyponatremia in the muscle cytoplasm and in turn precipitates a hypocalcemic induced muscle spasm. Clinically the body core temperature is normal. There is no evidence of systemic volume depletion. Laboratory chemistries may show hyponatremia or hypokalemia. Usually there is no change in the serum chemistry levels of calcium.

Treatment consists of rest in a cooled environment with adequate rehydration by oral or intravenous (IV) isotonic fluids (0.9% NaCl). Massage and stretching of the involved muscles will diminish the pain and facilitate the return of the athlete to participation in the sport or game.

Heat Syncope

Heat syncope is another form of a heat-related injury in which the involved individual will experience a syncopal episode in response to volume depletion from sweating and peripheral vasodilation from the heat. The cumulative effect is a marked decrease in venous return, a subsequent diminishment in cardiac output, and ultimately cerebral perfusion pressure making it impossible to maintain consciousness. The mechanism of action is very similar to vasovagal syncope. Although this disorder is benign in itself, it is possible for the involved individuals to injure themselves when they fall. The typical setting is a Boy Scout or a band member who has been standing for a prolonged time in a summer parade. Clinically the core body temperature is normal. Generally there are no remarkable laboratory abnormalities. The attending clinician should closely evaluate the victim for injuries incurred as a result of the fall.

Treatment is confined to placing the patient in the Trendelenburg position and rehydration with oral or IV isotonic fluids.

Heat Exhaustion

Heat exhaustion is a syndrome consisting of weakness, fatigue, malaise, headache, nausea, vomiting, hyperventilation, mild altered mental status, and orthostatic symptoms. The common denominator to all of the symptoms is systemic volume depletion. If many young people start developing these symptoms while they are participating in group sports activities during warm weather, suspicion of heat exhaustion or heat stroke should arise. If this syndrome is not recognized early and treated aggressively, it can progress into heat stroke.

Clinically, the patients are diaphoretic and may be complaining of chills in addition to the previously mentioned symptoms. The core body temperature may be elevated but is less than 40° C (1,7). Laboratory studies will further support the evidence of volume depletion. Specific electrolyte abnormalities will vary based on whether there was a deficit in water or in salt (sodium).

The primary focus of treatment is volume replacement along with rest. Typically the administration of 1 to 2 fluid boluses of 20 cc/kg of IV isotonic fluids is most beneficial. The correction of specific electrolyte abnormalities (K+, Mg+) should be evaluated on an individual basis. Rapid cooling techniques are usually not required (1,7).

Heat Stroke

Heat stroke occurs when the body's heat loss mechanisms are unable to meet the environment's demands, which are overpowered and overwhelmed. The cardinal tenets of diagnosis are: (1) a history of heat exposure, (2) body core temperature greater than 40° C, and (3) altered mental status. Historically two forms of heat stroke have been described: (1) exertional heat stroke and (2) classic (nonexertional) heat stroke. Exertional heat stroke is the most common form of heat stroke occurring in the pediatric population, especially among aspiring athletes. Although rarely encountered, classic heat stroke can be found among children with sweat gland abnormalities, metabolic disorders (Table 38.4) and among those who take anticholinergic, sympathomimetic, or other predisposing drugs (Table 38.5).

PATHOPHYSIOLOGY OF HEAT STROKE AND ITS CLINICAL COMPLICATIONS
Cardiovascular System (CVS)

1. Cardiac output, heart rate, and cardiac work must increase dramatically as systemic vascular resistance falls and central venous pressure rises during exposure to hot humid environments (1,7).
2. Pulmonary edema may occur in normal hearts if they are unable to sustain the required increased performance.

Table 38.4 Predisposing factors to heat stroke

1. In normal, healthy humans
   a. Lack of acclimatization
   b. Salt and water depletion
   c. Heat intolerance
   d. Acute infection or fever
   e. Mild to moderate obesity
2. Commonly associated disease states
   a. Cardiovascular, i.e., congestive heart failure
   b. Endocrine disturbances
     1) Diabetes mellitus
     2) Thyrotoxicosis
     3) Addison's disease
3. Malnutrition
	4. Impaired sweat production
	   a. Miliaria
	   b. Scleroderma
	   c. Sweat gland injury
	     1) Postthermal burn
	     2) Postbarbiturate poisoning
	     3) Postheat-stroke
	   d. Sweat gland obstruction
	   e. Ectodermal dysplasia
	   f. Cystic fibrosis
	5. Autonomic dysfunction (Shy-Drager syndrome)
	6. Schizophrenia
	7. Potassium deficiency
	8. Drugs use (56 percent of drugs are known to predispose to heat injury)

3. Patients with congestive heart failure are unable to increase their heart rates and cardiac output as well as noncardiac subjects do, and some experience a fall in cardiac output. Symptoms of congestive heart failure (CHF) or angina at rest can occur in such settings (1,7).
4. Dynamic cardiac states (*hypotension-poor prognosticator*)
   a. Hyperdynamic patients
      (1) High cardiac index, moderately decreased blood pressure (BP), and low peripheral vascular resistance
      (2) Cooling results in a return of the cardiac index to normal, a rise in BP, and a progressive increase in systemic vascular resistance (SVR).
   b. Hypodynamic patients
      (1) Present with cyanosis, marked hypotension, a low cardiac index, and markedly elevated central venous pressure (CVP)
      (2) These patients may respond to isoproterenol infusion.

Table 38.5 Drugs increasing the risk of heat stroke

1. Drugs impairing heat dissipation
   a. Anticholinergics
   b. Antihistamines
   c. Phenothiazines
   d. Tricyclic antidepressants
   e. Monoamine oxidase (MAO) inhibitors
   f. Diuretics
   g. Vasoconstrictors
   h. Beta-adrenergic blockers
   i. Cocaine
	2. Drugs increasing heat production
	   a. Phencyclidine (PCP)
	   b. Lysergic acid diethylamide (LSD)
	   c. Amphetamines
	   d. Cocaine
	   e. Tricyclic antidepressants
	   f. Lithium Carbonate
	   g. Drug withdrawal syndromes (ethanol, barbiturates, benzodiazepines, sedative-hypnotics)

c. Either hemodynamic alteration may occur in young healthy persons with exertional heat stroke and in elderly patients with classic heat stroke, but the hyperdynamic state is more common.
5. Structural changes may occur in the myocardium of heat-stroke victims (1,7).
6. Arrhythmias occur often, particularly during the cooling phase. Electrocardiogram (EKG) abnormalities include diffuse T-wave and ST-segment abnormalities, conduction defects, ventricular ectopy, and tachyarrhythmias. Because severe metabolic acidosis and hyperkalemia are usually present (particularly in exertional heat stroke), digitalis should be used only with extreme caution (1,7).

Central Nervous System

1. Victims are usually comatose or display profound disorientation; mental status changes usually respond to cooling. Prolonged coma after cooling is a poor prognostic indicator.
2. Pupillary abnormalities are common, including wide dilated pupils in patients who recover.
3. Grand mal seizures occur during the cooling period.
4. Neurologic sequela include peripheral neuropathies, profound cerebellar dysfunction (ataxia, nystagmus, dysmetria, dysarthria), dementias, diminished intellectual function, and hemiparesis (1,7).
5. CNS damage with combinations of cerebral edema, petechial hemorrhage, and marked deterioration or disappearance of purkinje cells in the cerebellum are universal changes in fatal cases.

Renal Function

1. Acute renal failure occurs in exertional heat stroke (30 percent) and more rarely in classic heatstroke (5 percent) (1,7).
2. Several reports suggest that acute oliguric renal failure occurs in association with intense physical work in hot climates without clinically apparent hyperpyrexia.
3. Nearly all exertional heat-stroke patients have mild proteinuria and active urinary sediment. These patients are dehydrated and hyperuricemic, excrete an acid urine, and may develop a uric acid nephropathy. Rhabdomyolysis with subsequent nephrotoxic myoglobinuria in the concentrated acid urine of a heat-stroke victim can result in acute tubular necrosis (ATN).
4. A glomerular injury secondary to disseminated intravascular coagulation (DIC) can occur.
5. Hypokalemic tubular damage, glomerular filtration rate, and renal plasma flow depression may occur in some patients.

6. Early intervention with osmotic agents can prevent acute renal failure in exertional heat-stroke patients.
7. Urinalysis
   a. Urine is isotonic to plasma, the urine/plasma concentration ratio for urea nitrogen is less than 5:1, and urinary sodium is high. The development of ATN is very probable.
   b. Treatment with IV furosemide should be given in conjunction with mannitol to initiate a diuresis to prevent oliguric renal failure.

Liver

1. Core (rectal) temperature may underestimate temperature in the liver during hard work. In a study of unacclimatized men working for 1 hour in temperate heat at a workload of 50 percent maximal O_2 utilization, hepatic venous temperature rose to 41.6° C while rectal temperature was documented at only 40° C.
2. Hepatocellular necrosis with marked evaluations in serum glutamic-oxaloacetic transaminase (SGOT), jaundice, and disturbances in synthesis of clotting protein occurs.
3. These chemical abnormalities usually peak in 48 to 72 hours.
4. SGOT levels greater than 1000 in the first 24 hours after insult connotes a poor prognosis.

Pancreas

1. Thrombocytopenia usually occurs in the first 24 hours and becomes most profound in 2 to 3 days. Complete recovery occurs in one week.
2. DIC is a major cause of severe hemorrhage and late death in heat-stroke survivors.
3. This is a leukocytosis (white blood count [WBC] greater than 11,000); blood glucose is increased.

Skeletal Muscle Injury

1. In exertional heat stroke or heat stroke associated with hyperkinetic agitation, muscle damage occurs with secondary elevations of serum creatinine phosphokinase (CPK) and myoglobinuria.
2. Frank rhabdomyolysis and subsequent sequestration of fluid into an injured muscle can be severe enough to cause shock, acute myoglobinuric renal failure, and serious hyperkalemia.

Sweat Gland Injury

1. Sweat gland necrosis may follow heat stroke, and impaired sweating may persist.

2. Patients with this sequela are prone to repeated bouts of heat illness because of their lessened ability to dissipate heat load.

TREATMENT OF HEAT STROKE

1. Secure access to the circulation and respiratory systems is established; IV lines sufficient to withstand cardiopulmonary resuscitation (CPR) and an endotracheal tube should be placed (oxygen, monitor, IV).
2. Insert rectal probe into the rectal ampulla to provide continuous core monitoring of the core temperature.
3. Immediate *cooling*
   a. This is the most important aspect of therapy.
   b. Restrictive clothing should be removed prior to transport if possible.
   c. The goal is to decrease the temperature rapidly to 102° F.
   d. *Ice bath*
      (1) Difficulties include getting obese patients in and out, monitoring the patient, performing CPR, and applying direct current (DC) countershock.
      (2) Application of extremity rubbing to prevent vasoconstriction has not proved to be adequate.
      (3) The ice bath is extremely uncomfortable for the patient.
   e. *Body cooling unit*   The unit sprays finely atomized water under pressure at 15° C (59° F) over the whole nude body surface from above and below and blows linear air currents (air warmed to 45° to 48° C) over the body at 30 m/min. This keeps the skin temperature above 30° C, maintaining the cutaneous vasodilatation needed to ensure a high rate of heat loss from the body core to the skin while still allowing evaporative cooling.
   f. In case of seizures, use benzodiazepine, phenytoin or barbiturates.
   g. Prevent shivering, as it can generate a considerable amount of heat. Treatment with chlorpromazine has been recommended in the past but may produce hypotension, usually in the more seriously ill patients. Phenothiazines can impair heat dissipation, cause seizures (lower the seizure threshold), and cloud an already obtunded sensorium.
   h. Monitor the rectal temperature continually, even after the patient has been cooled. If cooling is excessive, the patient may become hypothermic.
   i. Be conservative in salt and water administration during cooling. Cooling alone may restore blood pressure to normal by causing a translocation of this fluid to the central circulation. Patients with exertional heat stroke may have a large fluid deficit.
   j. Continuous cardiac monitoring is necessary because of the common occurrence of atrial and ventricular arrhythmias.
   k. Baseline labs should include: extended chemistry panel, arterial blood gas (ABG), complete blood count (CBC), platelets, prothrombin time

(PT), partial thromboplastin time (PTT), lactic acid level, urinalysis, and urine myoglobin level.

l. Sodium bicarbonate should only be administered when severe acidosis is present, monitoring carefully for signs of induced hypocalcemia.

m. Hypotension usually responds to cooling but may require fluids and a pressor agent. Due to vasoconstriction, agonists should be avoided. Dobutamine and isoproterenol are the preferred ionotropes.

NEUROLEPTIC MALIGNANT SYNDROME

Neuroleptic malignant syndrome (NMS) is a rare, life-threatening, idiosyncratic reaction to neuroleptic medications. More specifically, phenothiazenes, thioxanthenes, butyrophenones (especially haloperidol), tricyclic antidepressants, and lithium have been identified as causative agents (8,9). The central clinical manifestations are altered mental status, extreme hyperthermia, muscle rigidity, and instability of the autonomic nervous system. Surprisingly this lethal idiosyncratic reaction can occur at any time during therapeutic use or regular abuse of these neuroleptic drugs. The occurrence of NMS, however, is more apt to transpire after the initiation of use/abuse or after an increase in the dosage. Furthermore NMS may present after the sudden discontinuation of dopamine agonist antiparkinsonian drugs. This phenomenon has lead to the speculation that NMS may be a result of dopamine antagonism (8,9).

Clinical declaration of NMS centers around autonomic and central nervous system volatility. A hallmark in the diagnosis is hyperpyrexia. Core temperatures commonly exceed 41° C. The changes in mental status often start with agitation and confusion and progress to coma. Muscle hypertonicity is reflected as a severe, recalcitrant, dystonic reaction consisting of oculogyric crisis, opisthotonos, torticollis, laryngeal spasm, and facial grimacing. The sustained autonomic discharge is expressed by tachycardia, diaphoresis, urinary incontinence, tremors, and vacillating blood pressure. The marked hyperthermia is felt to result possibly from blockade of the thermoregulatory center.

Complications of NMS include rhabdomyolysis, renal failure, coagulopathies, disseminated intravascular coagulation, cardiac arrhythmias, pulmonary edema, pulmonary embolism, seizures, and acute respiratory failure. Consequently the mortality rate is reported to be high (5 to 30 percent) (8,9). It is apparent that the likelihood of a good outcome is dependent on rapid recognition and aggressive treatment.

Besides the universal standards of supportive management consisting of airway, breathing, and circulation (ABCs), successful treatment has to address the normalization of body temperature, rehydration, and cessation of muscle rigidity. In addition, it should be realized that despite discontinuation of the offending neuroleptic agent, NMS can last from 5 to 10 days.

The key feature of NMS management is muscle relaxation. The reversal of muscle rigidity facilitates the cooling rate as well as diminishing rhabdomyolysis. Benzodiazepines may be helpful, but it is not uncommon for pancuronium or dantrolene to be required. The use of pancuronium necessitates intubation. The employment of dantrolene does not require any special supportive measures. IV dantrolene can be administered starting at 1 mg/kg (rapid push) and continued until symptoms subside or until the cumulative maximum dose of 10 mg/kg is reached. Also dantrolene is commonly used in the treatment of malignant hyperthermia.

REFERENCES

1. Yarbrough BE, Hubbard RW. Heat-related illness. In Auerbach PS, Geehr ED, eds. Management of wilderness and environmental emergencies, 2d ed. 1989;124–125.
2. Stitt JT. Fever versus hyperthermia. Fed Proc 1979;38:39–43.
3. Henretig FM. Fever. In Fleisher GR, Ludwin S, eds. Textbook of pediatric emergency medicine, 2d ed. Baltimore: Williams and Wilkins, 1988;163–164.
4. Glowes GHA, O'Donnell TF. Current concepts: Heat stroke. New Engl J Med 1974;291:564.
5. Ellis FP. Mortality from heat illness and heat aggravated illness in the United States. Environ Res 1972;5:1–58.
6. Robertshaw D. Factors in heat stroke. In Khogali M, Kales JRS, eds. Heat stroke and temperature regulation. Sydney, Aus.: Academic Press, 1983.
7. Stewart CE. Environmental emergencies. Baltimore: Williams and Wilkins, 1990.
8. Levenson JL. Neuroleptic malignant syndrome. Am J Psych 1985;142:1137.
9. Rosenberg MR, Green M. Neuroleptic malignant syndrome: Review of response to therapy. Arch Intern Med 1989;19:27.

Index

Abdominal pain, 275–282
    clinical presentation of, 276, 277
    differential diagnosis of, 276–278
    laboratory evaluation of, 279–280
    management of, 280–282
    pathophysiology of, 275–276
    physical examination in, 278–279
    in right lower quadrant, **271**
Abdominal trauma, 157–167, 276
    child abuse and, 369
    computed tomography (CT) for, 159
    diagnostic peritoneal lavage (DPL) for, 159, 165–167
    initial assessment in, 158–159
    intravenous pyelography (IVP) for, 159
    laboratory evaluation of, **158**
    pathophysiology of, 157–158
    major multiple trauma with, 130, 138–139, 139–140
    specific injuries seen with, 160–165
Abuse. *See* Child abuse; Sexual abuse
Accidents. *See* Automobile accidents
Acquired immunodeficiency syndrome (AIDS), 375
Acute chest syndrome (ACS), 334
Adolescence
    abdominal pain in, 27, 282
    asthma in, 37
    dysrhythmias in, **90**
    poisoning in, 112
    wheezing in, **35**
Adrenal insufficiency, 315–322
    clinical manifestations of, 316–317
    diagnosis of, 320–321
    differential diagnosis of, 317–320
    idiopathic autoimmune adrenalitis with, 319–320
    infection and, 318–319
    treatment of, 321–322
Adrenocorticotropin (ACTH), 315, 316, 317, 319, 320–321
Adult respiratory distress syndrome (ARDS), 77, 80
Advanced life support (ALS), 3, 361, 362
Afterload
    congestive heart failure and, 95
    shock and, 76, 82–83
Airway management, 21–64
    cardiopulmonary resuscitation and, 4–6
    diabetic ketoacidosis (DKA) and, 308
    emergency medical service (EMS) response to, 362
    gastrointestinal bleeding and, 246
    major multiple trauma and, 132–133
    snakebite poisoning and, 381–382
    status epilepticus and, 225
    thoracic trauma and, 169–170
Airway obstruction, acute, 23
    asthma and, 33–34, 35
    causes of, 27
    foreign body aspiration and, 57–59
    See also Croup; Epiglottitis
Albuterol, with asthma, **38**, 40
Amrinone, and shock, **82**
Analgesics, in sickle cell disease, 331–332
Anemia
    oncologic emergencies with, 340
    sickle cell disease and, 328, 333, 334

Italic equals figure reference. Bold equals table reference.

425

Animal bites. *See* Mammalian bites
Anoxia, cardiac arrest with, 3
Antibiotic therapy
    mammalian bites with, 397
    sickle cell disease and, 329–330
Anticonvulsant medications, 226–228, **229**
Antidiuretic hormone, syndrome of inappropriate secretion of (SIADH), 346
Antidotes for poisoning, 107, 109, 110, **111**
Antivenin, 388–390
Aorta, trauma injuries to, 165, 176–177
Apgar scores, 14, **15**
Aplasia, 189
Aplastic crises, in sickle cell disease, 334
Apnea
    neonatal asphyxia with, 12, 17
    respiratory syncytial virus (RSV) infection with, 44
Appendicitis, acute, 267–273, 275
    abdominal pain with, 267, 268, 271, 275, 278
    clinical presentation of, 267–271
    complications of, 269
    diagnostic rules for, 279
    differential diagnosis of, 269, 271–272
    laboratory evaluation of, 269
    leukemia with, 346–347
    management of, 272, 273
    pathophysiology of, 267
    physical examination in, 268–269
    radiologic examination in, 269–271
Arm fractures, 130, 139, 140
Arthritis. *See* Septic arthritis, acute
Asphyxia
    clinical presentation of, 13–14
    evaluation of newborn for, 14
    laboratory evaluation of, 15
    management of, 15–19
    pathophysiology of, 11–13
    traumatic, 178
Asthma, 33–41
    clinical presentation of, 34–35
    differential diagnosis of, 35, 42–43, 52, 61
    disposition of, 41
    evaluation of, 35–36
    history in, 36–37
    management of, 37–40
    pathophysiology of, 33–34

pharmacologic basis of, 34
    risk factors for, 36–37
Asystole, 7, 8, 9, 87, **88**
Atlantoaxial instability, 189, *194*
Atlantoaxial rotary fixation (AARF), 195–196, 200, *201, 202, 203*, 205
Atlas fracture, 205
Atrial tachyarrythmias, 96, 100
Atropine, in cardiopulmonary resuscitation, 8, 9
Automobile accidents
    abdominal trauma with, 157, 161, 162, 163, 165
    emergency medical service (EMS) system and, 359, 360
    head trauma with, 143
    major multiple trauma in, 130
    spinal cord injuries in, 185, 186, 193
    thoracic trauma with, 169, 171, *173, 174*, 175, 176, 178
Avulsion fracture, 192

Back injuries. *See* Spine injuries
Bacteremia
    fever in, **352**, 354
    meningitis with, 233
Bacterial infections
    acute abdominal pain with, 276
    acute meningitis with, 233
    acute osteomyelitis with, 117, 118, 121
    acute septic arthritis with, 122, 123, 125
    airway obstructions with, 23
    orchitis with, 299
    pneumonia with, 339
    septic shock with, 74, 75
    sickle cell disease with, 329
Battle sign, 147
Bell clapper deformity, 293
Benzodiazepines
    asthma and, 40
    shock and, 83
Beta-agonist therapy
    asthma with, 40, 43
    bronchiolitis with, 43–44
Bites
    child abuse and, 368
    See also Mammalian bites; Snakebite poisoning
Bleeding. *See* Gastrointestinal bleeding; Hemorrhage

Bone injuries
    major multiple trauma with, 130, 140
    See also Fractures *and specific fractures*
Bone infections
    workup for, 120
    See also Osteomyelitis, acute; Septic arthritis, acute
Bowel
    acute appendicitis and, 269, 270
    blockage of. *See* Intussusception
    inguinal hernia and, 298
Bradycardia
    cardiopulmonary resuscitation for, 7, 8, 9
    shock and, 75-76
Brain death, 210
Brain injuries
    computerized axial tomography (CT) of, 153-154, 154-155
    head trauma and, 144-145, 147-149, 150
    shock and, 76-77
    status epilepticus and, 224
Breathing
    emergency medical service (EMS) response to, 362
    major multiple trauma and, 133-134
Bretyllium
    cardiopulmonary resuscitation with, 8, 9
    tachycardia and, 93
Bronchiolitis, 41-44
    assessment of, 43
    clinical presentation of, 42-43
    differential diagnosis of, 42-43
    epidemiology and pathology of, 41-42
    treatment of, 43-44
    wheezing in, 34, 35
Bronchitis, chronic, 35
Bronchodilator therapy
    asthma and, 37-39, 40, 41
    foreign body aspiration and, 61, 62
    respiratory failure and, 54
Bronchopulmonary dysplasia (BDP), 42
Bronchoscopy, with foreign body aspiration, 61-62
Bronchospasm, 42, 61
Bronchus
    foreign body aspiration and, 57
    trauma to, 175
Bruises, in child abuse, 368

Burns, and child abuse, 368
Burst fracture, 192-193

Cancer, 337. *See also* Oncologic emergencies
Cardiac arrest, 87
    cardiopulmonary resuscitation for. *See* Cardiopulmonary resuscitation
    clinical presentation in, 3-4
    coma and, 210
    diabetic ketoacidosis (DKA) and, 306
    pathophysiology of, 3
Cardiac contusion, 176
Cardiac dysrhythmias. *See* Dysrhythmias
Cardiac index (CI), 67, 68
Cardiac output, 68, 69, 75, 83
Cardiac function, and shock, 75, 79
Cardiogenic shock, 70, 71, **72**, 73
    effects of, 76
    management of, 79, 80, 81, 82
Cardiopulmonary resuscitation (CPR), 3-10
    airway establishment and ventilation in, 4-6
    cardiac rhythm assessment in, 6-8
    compression/ventilation standards for, 5
    drug therapy in, 8-9
    guidelines for stopping, 9-10
    hypothermia and, 409
    team used in, 4
    venous access obtained in, 6
Cardiovascular system
    heat stroke and, 417-419
    hypothermia and, 404-405
    snakebite poisoning and, 382, 383
Cardioversion, and tachycardia, 92-93
Carotid artery, with skull fracture, 146
Cat bites. *See* Mammalian bites
Cellulitis
    fever in, **352**, 354
    oncologic emergencies with, 344
Central nervous system (CNS), 183-240
    heat stroke and, 419
    shock and effects on, 76-77, 81
    snakebite poisoning and, 382, 383
    trauma to, 130, 137
    See also Spine injuries
Cerebrospinal fluid (CSF)
    coma and, 209-210
    meningitis and, 234, **235**, 239
    status epilepticus and, 225
    trauma injuries and leak of, 137, 145, 147

Cervical spine
  fractures of, 191–193, 206
  wedged appearance of, 189, 192, *193*
Chance fracture, 193, 206
Chemotherapy, fever with, 353
Chest compression, in neonatal resuscitation, 18
Chest injuries, trauma with, 138
Chest roentgenography
  foreign body aspiration on, *60*, 61
  respiratory failure on, 53
Chicken pox, 345
Child abuse, 367–371
  abdominal injury in, 369
  burns and, 368
  dating of bruises in, 368
  differential diagnosis of, 269
  emergency medical service (EMS) response to, **360**
  fractures and, 368–369
  gastrointestinal bleeding and, 243
  head injury in, 369–370
  mandatory reporting of, 367
  poisoning and, 103
  trauma and, 130, 157, 161, 162, 169, 171
Chlamydia, 375
Circulation assessment
  cardiopulmonary resuscitation with, 6
  neonatal resuscitation with, 17
Circulation problems
  congestive heart failure and, 95
  emergency medical service (EMS) response to, 363–364
  neonatal asphyxia with, 13
Closed-head trauma, 151
Cloudy sensorium, 210
CNS. *See* Central nervous system (CNS)
Coagulation, and shock, 78, 84
Colon obstruction. *See* Intussusception
Coma, 209–218
  clinical presentation of, 210–213
  differential diagnosis of, 213–214
  emergency medical service (EMS) response to, 364
  laboratory evaluation of, 215–216
  management of, 216–218
  pathophysiology of, 209–210
  physical examination in, 215
  rapid neurologic assessment in, 212, **213**

Compensated shock, 69–70
Compression fracture, 192, 193, *199*, *200*, 206
Computerized tomography (CT)
  abdominal trauma on, 159, 161, *162*, 163, *164*
  head trauma on, 153–154, 154–155
  major multiple trauma and, 139–140
  spine injuries on, 199–200
Concussion
  myocardial, 176
  skull, 150
Condyloma acuminata, 375
Congenital adrenal hyperplasia (CAH), 316, 317–318, 320
Congenital heart disease, 73
Congestive heart failure, 95–100
  differential diagnosis of, 96–97
  laboratory evaluation of, 98
  management of, 98–100
  pathophysiology of, 95–96
  rapid cardiopulmonary assessment in, 98, **99**
  rhythm disturbances in, 95, 100
Contractility, and shock, 76, 81–82
Convulsive status epilepticus, 221–230
  clinical presentation of, 224
  differential diagnosis of, 224
  history of, 224–225
  laboratory and radiologic evaluation of, 225
  management of, 225–230
  pathophysiology of, 222–224
  physical examination for, 225
Corticosteroids
  asthma with, 39
  meningitis and, 236–237
  shock and, 84–85
Cough
  asthma with, 33, 34–35
  bronchiolitis and, 41
  croup with, 27, **29**, 51
  foreign body aspiration with, 59, 61
Cranial nerves
  coma and, 212, **213**
  skull fracture and, 146–147
Critical oxygen availability, 67
Croup, 23–32, 51
  clinical presentation of, 25
  croup score in, 27, **29**

differential diagnosis of, 25–27
  fever in, **352**
  laboratory evaluation of, 25
  management of, 27–29
  pathophysiology of, 23–25
CSF. *See* Cerebrospinal fluid (CSF)
CT. *See* Computerized tomography (CT)
Cushing's ulcers, 346
Cyanosis
  congestive heart failure and, **97**, 98
  respiratory distress and, 52

Dactylitis, 331
Dance's sign, 251
Decerebrate posturing, 211
Decorticate posturing, 211
Dehydration, 285–292
  assessing severity of, 287
  child abuse with, 367
  clinical presentation of, 287
  diabetic ketoacidosis (DKA) with, 303, 304, 305, 310
  differential diagnosis of, 288
  hypertrophic pyloric stenosis with, 260, 263
  laboratory evaluation of, 288
  management of, 289–292
  pathophysiology of, 285–287
Diabetic ketoacidosis (DKA), 303–313
  clinical presentation of, 304–306
  differential diagnosis of, 306–307
  laboratory evaluation of, 307–308
  management of, 308–313
  pathophysiology of, 303–304
Diagnostic peritoneal lavage (DPL), 159, 165–167
Diaphragm, trauma to, 175–176
Diazepam, with status epilepticus, 226–228, **229**
Digoxin
  congestive heart failure and, 99
  tachycardia and, 92–93
Diphtheria and tetanus toxoids and pertussis vaccine (DTP) immunization, 352
Dislocations, spinal, 194–195
Distributive shock, 71, 72, 73–74
Diuretic therapy, in congestive heart failure, 99–100
Diving reflex, 13, 92
Dobutamine, and shock, **82**, 83

Dog bites. *See* Mammalian bites
Dopamine
  cardiopulmonary resuscitation with, 8
  neonatal resuscitation with, **19**
  shock and, 81–82, **82**, 83
Down's syndrome, 189, *194*
Drowning
  emergency medical service (EMS) response to, **360**
  hypothermia from, 411
Drug therapy
  asthma and, 37–39
  cardiopulmonary resuscitation with, 8–9
  neonatal resuscitation with, 18–19
  See also specific drugs
Drug toxicity, and poisoning, 103–104
Dwarfism, 189
Dysrhythmias, 87–93
  cardiopulmonary resuscitation for, 6–8
  classification of, based on heart rate, 87, 88
  clinical assessment of, 88–89
  congestive heart failure with, 96, 100
  pathophysiology of, 87–88
  poisoning and, 108
  therapy for, 92–93

Ear injuries, with trauma, 137
Edema
  scrotal, 299–300
  snakebite poisoning and, 383–384
Electrocardiogram (EKG)
  congestive heart failure on, **97**, 98
  tachycardia on, 91
Electrolyte problems, 285–292
  acute adrenal insufficiency and, 321
  clinical presentation of, 287
  dehydration related to, 287
  diabetic ketoacidosis (DKA) and, 310
  differential diagnosis of, 288
  laboratory evaluation of, 288
  management of, 289–292
  pathophysiology of, 285–287
Electromechanical dissociation (EMD), 7, 9, 87, 88, 89
Emergency department approved for pediatrics (EDAP), 365
Emergency departments
  child abuse reporting and, 367, 370–371
  sexual abuse and, 373, 376

Emergency departments (*continued*)
  snakebite poisoning and, 384–387
Emergency medical service (EMS) system, 359–366
  access to care and, 364–365
  airway/breathing in, 362
  circulatory compromise and, 363–364
  components of, 359, **360**
  enhanced 911 telephone access to, 365
  epidemiology of, 359–360
  neurological compromise and, 364
  pediatric focus of, 360–361
  spinal immobilization with, 363
  training in, 361–362
Emergency medical technicians (EMTs), 361, 366
Emesis, in poisoning, 109
Encephalitis, 215, 237, **238**
Encephalopathy, and cancer, 347
Endotracheal (ET) intubation
  cardiopulmonary resuscitation with, 4–5, 10
  epiglottitis and, 32
  equipment used in, 5
  neonatal resuscitation with, 18
Eosinophilic granuloma, 190, *196*
Epididymitis, 294–295
Epidural hematoma, 147–148
Epiglottitis, 23–32
  clinical presentation of, 25
  differential diagnosis of, 25–27
  laboratory evaluation of, 25
  management of, 30–32
  pathophysiology of, 23–25
  radiologic evaluation of, 25, 27, 28
Epinephrine
  asthma and, 34, 37, **38**, 40
  cardiopulmonary resuscitation with, 8–9, 10
  croup therapy with, 29
  neonatal resuscitation with, **19**
  shock and, 81, **82**, 83
Esophagus
  oncologic emergencies with, 346
  trauma to, 177
Extremities, multiple trauma to, 130, 139, 140
Eye injuries, and trauma, 136–137

Failure to thrive, 367

Fever, 351–358
  clinical presentation of, 351–353
  diagnostic categories in, **352**, 353
  immunocompromised children and, 353–354
  infants under two to three months of age and, 353
  laboratory evaluation in, 353
  management of, 354–356
  occult bacteremia and, 354
  oncologic emergencies with, 344
  parental education on, 356–358
  septic shock with, 74
  site for temperature measurement in, 351
First aid, and poisoning, 106–107
Flail chest, 174–175
Flexion-distraction injuries, 193, 206
Fluid therapy
  abdominal pain and, 280
  acute adrenal insufficiency and, 321–322
  dehydration and electrolyte problems and, 290–291
  diabetic ketoacidosis (DKA) and, 310, 313
  hypovolemic shock and, 79–80
  poisoning treatment with, 108
  trauma and, 134, 174
Foley catheter, 136
Foreign body aspiration, 57–62
  age and object nature and location in, 57, **58**
  clinical manifestations of, 59–61
  differential diagnosis of, 51, 52
  management of, 61–62
  pathophysiology of, 57–59
Fracture-dislocations, spinal, 194–195
Fractures
  child abuse and, 368–369
  differential diagnosis of, 121
  major multiple trauma and, 130, 139–140
  See also specific fractures

Gastric tube, in trauma resuscitation, 136
Gastroenteritis
  abdominal pain with, 276
  fever in, **352**
Gastrointestinal bleeding, 243–247
  clinical presentations of, 244–245
  common causes of, by age group, 244, **245**

laboratory evaluation of, 245–246
pathophysiology of, 243–244
treatment of, 246–247
Gastrointestinal tract, 241–282
dehydration and, 288
oncologic emergencies with, 346–347
shock and, 77, 84
Genitalia, trauma to, 139, 164–165
Glasgow Coma Scale (GCS), 134–135, **135**, 153, 364
Glucose
cardiopulmonary resuscitation with, 8, 9
diabetic ketoacidosis (DKA) and, 304, 306, 310–311
Gonorrhea, 375
Granulocytopenia, 344
Growth plate fractures, 188, *191*
Gunshot wound, 130, 149–150, *151*, 165, 175

Hangman's fracture, 192, *198*, 205
Head trauma, 143–156
cerebrospinal fluid leak with, 147
child abuse with, 369–370
clinical presentation of, 152
closed-head injury with, 151
concussion with, 150
emergency medical service (EMS) response to, 362
history in, 153
laboratory evaluation of, 153
major multiple trauma with, 130, 136
management of, 154–155
mass lesions with, 147–149
pathophysiology of, 143–151
penetrating injury in, 149–150
physical examination in, 153
radiographic evaluation of, 153–154
scalp lacerations with, 143–144
skull fracture with, 144–147
Heart. *See* Cardiac *entries*
Heat cramps, 416
Heat exhaustion, 417
Heat injuries, 413–423
environmental factors in, 413–417
pathophysiology of thermoregulation and, 415–416
Heat stroke
pathophysiology of, 417–421
treatment of, 421–422

Heat syncope, 416–417
Hematogenous osteomyelitis. *See* Osteomyelitis, acute
Hematomas
duodenal, 162
epidural, 147–148
renal injuries with, 163
retroperitoneal, 165
subdural, 148–149
subgaleal, 144
supraclavicular, 176
Hemolytic anemia, 328
Hemopericardium, 177
Hemorrhage
abdominal trauma with, 157–158
adrenal, 318–319
gastrointestinal. *See* Gastrointestinal bleeding
major multiple trauma and, 134
oncologic emergencies with, 340–343
shock and, 78
skull fracture with, 146
Hemothorax, 133–134, 172, *173*
Henoch-Schonlein syndrome, 299
Hernia
diaphragmatic, 175
inguinal, 278, 298–299
Herpes simplex encephalitis (HSE), 237, 238, 239
Herpes simplex virus (HSV), 237, 238, 375
Hip joint, septic arthritis in, 125
Hodgkin's disease, 337
Hospitals
emergency medical service (EMS) system and, 359, **360**
medical control/protocol development in, 366
triage in, 365
Human immunodeficiency virus (HIV) infection, 239, 337, 375
Hydrocele, 299
Hydrops fetalis, 19
Hypercalcemia, 345–346
Hypercapnia, with respiratory failure, 50, **51**, 54
Hyperglycemia
diabetic ketoacidosis (DKA) with, 303, 304, 306
septic shock with, 74
Hyperglycemic nonketotic coma, 306

Hyperleukocytosis, 343
Hyperphosphatemia, 345
Hyperpyrexia, 413
Hypertension
　poisoning and, 109
　thoracic trauma and, 176–177
Hypertonic dehydration, 286, 287, 290–291
Hypertrophic pyloric stenosis, 259–264
　clinical presentation of, 260–264
　pathophysiology of, 259–260
　treatment of, 261, 263–264
　ultrasound of, 259, 261, 262
Hyperuricemia, 345
Hypocalcemia, 345
Hypoglycemia, and diabetic ketoacidosis (DKA), 304, 306–307
Hyponatremia, with diabetic ketoacidosis (DKA), 306, 308
Hypoplasia, 189
Hypotension
　acute adrenal insufficiency and, 317
　poisoning and, 108
　shock and, 67
Hypothermia, 403–412
　laboratory evaluation of, 406–407
　management of, 407–409
　pathophysiology of, 404–405
　physical examination for, 406
　physiology of, 403–404
　predisposing conditions for, 405–406
　prevention of, 411
　rewarming techniques in, 409–411
　septic shock with, 74
Hypotonic dehydration, 286, 287, 290–291
Hypovolemic shock, 71, 72, 72
　abdominal trauma with, 158
　causes of, 72
　effects of, 76
　major multiple trauma and, 134
　management of, 79–80
Hypoxemia
　dysrhythmias with, 87
　respiratory failure with, 48–50, 51, 52, 55
Hypoxia
　asthma with, 35, 36, 40
　bronchiolitis with, 43
　dysrhythmias with, 88

Idiopathic autoimmune adrenalitis, 319–320
Immunodeficiency, fever in, 353–354
Immunotherapy, and septic shock, 85
Infections
　acute adrenal crisis of, 318–319
　airway obstructions with, 23
　hyperthermia and, **414**
　mammalian bites and, 394–395, 396
　oncologic emergencies with, 343–345
　sickle cell disease with, 329–330
Influenza viruses, and croup, 24–25
Inguinal hernia, 278, 298–299
Insulin, and diabetic ketoacidosis (DKA), 303, 305, 310–311, 313
Intestines
　abdominal trauma with injuries to, 162
　oncologic emergencies with, 346
　See also Intussusception
Intracranial pressure (ICP)
　coma and, 209–210, 211, 214
　head trauma and, 154, *155*
　meningitis and, 234
Intravenous pyelography (IVP), with abdominal trauma, 159, 163
Intussusception, 249–255
　abdominal pain with, 276–278
　clinical presentation of, 250–251
　differential diagnosis of, 252
　epidemiology of, 250
　laboratory evaluation of, 252
　management of, 253–255
　physical examination for, 251–252
　radiologic evaluation of, 252–253
　types of, 249–250
Isoproterenol
　asthma and, **38**, 40
　shock and, 82

Jefferson fracture, 192, *197*, 205
Joints
　trauma and injuries to, 130, 140
　work-up for infections of, 120
　See also Osteomyelitis, acute; Septic arthritis, acute

Ketamine, with asthma, 40
Ketoacidosis, diabetic. *See* Diabetic ketoacidosis (DKA)

Kidneys
  abdominal trauma with injuries to, 163
  shock and, 77, 83
Kussmaul breathing, 305, 307

Larynx, and foreign body aspiration, 57, 59, 62
Lavage
  abdominal trauma and, 159, 165–167
  poisoning and, 109–110
Leg fractures, 130, 139, 140
Leukemia, and oncologic emergencies, 340, 343, 346–347
Leukocytosis, in oncologic emergencies, 343
Lidocaine
  cardiopulmonary resuscitation with, 8, 9
  tachycardia and, 93
Ligamentous disruption, spinal, 206
Limb fractures, 130, 139, 140
Liver
  heat stroke and, 420
  shock and, 78
  trauma with injuries to, 161, 171
Lorazepam, with status epilepticus, 226, **229**
Lown-Ganong-Levine (LGL), 91
Lumbar puncture (LP) studies
  coma and, 215
  meningitis and, 234, 239
  status epilepticus and, 225

Major multiple trauma, 129–140
  airway maintenance in, 132–133
  bleeding in, 134
  breathing and, 133–134
  diagnostic studies in, 139–140
  disability in, 134–135
  ears in, 137
  evaluation of extremities in, 135, 139
  eyes in, 136–137
  Foley catheter in, 136
  gastric tube in, 136
  guidelines in, 131, **132**
  patient dispositions in, 140
  patterns of injury in, 130
  pediatric trauma score in, 130, **131**
  primary survey and resuscitation in, 131–136
  response to injury event in, 130–131
  secondary survey in, 136–139
  team in, 129
Mammalian bites, 393–399
  diagnosis of, 395–396
  epidemiology of, 393
  management of, 396–397
  pathophysiology of, 394–395
  prevention of, 397–399
  rabies treatment in, 397, **398**
  tetanus prophylaxis in, 397, **398**
Management algorithms and guidelines
  acute abdominal pain, *281*
  acute appendicitis, *272*
  acute hematogenous osteomyelitis, *122*
  acute scrotum, *296*
  acute septic arthritis, *125, 126*
  cardiopulmonary resuscitation, *7*
  coma, **216, 217**
  croup, *30*
  diabetic ketoacidosis (DKA), *309*
  dysrhythmias, *88, 89*
  epiglottitis, *31*
  head trauma, *152, 155*
  hypothermia, *408*
  intussusception, *254*
  major multiple trauma, *133*
  neonatal resuscitation, *15, 16*
  snakebite poisoning, *385*
  spine injuries, *204*
  status epilepticus, **227**
  superior vena cava syndrome, *339*
Measles, 345
Meckel's diverticulum, 243, 246, 250, 276
Mediastinitis, 177
Medications. See Drug therapy and *specific medications*
Megaloblastic crises, in sickle cell disease, 334
Meningitis, 215, 233–237
  clinical presentation of, 234
  differential diagnosis of, 234
  fever in, **352**, 354, 355
  laboratory evaluation of, 234–236
  management of, 236–237
  pathophysiology of, 233–234
Metabolic acidosis
  dehydration and, 288, 292
  diabetic ketoacidosis (DKA) and, 307
Methylprednisolone, in asthma, 39
Motor vehicle accidents. See Automobile accidents

Mouth injuries, with trauma, 137
Mumps orchitis, 299
Munchausen syndrome, 370–371
Myelogenous leukemia, acute, 343
Myocardial concussion, 176
Myocardiopathy, and neonatal resuscitation, 19

Narcan, neonatal resuscitation with, **19**
Neck injuries
 spinal cord injuries with, 186
 trauma and, 138
Neisseria gonorrhea, 375
Neonatal resuscitation, 11–19
 Apgar score evaluation in, 14, **15**
 chest compression used in, 18
 clinical presentation in, 13–14
 endotracheal (ET) intubation in, 18
 equipment used in, **14**
 goals of, 15
 high-risk conditions in, 11, **12**
 laboratory evaluation of, 15
 management algorithm in, 15, *16*
 medications during, 18–19
 pathophysiology of asphyxia in, 11–13
 thermal environment in, 15–17
 ventilation and circulation in, 17
Neurocentral synchondroses, 188, *189*
Neuroleptic malignant syndrome (NMS), 422–423
Neurologic dysfunction
 emergency medical service (EMS) response to, 364
 hypothermia and, 405
 neonatal asphyxia with, 13
 sickle cell disease and, 334–336
Neurologic evaluation
 coma and, 212, **213**
 spine injuries and, 198
Neutropenia, and cancer, 344, 34
Nitroglycerine, and shock, **82**
Nitroprusside, and shock, **82**, 83
Non-Hodgkin's lymphoma, 337
Norepinephrine
 asthma and, 34
 shock and, 81, **82**, 83
Nose injuries, with trauma, 137

Obstructive shock, 71, **72**
Oculovestibular reflex, 212

Odontoid process, 188, 189–193, 205–206
Oncologic emergencies, 337–348
 cardiorespiratory system and, 337–340
 gastrointestinal emergencies with, 346–347
 hematopoietic system and, 340–343
 infectious complications with, 343–345
 metabolic emergencies with, 345–346
 neurologic emergencies with, 347
Open chest, 172
Orchitis, 299
Osmolar gap, 105, **106**
Osteomyelitis, acute, 117–122
 acute septic arthritis with, 122
 clinical presentation of, 118
 differential diagnosis of, 121, 124
 laboratory evaluation of, 119–120
 management of, 121, *122*
 pathophysiology of, 117–118
 radiographic bone changes in, 119
 sickle cell disease and, 329
 work-up of bone and joint infections in, 120
Otitis media, fever in, **352**
Oxygen availability, and shock, 67–69, 77
Oxygen extraction ratio, 67, 68
Oxygen therapy
 asthma with, 40
 cardiopulmonary resuscitation with, 8
 croup and, 28, 29
 epiglottitis and, 31
 major multiple trauma and, 134
 neonatal resuscitation with, 17
 respiratory failure and, 53–54
 shock and, 83
Oxygen uptake, 67, 68

Pain
 abdominal. *See* Abdominal pain
 acute appendicitis with, 267, *268*, 271, 275, 278
 acute osteomyelitis with, 118
 coma and response to, 211
 diabetic ketoacidosis (DKA) with, 305
 intussusception with, 250–251
 scrotal, 293, 294
 sickle cell disease and, 330–333
 spinal cord injuries with, 186
Pancreas
 abdominal trauma with injuries to, 161
 heat stroke and, 420

Parainfluenza virus, and croup, 24
Paraldehyde, with status epilepticus, 228, **229**
Paramedics, 361, 366
Parietal pain, 275
Paroxysmal atrial tachycardia (PAT). *See* Supraventricular tachycardia (SVT)
Pediatric critical care center (PCCC), 365
Pelvic fractures, 130, 163, 165
Penetrating trauma, 130, 149–150, 165, 172, 175
Pericardiocentesis, 178–179, *180*
Peritonitis, 162, 269, 279, 281
Phenobarbital, with status epilepticus, 228, **229**
Phenytoin, with status epilepticus, 228, **229**
Pleural effusions, 172, *173*, 338–339
Pneumocystis carinii pneumonia, 339
Pneumonia
  fever in, **352**, 354
  foreign body aspiration with, 61
  oncologic emergencies and, 339, 345
Pneumothorax, 130, 133, 171–172
Poisoning, 103–112
  antidotal therapy in, 110, **111**
  assessment of severity of, 103
  child abuse and, 370
  demographics in, 103–104
  diagnosis in, 103, 104–106
  emergency medical service (EMS) response to, **360**
  first aid in, 106–107
  history in, 104
  laboratory evaluation of, 105–106
  patient disposition in, 112
  physical exam in, 104–105
  radiographic evaluation in, 106, **107**
  snakebites and. *See* Snakebite poisoning
  stabilization and support in, 107–109
  toxicological therapy in, 109–112
  toxidromes in, 105
Potassium
  dehydration and loss of, 288
  diabetic ketoacidosis (DKA) and, 306, 311–312
  tumor lysis syndrome and, 345
Preload
  congestive heart failure and, 95
  shock and, 76, 79–80
Primary apnea, 12

Propranolol, and tachycardia, 92
Pseudoparalysis, 123
Pseudosubluxation, 188, *192*
Pulmonary system
  contusions to, 173, *174*
  oncologic emergencies involving, 339–340, *341*
  snakebite poisoning and, 382, 383
  shock and, 77, 83
  sickle cell disease and, 329
Pulsus paradoxus, 177

Rabies, 395, 397, **398**
Racoon sign, 147
Radiological evaluation
  abdominal pain with, 280
  acute appendicitis on, 269–271
  acute osteomyelitis on, 119–120
  acute septic arthritis on, 123, *124*
  intussusception and, 252–253
  major multiple trauma and, 139
  poisoning on, 106, **107**
  spine injuries on, 199
  See also Chest roentgenography
Rapid cardiopulmonary assessment, 98, **99**
Rectum
  cancer and, 347
  fever temperature measurement and, 351, 357
  trauma injuries to, 139, 164–165
Referred pain, 275
Renal function
  heat stroke and, 419–420
  shock and, 77, 83
  snakebite poisoning and, 383
Respiratory distress
  asthma with, 33, 35, 40
  bronchiolitis and, 41–42, 43
  congestive heart failure with, 96, 98
  emergency medical service (EMS) response to, **360**
  hypothermia and, 405
  oncologic emergencies and, 339
  pathophysiology of, 47
  poisoning and, 107–108
  status epilepticus with, 223
Respiratory failure, 47–55
  asthma with, 33
  causes of, **49**
  clinical presentation of, 50–52

Respiratory failure *(continued)*
　coma and, 210
　congestive heart failure with, 96
　foreign body aspiration with, 59, 62
　laboratory evaluation of, 52–53
　management of, 53–54
　pathophysiology of, 47–50
　shock and, 83
Respiratory syncytial viruses (RSV), 24, 41, 42, 43, 44
Respiratory tract infections, and croup, 24–25
Resuscitation
　major multiple trauma and, 131–136
　See also Cardiopulmonary resuscitation; Neonatal resuscitation
Reye's syndrome, 212
Rhinitis, 48
Rhythm disturbances. *See* Dysrhythmias
Ribavirin, and bronchiolitis, 44
Rib fractures, 130, 171, 173, 370
Risk factors
　asthma and, 36–37
　neonatal resuscitation and, 11, **12**
Rubeola, 345

Scalp
　bite wounds to, 396
　lacerations of, 143–144, 153
Scrotum, acute
　edema and, 299–300
　epididymitis and, 294–295
　hydrocele and, 299
　inguinal hernia and, 298–299
　management algorithm for, *296*
　orchitis and, 299
　pain in, 293, 294
　testicular torsion and, 293–294
　torsion of testicular appendages and, 298
　tumors of, 300
Secondary apnea, 12
Seizures
　coma and, 212, 213
　diabetic ketoacidosis (DKA) with, 307
　emergency medical service (EMS) response to, 364
　fever with, 358
　poisoning and, 109
　sickle cell disease with, 335
　status epilepticus with, 224

Septic arthritis, acute, 117, 122–126
　acute hematogenous osteomyelitis with, 122
　clinical presentation of, 123
　differential diagnosis of, 118, 121, 124
　laboratory evaluation of, 123–124
　management of, 124–125
　pathophysiology of, 123
Septic shock, 69, 71, **71**, 74
　management of, 78–79, 80, 85
　oncologic emergencies with, 344
　pathogens causing, **75**
Sexual abuse, 373–376
　conditions mistaken for, 376
　history in, 373
　physical examination in, 374
　sexually transmitted disease with, 374–375
　trauma with, 164–165
Sexually transmitted disease, 165, 374–375
Shaken baby syndrome, 130, 370
Shock, 67–85
　abdominal trauma with, 157–158
　classification of, 71–74
　clinical presentation of, 75–78
　coma and, 211
　dehydration and, 289
　emergency medical service (EMS) response to, **360**
　gastrointestinal bleeding and, 244
　major multiple trauma and, 134
　management of, 78–85
　oxygen deprived variables in, 67–69
　pathophysiology of, 67–70
　stages of, 69–70
Sickle cell anemia, 327
Sickle cell beta thalassemia (Sβ thal), 327
Sickle cell disease (SCD), 327–336
　clinical presentation of, 329–336
　diagnosis of, 328
　fever in, 354
　pathophysiology of, 328–329
Sickle cell hemoglobin C disease (Hb SC disease), 327, 333, 336
Sickle cell trait, 327
Sinus tachycardia (ST), 79, **88**
Skull fractures
　basilar, 146–147
　child abuse with, 369–370
　depressed, 145–146

multiple trauma with, 130, 136, 139, 140
simple, 144–145
Snakebite poisoning, 379–390
   antivenin and, 389–390
   clinical presentation with, 383–384
   epidemiology of, 379–380
   laboratory evaluation in, 387
   location of bite and, 381–382
   management of, 384–389
   pathophysiology of, 381–383
   snake identification in, 380–381
Sodium bicarbonate
   cardiopulmonary resuscitation with, **8**, **9**
   diabetic ketoacidosis (DKA) and, 312
   neonatal resuscitation with, **19**
Soft tissue injury, with spine trauma, 196
Somagyi phenomenon, 304
Spine injuries, 185–206
   cancer and, 347
   cervical fractures with, 191–193
   clinical presentation of, 186–188
   differential diagnosis of, 188–190
   emergency medical service (EMS) response to, 363
   history in, 196–197
   immobilization in, 363
   incidence of, 185
   major multiple trauma with, 130, 131
   management of, 201–206
   neurologic evaluation in, 198
   pathophysiology of, 185–186
   physical examination in, 197–198
   radiographic and CT studies in, 199–201
   spinal cord injuries without radiographic abnormality (SCIWORA), 186, 201, 205
   spine trauma in, 190–198
Spleen
   sickle cell disease and, 333–334
   trauma with injuries to, 160–161, 171
Status asthmaticus, 40
Status epilepticus
   categories of, 221
   differential diagnosis of, 224
   emergency medical service (EMS) response to, **360**
   epidemiology of, 221–222
   etiologies of, 221, **222**
   systemic complications of, 222, **223**
   See also Convulsive status epilepticus

Steeple sign, 27, *28*
Steroids. *See* Corticosteroids
Stress ulcers, 346
Stridor, with respiratory failure, 51
Stroke volume, 75
Subdural hematoma, 148–149
Subgaleal hematoma, 144
Sunset sign, 212
Superior mediastinal syndrome, 337–338
Superior vena cava syndrome (SVCS), 337–338, *339*
Supraclavicular hematoma, 176
Supraventricular tachycardia (SVT), **88**, 89–91
   cardiopulmonary resuscitation for, 6
   clinical presentation in, 91
   electrocardiogram in, 91
   treatment of, 92–93
Syndrome of inappropriate secretion of antidiuretic hormone (SIADH), 346

Tachycardia
   cardiopulmonary resuscitation for, 6
   shock and, 75, 79
Tamponade, 138
Teams
   cardiopulmonary resuscitation with, 4
   diabetic ketoacidosis (DKA) treatment and, 313
   trauma, 129
Terbutaline, with asthma, **38**, 40
Testicles
   torsion of, 293–294, 297
   torsion of appendix of, 298
Tetanus prophylaxis for bites, 397, **398**
Theophylline
   asthma and, 36, 39
   bronchiolitis and, 44
Thoracic trauma, 169–180
   initial approach to, 169–171
   laboratory evaluation of, **170**
   specific injuries seen in, 171–178
   special procedures in, 178–180
Thoracolumbar spine, 193, *200*, 206
Tidal volume, and respiratory failure, 47–48, 51–52
Todd's paresis, 214
Toxicologic assays
   coma and, 215
   poisoning and, 105, **106**

Toxic substances
  head trauma and, 152
  See also Poisoning
Toxidromes, 105
Trachea
  foreign body aspiration and, 57, 59, 62
  trauma to, 175
Tracheostomy
  cardiopulmonary resuscitation with, 5
  foreign body aspiration and, 61
Training, in emergency medical service (EMS) system, 361–362
Trauma
  acute appendicitis and signs of, 269
  child abuse with, 367
  shock and, 69
  spinal cord injuries with, 188, 190–198
  See also Abdominal trauma; Head trauma; Major multiple trauma; Thoracic trauma
Triage, 365
Trichomonas vaginalis, 375
Tuberculosis, 319
Tuberculous granuloma, 337
Tube thoracostomy, 178, *179*
Tumor lysis syndrome, 345
Typhlitis, acute, 346

Uncompensated shock, 70, 72
Universal antidote, 107
Upper respiratory tract infections
  croup and, 24–25
  intussusception with, 250
  respiratory failure and, 48
Ureter, abdominal trauma with injuries to, 163
Urinary tract
  infection of, 295, 329, **352**
  trauma and injuries to, 163–164, 165

Valproic acid, with status epilepticus, 228, **229**
Varicella, 345
Vaso-occlusion, in sickle cell disease, 328–329
Vasopressor effect, 81
Vasopressors, and shock, 81–82
Vehicular accidents. See Automobile accidents
Venereal warts, 375

Venous access
  cardiopulmonary resuscitation and, 6
  major multiple trauma and, 134
  thoracic trauma and, 170
Ventilation
  cardiopulmonary resuscitation and, 4–6
  croup and, 29
  neonatal resuscitation with, 17
  respiratory failure and, 47–50, 52–53
Ventricular fibrillation, 87, **88**
  cardiopulmonary resuscitation for, 3, 6–8, 9
Ventricular tachycardia (VT), **88**
  cardiopulmonary resuscitation for, 6
  congestive heart failure and, 96, 100
Verapamil, and tachycardia, 92
Vertebra plana, 190, *196*
Viral croup. See Croup
Viral infections
  abdominal pain with, 276
  airway obstructions with, 23
  bronchiolitis and, 41
  diabetic ketoacidosis (DKA) and, 303
  fever in, 355
  intussusception with, 250
  meningitis and, 237
  oncologic emergencies with, 345
  septic shock with, 74, 75
Visceral pain, 275
Volvulus, acute, 276, 280
Vomiting
  acute appendicitis with, 267, 268
  diabetic ketoacidosis (DKA) with, 304, 305
  hypertrophic pyloric stenosis with, 259, 260

Warts, venereal, 375
Wet-brain syndrome, 338
Wheezing
  asthma with, 34
  bronchiolitis with, 34, 41, 42
  differential diagnosis of, 35, 52
  foreign body aspiration with, 59, 61
Whiplash injury, 196
Whole bowel irrigation, 110
Wolff-Parkinson-White (WPW), 89

X-ray evaluation. See Chest roentgenography; Radiographic

RJ 370 .S96 1993

Synopsis of pediatric
  emergency care

NO LONGER THE PROPERTY
OF THE
UNIVERSITY OF R. I. LIBRARY